Study Guide for deWit's

Medical-Surgical Nursing: Concepts and Practice

4th Edition

HOLLY K. STROMBERG, RN, BSN, MSN, PHN

Alumnus CCRN
Professor Emeritus of Nursing
Allan Hancock College;
Clinical Educator
Marian Regional Medical Center
Santa Maria, California

ELSEVIER

ELSEVIER

3251 Riverport Lane
St. Louis, Missouri 63043

Study Guide for deWit's Medical-Surgical Nursing: Concepts and Practice
Fourth Edition

ISBN: 978-0-323-60953-1

Notices

Knowledge and best practice in this field are constantly changing. As new research and experience broaden our understanding, changes in research methods, professional practices, or medical treatment may become necessary.

Practitioners and researchers must always rely on their own experience and knowledge in evaluating and using any information, methods, compounds, or experiments described herein. In using such information or methods they should be mindful of their own safety and the safety of others, including parties for whom they have a professional responsibility.

With respect to any drug or pharmaceutical products identified, readers are advised to check the most current information provided (i) on procedures featured or (ii) by the manufacturer of each product to be administered, to verify the recommended dose or formula, the method and duration of administration, and contraindications. It is the responsibility of practitioners, relying on their own experience and knowledge of their patients, to make diagnoses, to determine dosages and the best treatment for each individual patient, and to take all appropriate safety precautions.

To the fullest extent of the law, neither the Publisher nor the authors, contributors, or editors, assume any liability for any injury and/or damage to persons or property as a matter of products liability, negligence or otherwise, or from any use or operation of any methods, products, instructions, or ideas contained in the material herein.

Previous editions copyrighted 2017, 2013, and 2009.

ISBN: 978-0-323-60953-1

Senior Content Strategist: Nancy O'Brien
Content Development Manager: Lisa Newton
Senior Content Development Specialist: Laura Selkirk
Publishing Services Manager: Julie Eddy
Senior Project Manager: Tracey Schriefer

Printed in the United States of America

Last digit is the print number: 9 8 7 6 5 4 3 2 1

Working together
to grow libraries in
developing countries

www.elsevier.com • www.bookaid.org

To the Student

This Study Guide has been constructed to help you achieve the objectives of each textbook chapter and establish a solid base of knowledge in medical-surgical nursing. The exercises in this guide reinforce the material presented in the textbook and in class. Additional *Interactive Review Questions for the NCLEX® Examination* and *Interactive Exercises and Activities* are available on the Evolve website (evolve.elsevier.com/deWit/medsurg). These exercises and activities will assist you to develop solid critical thinking and priority-setting skills, and some require you to call upon and synthesize previously learned information to reach an answer. Completing the exercises will help you succeed on the NCLEX® examination.

In an effort to assist limited English proficient (LEP) students in mastering communication in English, a section has been included in each chapter called *Steps Toward Better Communication*. The exercises in this section are aimed at improving communication while reinforcing the content of the chapter. The exercises have been constructed so that they will be helpful to English proficient students as well.

STUDY HINTS FOR ALL STUDENTS

- *Ask questions!* There are no bad questions. If you do not know something or are not sure, you need to find out. Other people may be wondering the same thing but may be too shy to ask. The answer could mean life or death to your patient, which certainly is more important than feeling embarrassed about asking a question.
- *Make use of chapter objectives.* At the beginning of each chapter in the textbook are objectives that you should have mastered when you finish studying that chapter. Write these objectives in your notebook, leaving a blank space after each. Fill in the answers as you find them while reading the chapter. Review to make sure your answers are correct and complete, and use these answers when you study for tests. This should also be done for separate course objectives that your instructor has listed in your class syllabus.
- *Locate and understand key terms.* At the beginning of each chapter in the textbook are key terms that you will encounter as you read the chapter. Page numbers are provided for easy reference and review, and the key terms are in bold, blue font the first time they appear in the chapter. Phonetic pronunciations are provided for terms that might be difficult to pronounce.
- *Review Key Points.* Use the Key Points at the end of each chapter in the textbook to help you review for exams.
- *Get the most from your textbook.* When reading each chapter in the textbook, look at the subject headings to learn what each section is about. Read first for the general meaning, then reread parts you did not understand. It may help to read those parts aloud. Carefully read the information given in each box and table and study each figure and its caption.
- *Follow up on difficult concepts.* While studying, put difficult concepts into your own words to see if you understand them. Check this understanding with another student or the instructor. Write these in your notebook.
- *Take useful notes.* When taking lecture notes in class, leave a large margin on the left side of each notebook page and write only on right-hand pages, leaving all left-hand pages blank. Look over your lecture notes soon after each class, while your memory is fresh. Fill in missing words, complete sentences and ideas, and underline key phrases, definitions, and concepts. At the top of each page, write the topic of that page. In the left margin, write the key word for that part of your notes. On the opposite left-hand page, write a summary or outline that combines material from both the textbook and the lecture. These can be your study notes for review. If a handout of the presentation has been provided, use the right hand column for note taking and highlight key terms and concepts on the slides. After class, use the notes to write out or type up an outline of the presentation and highlight terms, concepts and topics.
- *Join or form a study group.* Form a study group with some other students so you can help one another. Practice speaking and reading aloud, ask questions about material you are not sure about, and work together to find answers.

- *Improve your study skills.* Good study skills are essential for achieving your goals in nursing. Time management, efficient use of study time, and a consistent approach to studying are all beneficial. There are various study methods for reading a textbook and for taking class notes. The library staff can be a helpful resource in finding instruction in study skill techniques.

ADDITIONAL STUDY HINTS FOR STUDENTS WHO USE ENGLISH AND A SECOND LANGUAGE (ESL)

- *Find a first-language buddy.* ESL students should find a first-language buddy—another student who is a native speaker of English and is willing to answer questions about word meanings, pronunciations, and culture. Maybe your buddy would like to learn about your language and culture. This could help in his or her nursing experience as well.
- *Expand your vocabulary.* If you find a nontechnical word you do not know (e.g., *drowsy*), try to guess its meaning from the sentence (e.g., *With electrolyte imbalance, the patient may feel fatigued and drowsy*). If you are not sure of the meaning, or if it seems particularly important, look it up in the dictionary.
- *Keep a vocabulary notebook.* Keep a small alphabetized notebook or address book in which you can write down new nontechnical words you read or hear along with their meanings and pronunciations. Write each word under its initial letter so you can find it easily, as in a dictionary. Or use a handheld electronic device for recording your vocabulary list. For words you do not know or for words that have a different meaning in nursing, write down how they are used and sound. Look up their meanings in a dictionary or ask your instructor or first-language buddy. Then write the different meanings or usages that you have found in your book, including the nursing meaning. Continue to add new words as you discover them. For example:

  –Primary—Of most importance; main (e.g., the primary problem or disease); The first one; elementary (e.g., primary school)

  –Secondary—Of less importance; resulting from another problem or disease (e.g., a secondary symptom); The second one (e.g., secondary school ["high school" in the United States])

PRONUNCIATION NOTES

The pronunciation of words in the *Vocabulary Building Glossary* in each chapter in this guide is shown by a simple respelling. It follows the pronunciation guide in Miller-Keane *Encyclopedia and Dictionary of Medicine, Nursing, and Allied Health, 7th edition* (Saunders, 2006):

- Long Vowels: "Long" vowels (a, e, i, o, u, y) are pronounced with the sound of the name of the letter.
  1. An unmarked vowel ending a syllable is long *(ba' be=baby)*.
  2. A long vowel in a syllable ending with a consonant is marked with a long symbol or macron (ˉ) *(be hāv'yer)*.
- Short Vowels: "Short" vowels have varying pronunciations.
  3. An unmarked vowel in a syllable ending with a consonant is short *(ab dukt' = abduct)*.
  4. A short vowel at the end of a syllable is marked with a short mark or breve (˘) *(lip ĭ do' sis)*. Sometimes, the vowel is followed by a silent *h* instead of using the breve *(lip ih do' sis)*.
  5. Some sounds are represented by two letters:
     ah': In stressed syllables, *ah* represents the "a" sound heard in father *(fah' ther)*.
     ah: In unstressed syllables, *ah* represents the "a" sound heard in sofa *(so' fah)*. (It often sounds like *uh*. This sound, called a *schwa*, is represented in many dictionaries by an upside-down *e*. Many people pronounce any unaccented vowel as a schwa.)
     aw: The *aw* in paw.
     oi: The *oi* in oil.
     oo: The *oo* in food.
     ou: The *ou* in out.
  6. A stressed syllable is indicated by an accent mark (') at the end of the syllable.

Good luck!

Holly K. Stromberg
Susan C. deWit

To the Instructor

The *Study Guide for Medical-Surgical Nursing: Concepts & Practice* is designed to reinforce the students' understanding of terms and concepts presented in the text. It will assist them in setting priorities, applying the nursing process, thinking critically, making good judgments and decisions, communicating therapeutically, and meeting chapter objectives. Answers are provided (for instructors only) on the Evolve website.

ORGANIZATION OF THE TEXT

Included are a wide variety of exercises, questions, and activities. Most chapters include *Terminology, Short Answer, Review Questions for the NCLEX® Examination, Critical Thinking Activities,* and a special section called *Steps Toward Better Communication* written by a specialist in English as a second language. Other sections that appear where appropriate are *Completion, Identification, Review of Structure and Function, Priority Setting,* and *Application of the Nursing Process.* Additional interactive activities and exercises are provided on the Evolve website for the textbook.

DESCRIPTION OF EXERCISES

The exercises are as follows:

- **Terminology** – Reinforce correct use of words from the chapter terms list with matching and/or fill-in-the-blank questions.
- **Short Answer** – List brief answers to reinforce knowledge and assist students to meet the chapter objectives.
- **Review Questions for the NCLEX® Examination** – Multiple choice and alternate item format questions are based on real-life situations and require knowledge, synthesis, analysis, evaluation, and application.
- **Critical Thinking Activities** – Brief scenarios and questions foster problem-solving skills in nursing care which may be practiced individually or in study groups.
- **Completion** – Reinforce chapter content with fill-in-the-blank questions.
- **Identification** – Identify appropriate steps in a process or procedure or verify normal or abnormal laboratory values.
- **Review of Structure and Function** – Re-examine anatomy and physiology of the body system pertinent to the text chapter.
- **Priority Setting** – Analyze information and make decisions to set priorities within tasks or clinical situations.
- **Application of the Nursing Process** – Apply critical thinking skills and the steps of the nursing process to real-life patient care.

STUDENTS WITH LIMITED ENGLISH PROFICIENCY

Because so many students from other countries where the primary language is not English are entering nursing programs in the United States and Canada, we have enlisted the aid of a specialist in English as a Second Language who has worked with many health care occupation students. She helped construct the exercises in the *Steps Toward Better Communication* within each chapter. Her letter to you follows. I hope you find this section helpful to your students with limited English proficiency.

STEPS TOWARD BETTER COMMUNICATION

Imagine yourself back in nursing school—trying to read the texts and understand the lectures in Spanish or German. Students studying in a language that is not their native language face not only the challenge of learning the medical and physiologic lessons that are required of all nursing students, but they must also decipher and use a language whose nuances and grammar are unfamiliar to them. In order to ease some of that burden, we've attempted to simplify and regularize the language of *Medical-Surgical Nursing: Concepts & Practice* and the study guide, and to explain some of the colloquial uses of English that occur.

A major part of the nursing process could be described as "knowing your patient inside and out," and one key to that knowledge is being able to accurately and sensitively communicate with the patient and colleagues. To this end, after the regular exercises, we added a section for the ESL student titled *Steps Toward Better Communication*, which offers help in pronunciation, vocabulary building, and use of grammatical issues such as verb tense, and encourages asking for help and clarification. In addition, a section on understanding cultural nuances and mannerisms helps student face real-life situations and clarify feelings. Another section offers facility in appropriately asking questions and carrying on conversations.

A note about pronunciation: we assume that the important medical terms will be used and modeled correctly by the instructor. In terms of conversation, intelligibility rather than native-like accuracy should be the goal. Correct stress is the major determining factor in how easily a person can be understood. Therefore, we chose to indicate stressed syllables in words and phrases, rather than giving phonetic pronunciations that students often find difficult to understand.

Description of Exercises
The following exercises appear in the *Steps Toward Better Communication* section as appropriate.
- *Vocabulary Building Glossary* – explains and defines idiomatic or unusual use of non-medical terms used in the chapter and indicates the stressed syllables for capitalizing them.
- *Completion Sentences* – offer opportunities to use the words presented in the Glossary, often in different context than they are used in the text, thereby offering yet another way to increase vocabulary.
- *Vocabulary Exercises* – use words from the chapter in various ways to increase ease of understanding.
- *Word Attack Skills* – deal with word segments, suffixes, prefixes, and types of words to help the student learn to decode new words and their usage.
- *Pronunciation Skills* – offer practice in pronouncing difficult terms as well as phrases and sentences, with emphasis on stress and intonation.
- *Grammar Points* – are made occasionally, especially when there is a recurring point raised by the chapter, such as the use of the past tense in taking case histories.
- *Communication Exercises* – encourage communicative interchange, writing, and dialogues that might actually be used by a practicing nurse. The value of this section is enhanced if students can be paired in first- and second-language speaker combinations, giving each the opportunity to experience the other's accent and offering the possibility for cross-cultural exchange. Answers to the Communication Exercises are provided in the TEACH Instructor Resources on the Evolve website for the text, and could be printed out for student use.
- *Cultural Point(s)* – present explanations and questions about issues and customs that may differ across the cultures represented in the class, and in the prospective patient community. They can explain the normative culture in which the individual will be working, while at the same time, acknowledge and validate an individual's cultural differences.

In preparing these materials, I have drawn on my teaching experience of practicing and aspiring health care personnel. I have found them to be dedicated and eager to improve their own lives while helping others. I have learned much from them about hard work, perseverance, humor, and what they need in order to do a better job. My colleagues in teaching English and nurses with whom I have worked have been helpful with ideas for teaching projects, indicating language areas needing to be addressed, and offering suggestions and solutions for problems. However, any omissions and errors are my own.

I have been impressed with the similarity between learning language skills and nursing skills. Both require access to academic knowledge, but mastery occurs with hands-on practice and experience. The exercises are geared to provide this opportunity. Encourage your students to interact as often as possible. Look at each lesson with the question, "How can I structure this lesson so the students will have to generate their own language to complete the exercise?" Offer real-life challenges and tasks for speaking and communicative interaction with other students, colleagues, and patients whenever possible. An encouraging, open, and interactive classroom is the best setting for language learning and improvement. I wish you well in working with this special group of people.

Gail C. Boehme, ESL Consultant

Illustration Credits

Chapter 10
From VanMeter, K.C., Hubert, R.J. (2016). *Microbiology for the Healthcare Professional* (2nd ed.). St. Louis: Elsevier.

Chapter 17
From Waugh, A., Grant, A. (2018). *Ross and Wilson Anatomy and Physiology in Health and Illness* (13th ed.). St. Louis: Elsevier.

Chapter 19
From Aehlert, B. (2018). *ECGs Made Easy* (6th ed.). St. Louis: Mosby; Aehlert, B. (2002). *ECGs Made Easy* (2nd ed.). St. Louis: Mosby.

Chapter 29
Modified from Williams, P.A. (2018). *deWit's Fundamental Concepts and Skills for Nursing* (5th ed.). Philadelphia: Saunders.

Chapter 33
Modified from Lewis, S.L., Bucher, L., Heitkemper, M.M., & Harding, M.M. (2017). *Medical-Surgical Nursing: Assessment and Management of Clinical Problems* (10th ed.). St. Louis: Mosby.

Chapter 34
Modified from Ignatavicius, D.D., & Workman, M.L. (2018). *Medical-Surgical Nursing: Concepts for Interprofessional Collaborative Care* (9th ed.). Philadelphia: Saunders.

Contents

Caring for Medical-Surgical Patients

Answer Key: Review the related chapter to answer these questions. A complete answer key was provided to your instructor.

SHORT ANSWER

Directions: Provide the answers to the following questions.

1. List settings in which you might seek employment after graduation.
   a. _Labor + delivery_
   b. _Social service agency_
   c. _school nurse_

2. List four functions of the LPN/LVN.
   a. _Promote/maintain health_
   b. _prevent disease_
   c. _assist with rehabilitation_
   d. _assist with end of life_

3. List three overarching goals in the U.S. *Healthy People 2020* agenda.
   a. _Create social/economic environments that promote health/well being_
   b. _Promote healthy behaviors among all ages_
   c. _Engage leadership to create policies to improve health_

Nursing Roles and Responsibilities

Directions: Provide the answers to the following questions.

1. List the six specific roles of the LPN/LVN.
   a. _Educator_
   b. _Advocate_
   c. _Caregiver_
   d. _Leader_
   e. _Delegator_
   f. _Collaborator_

2. What are the five rights of delegation according to the *ANA and NCSBN Joint Statement on Delegation*?

    a. Right person

    b. Right task

    c. Right Circumstance

    d. Right Supervision

    e. Right communication

3. Identify five nursing competencies related to quality and safety.

    a. Provide patient-centered care

    b. Collaborate with the healthcare team

    c. Use information in patient care

    d. implement evidence-based practice

    e. use quality improvement in patient care

4. List at least five examples of patient teaching activities performed by the LPN/LVN.

    a. reinforce discharge instructions

    b. provide info about community resources

    c. teach self-care activities to promote rehabilitation

    d. teach how to take medication

    e. teach about nutrition

COMPLETION

Directions: Fill in the blanks to complete the statements.

1. The key pieces of informatics are Communication, documentation electronic data access, and data utilization.

2. Capitation involves a set monthly fee charged by the provider of health care services for each member of the insurance group for a specific set of services.

3. A(n) advocate stands up for patients' rights and intervenes in their best interests.

4. A continuous quality improvement program sets Standards for care.

5. The driving force today in all health care facilities is Cost containment

SHORT ANSWER

Dealing with Different Patient Behaviors

Directions: After reviewing the document "Nursing Interventions for Patients with Difficult Behaviors" on the website for your textbook, read the clinical scenario and answer the questions that follow.

Scenario A: Ms. Gay, age 78, has been hospitalized with a broken hip. She is very quiet, does not seem to want to be touched, and responds with "I'm just fine" when asked if she is worried about anything.

1. Ms. Gay's behavior is typical of anxiety or fear and is an expression of a need for _safety + security_.

2. Write four appropriate nursing interventions to help meet Ms. Gay's needs and establish a trusting relationship.
   a. _reduce environmental stress/disorder_
   b. _limit the number of staff caring for patient_
   c. _instill confidence_
   d. _provide routine/consistent_

Scenario B: Mr. Parsons has had one arm amputated as a result of injuries suffered in a farming accident. He has supported his wife and three small children by working as a farmer. During his hospitalization, Mr. Parsons has become increasingly abusive and critical and has threatened to report his nurse on several occasions.

1. Mr. Parsons' behavior probably indicates feelings of _anger_ and _frustration_.

2. His hostile behavior is an expression of a need to _be in control of his situation_.

3. Write three appropriate nursing interventions to satisfy Mr. Parsons' needs and modify his behavior.
   a. _encourage physical activity_
   b. _allow him to talk about his anger_
   c. _allow him to take action about his care_

Scenario C: Ms. Stinson has become manipulative with the nursing staff. She is demanding and attempts to bargain to get out of what she is supposed to do for rehabilitation after her stroke. She insists that she get something other than the broiled fish for dinner, stating that she wants pot roast, mashed potatoes, and gravy. She announces that she will not walk in the halls anymore until she gets something "decent" to eat.

1. List four nursing interventions and approaches that might help in dealing with Ms. Stinson's behavior.
   a. _Talk to her & ask if something else is wrong_
   b. _Tell her that you can check with the kitchen_
   c. _Request dietary consult_
   d. _Explain she's making progress even if it's slow_

PRIORITY SETTING

Directions: Read the scenario and prioritize as appropriate.

Scenario: You are caring for five patients. They have various needs that you must address. Prioritize the order in which you will assist these patients with their needs.

_3_   a.   Ms. Bora is calling for assistance to the bathroom. She is capable of managing this for herself but she routinely calls for assistance for many tasks that she can do for herself.

_2_   b.   Mr. Fogel has locked himself in the bathroom. The nursing assistant is speaking to him through the door but he "wants some time to himself."

_1_   c.   Mr. Ahrens had abdominal surgery 2 days ago and states he is in pain.

_5_   d.   Ms. Schott wants you to immediately call her doctor because she wishes to go home.

_4_   e.   Mr. McGinnis refuses to get out of bed to sit in the chair per orders. The nursing assistant has tried to encourage him but he just gazes off and then starts crying.

REVIEW QUESTIONS FOR THE NCLEX® EXAMINATION

Directions: Choose the best answer(s) for the following questions.

1. The RN charge nurse delegates hanging total parenteral nutrition (TPN) solution on a patient to the LPN/LVN. Before delegating this task, the RN should: *(Select all that apply.)*
   1. verify that the state nurse practice act allows LPN/LVNs to perform this procedure.
   2. question the LPN/LVN about his or her ability to perform the procedure.
   3. remind the LPN/LVN about the need for strict asepsis for the procedure.
   4. state when the solution should be hung.
   5. ask for a report on the patient's glucometer blood glucose level.

2. The doctor asks the LPN/LVN student to hang a unit of blood on a patient who has suddenly become very critical. The best action would be to:
   1. follow the doctor's orders because of the emergency situation.
   2. refuse to do it and explain that it is outside the scope of practice.
   3. immediately get an RN to assist the physician.
   4. obtain the equipment for the doctor, but tell him that he will have to hang the blood himself.

3. The nurse must be instrumental in helping contain the cost of health care. This can be accomplished by: *(Select all that apply.)*
   1. following policies for charging for supplies used in patient care.
   2. documenting patient care for reimbursement.
   3. reusing and recycling supplies whenever possible.
   4. organizing patient care for effective and efficient use of time.
   5. decreasing patient length of stay by recommending that patients leave.

4. The nurse is caring for a patient who is depressed about his health condition and he is concerned about how it will affect his ability to provide for his family. He tells the nurse, "I just don't know how my wife is going to cope if I die." What is the best response?
   1. "You are not going to die. For goodness' sake, cheer up! Don't be so pessimistic."
   2. "What makes you think you are going to die? Your prognosis is actually quite good."
   3. "Your wife is coming to see you today and you wouldn't want her to worry about this or about you."
   4. "It sounds like you are really worried about several issues. Let's talk about them."

5. Data for determination of evidence-based practice is derived from several areas including:
   1. professional organization standards.
   2. successful patient outcomes.
   3. National Patient Safety Goals.
   4. nursing unit–based research.

6. The doctor has just told the patient that she has a terminal illness. She is softly crying and the doctor instructs you to "take care of her." What would be the best immediate intervention to meet the spiritual needs of this patient?
   1. Offer to sit with her.
   2. Offer to call the hospital clergy.
   3. Offer to call family or friends.
   4. Offer to pray for her.

7. Measures that assist in developing a therapeutic relationship might include: *(Select all that apply.)*
   1. always follow through on obtaining requested information for the patient.
   2. talk encouragingly about the patient's physician.
   3. use an unhurried approach when interacting with the patient.
   4. always knock before entering the room.
   5. explain what you are going to do before performing any procedure.

8. Medicare will not pay for _____, a preventable hospitalized patient condition. *(Fill in the blank.)*
   1. new onset of diabetes
   2. wound dehiscence
   3. catheter-related urinary infection
   4. stage 2 pressure ulcer

9. Within the QSEN initiative, *patient-centered care* means: *(Select all that apply.)*
   1. the patient participates in care decisions.
   2. the patient's needs, values, and preferences are considered.
   3. assessment data are sought from the family.
   4. *Healthy People 2030* objectives are considered.
   5. coordinated care is delivered with respect.

CRITICAL THINKING ACTIVITIES

Scenario: You are caring for Mr. Huang, a young man who recently emigrated from a Southeast Asian country. You notice a strange bruising pattern on his back. When you question him about it, he appears to be embarrassed and just shakes his head. When you report the finding to the RN, she tells you that it may be from a culturally based home remedy known as "coin rubbing."

1. Nurses need to realize that individuals have the right to live according to personal beliefs and values as long as:

   those beliefs/values do not interfere with the rights of others + are legal

2. To meet patients' cultural needs, nurses need to:
   a. accept people as they are
   b. deliver high-quality care
   c. accept differences
   d. be open-minded

3.   How can you increase your cultural competence to prepare yourself for working with coworkers and patients from a variety of different cultural backgrounds?

Talk to classmates + learn about their culture

STEPS TOWARD BETTER COMMUNICATION

VOCABULARY BUILDING GLOSSARY

Term	Definition
signif'icant others	important people in the life of the patient; may include family, loved ones, and close friends
collab'orative (co lab' ah ra tive)	working together
pre'mium (pree' mee um)	amount patients pay for insurance coverage
fee'-for-service	amount paid to the doctor depending on the service given
em'pathy	understanding of another's feelings
feed'back	return information about actions or an idea
self-esteem'	one's own feelings of worth
eye contact	looking into a person's eyes while talking to him or her
compass'ion	caring
com'petence	knowing what to do and being able to do it
interact'ing	acting with each other; communicating
el'derly	polite term for people who are older than 65 years

COMPLETION

Directions: Fill in the blanks with the correct words from the Vocabulary Building Glossary to complete the statements.

1.   The LPN/LVN, the RN, the physician, and the respiratory therapist form a(n) _Collaborative_ team that provides the best and most efficient care for the patient.

2.   The patient's insurance was not valid because he forgot to pay the monthly _Premium_.

3.   The patient needed an explanation of _fee for service_ to understand that the insurance company would directly pay the doctor.

4.   When a patient is an adult and not married, you should inquire about _Significant others_ who are part of the patient's support system.

5.   To evaluate the effectiveness of your patient teaching, it is important to obtain _feedback_ from the patient.

6. Being able to feel _____*empathy*_____ helps you understand the patient and provide compassionate care.

VOCABULARY EXERCISE

1. The word **site** means "place." In this chapter, the places talked about are work sites, or places LPN/LVNs might work. On the job, you might talk about the **site** of the wound, or the **site** of the infection. Make two sentences using the word in the two different ways.

   The hospital has chosen a new site to build on.

   The police investigated the site of the crash.

Two other words with the same pronunciation are **sight** (verb): to see, or **sight** (noun): something to see, and **cite**: to quote or make reference to.

2. Complete the sentences using the correct word above: **site/sight/cite**

   a. It was quite a _____*sight*_____ to see Mr. Benson tangled in his oxygen tubes.

   b. This is the _____*site*_____ for the new clinic.

   c. When you write your paper, be sure to _____*cite*_____ your sources.

   d. The original _____*site*_____ of the infection is not known.

3. If medical personnel were *demeaning* and *aloof,* would that be good for the patient? Why or why not?

   No it's disrespectful.

SPECIAL VOCABULARY MEANINGS

Directions: Each language uses words or phrases as idioms that do not translate directly but are part of everyday speech. Explain in your own words the meaning of the idioms in quotation marks.

1. What does "bending the rules" mean? Slightly outside the rules — not doing anything really wrong

2. Why is "skyrocketing" a good description for the cost of health care? increasing in cost very quickly

3. What is meant by "unraveling… and stitched back together" with reference to the health care system? Coming apart + trying to put back together

4. Why would expensive and specialized medical care be called "boutique medicine"? Expensive or exclusive

CLINICAL SCENARIOS

Directions: Study the following scenarios and complete the indicated activities.

1. Ms. Bazan was admitted with weight loss, abdominal pain, and a diagnosis of "rule out cancer of the colon." She underwent a colonoscopy and a bone scan. A member of her church group has come to visit and stops you in the hall to ask if Ms. Bazan's tests show that she has cancer. You know that they did and that Ms. Bazan has been told her diagnosis. To protect your patient's privacy and confidentiality, which of the following is the *best* response?
    a. "You will have to speak to Ms. Bazan's doctor about that."
    b. "I really have no idea what the tests showed."
    c. "I cannot reveal the results of a patient's tests."
    d. "What did Ms. Bazan tell you?"

2. *Communication example:* Jane is talking with a nursing assistant. "Barry, I would like you to assist Mr. Januz with his range-of-motion exercises now. Put each joint of his affected arm through the range of motion five times. If he has discomfort, stop and let me know. I will be in room 212."

    Later, Jane checks with Barry about the task delegated. "Barry, how did the range-of-motion exercises go for Mr. Januz? Did he have any discomfort? Did you encounter any problems? How many times was each joint exercised?" Delegated task

3. Write out how you would delegate the following task and then describe how you would verify that the task was completed.

    Ms. Paul needs to be dangled and then ambulated twice on your shift. Ann, the nursing assistant working with you, is capable of performing this task.

    Ann I'd like you to dangle + then ambulate ms. Paul @ 10 AM + again at 1 PM. Sit her on the side of the bed with her feet on the floor for 3 minutes + if she's not dizzy help her stand. Please ambulate with a gait belt, walking to the end of the hall/back. If she experiences weakness or short of breath please come get me.

Critical Thinking and the Nursing Process

Answer Key: Review the related chapter to answer these questions. A complete answer key was provided to your instructor.

CRITICAL THINKING

1. In your own words, *critical thinking* is:_____

   _____.

2. List four characteristics of a critical thinker that you wish to improve in yourself.

   a. _____

   b. _____

   c. _____

   d. _____

3. How is clinical judgment developed? _____

   _____

4. How does the scientific method help a nurse to solve a problem? _____

   _____

5. List ways the LPN/LVN can specifically adhere to the NALPN Standards of Practice in regard to legal/ ethical status, practice, and continuing education *(one way for each)*: *(See https://nalpn.org/nalpn-practice-standards/ for the NALPN standards.)*

   a. _____

   b. _____

   c. _____

IDENTIFICATION

Phases of the Nursing Process

There are five major phases or components of the nursing process: assessment, nursing diagnosis, planning, implementation, and evaluation. Four of these apply to the LPN/LVN: data collection (assessment), planning, implementation, and evaluation.

Directions: For each nursing action, identify the name of the phase in which the action occurs.

1. _____   Noting whether the application of heat has relieved muscle pain

2. _____   Referring the patient and family to a community support group

3. _____   Setting a goal for prevention of damage to the skin from prolonged pressure

4. _____   Assisting a patient to turn, cough, and breathe deeply every 2 hours after surgery

5. _____   Changing the types of nourishing fluids offered to a patient to ones that he prefers

6. _____   Asking how often the patient normally has a bowel movement

7. _____   Looking at the laboratory report on a patient's chart to determine the results of a urinalysis

8. _____   Teaching a patient to administer his own insulin

COMPLETION

Directions: Fill in the blanks to complete the statements.

1. The nursing process is an orderly way of helping nurses _____ _____.

2. An example of how critical thinking, clinical reasoning, and clinical judgment are applied to the nursing process is _____ _____.

3. The focus of nursing should be on _____ patient needs, _____ nursing care, and _____ the plan.

4. Ongoing _____ is a necessary and important part of the nursing process.

5. Formulating the nursing care plan and writing outcome criteria are joint processes between the nurse and the _____.

Assessment (Data Collection)

Directions: Answer the following questions about the process of data gathering, which occurs during the assessment phase of the nursing process.

1. A patient history is obtained from what three sources?

   a. _____

   b. _____

   c. _____

2. An interview should be conducted in a(n) _____ and should take no longer than 20–30 minutes.

3. When interviewing an elderly patient, the nurse should _____ because the person probably has more health history information to relate and may speak slowly if ill.

4. Secondary sources for interview information when the patient is incapacitated might be

   _____, _____, _____, or

   _____.

5. Cultural values that may affect a patient's care or health practices are best assessed by asking about

   _____.

6. Part of a psychological assessment is determining how a patient reacts to _____ and then determining present _____ abilities.

7. One way to begin a spiritual assessment is to ask if _____ is important to the patient.

8. Your patient weighs 165 pounds. Convert the patient's weight to kilograms: _____ kg (*See Units Conversion Calculator on Evolve.*)

9. Your patient states she drinks 32 ounces of fluid a day. Convert the patient's fluid intake to milliliters: _____ mL (*See Units Conversion Calculator on Evolve.*)

SHORT ANSWER

LPN/LVN's Role and Use of the Nursing Process

Directions: Write a short essay answer for each question.

1. During the evaluation, you find that an intervention is not effective and the patient is not meeting the goal. What is the next step?

   _____

   _____

2. Explain why documentation of nursing care is important. *(Include at least three reasons.)*

_____

_____

_____

_____

_____

APPLICATION OF THE NURSING PROCESS

Directions: Provide the answers to the following questions.

Scenario A: The nursing diagnosis on the nursing care plan states, "Pain due to surgical incision." Nursing interventions include the following: "Monitor PCA morphine effectiveness; reposition every 2 hours; provide quiet environment and rest periods; offer distraction to minimize pain." The expected outcomes state, "Morphine will control pain effectively; patient says pain is not interfering with rest." What would be appropriate evaluation data to determine that these expected outcomes are being met?

_____

_____

_____

_____

_____

_____

Scenario B: Your home care patient who just had a knee replacement has considerable pain in the knee. The nursing care plan has a nursing diagnosis of Altered self-care ability due to knee pain. Write two expected outcomes for this problem relevant to this patient.

a. _____

b. _____

PRIORITY SETTING

Directions: Read each scenario and prioritize the needs for these patients.

Scenario A

1. Your patient has a complex health condition and as you are assessing the patient, you discover several problems. You realize that priorities of care are determined by a hierarchy of needs. Which problem has the highest level of need?
   a. Patient is vomiting and cannot retain meals.
   b. Blood pressure is elevated to 160/100 mm Hg.
   c. Respiratory rate is 32 breaths per minute.
   d. Patient has not had a bowel movement in 3 days.

Scenario B

1. Your patient is recovering from abdominal surgery. There are several important tasks that must be accomplished in the early part of the shift. It is 8:30 AM. What should be done first?
    a. Administer the AM oral medication for type II diabetes.
    b. Have the patient turn, cough, and deep-breathe with the incentive spirometer as scheduled.
    c. Get the patient up to the chair as ordered and make the bed.
    d. Obtain the medication ordered for pain that the patient has requested.

REVIEW QUESTIONS FOR THE NCLEX® EXAMINATION

Directions: Choose the best answer(s) for the following questions.

1. When approaching a clinical problem, an important characteristic of a critical thinker is to:
    1. rely on one's own family values in considering a problem.
    2. consider only data given in report.
    3. recognize one's own biases and limitations.
    4. read chart documentation and draw a conclusion.

2. To consider a problem using the nursing process, the nurse must: _____ *(List in order of priority.)*
    1. consider all possible alternatives as solutions to the problem.
    2. predict the likelihood of each outcome occurring.
    3. define the problem clearly.
    4. choose the alternative with the best chance of success and least chance of undesirable outcomes.
    5. consider the possible outcomes, both positive and negative, for each alternative.

3. The LPN/LVN contributes to the nursing care plan by:
    1. devising the problem statements/nursing diagnoses.
    2. collaborating with the RN on the problem statements/nursing diagnoses.
    3. independently choosing nursing diagnoses from a list.
    4. collaborating with the patient concerning the problems.

4. The focus of the planning step of the nursing process is:
    1. implementing nursing interventions.
    2. collecting data to determine appropriate nursing diagnoses.
    3. determining goals and identifying expected outcomes.
    4. revising interventions according to outcomes.

5. The most important part of writing expected outcomes for problem statements/nursing diagnoses is to:
    1. state the outcome so that it is measurable.
    2. include health promotion and resource management.
    3. make the outcome short-term.
    4. base it on objective patient data.

6. The nurse uses which technique to correctly palpate the abdomen?
    1. Depresses gently with the fingertips and thumb
    2. Uses a sweeping motion with the back of the hand
    3. Gently feels with the flat palmar surface of the fingers
    4. Warms the stethoscope bell before listening to four areas

7. The nurse is looking at the patient's chart and other documentation to determine when the patient received the last dose of blood pressure medication. Where would be the best place to locate this information?
   1. Physician's orders
   2. Medication reconciliation form
   3. Nurse's narrative notes
   4. Medication administration record

8. An increased number of white blood cells (WBCs) is most likely to be associated with:
   1. dehydration.
   2. improper diet.
   3. iron deficiency.
   4. infection.

9. The nurse knows that current vital signs are an important indication of what is happening at a given moment. In addition, vital signs should be correlated with which patient data?
   1. Trends of past readings
   2. Standardized normal readings
   3. The patient's ideal body weight
   4. Accuracy of the equipment

10. In the collaborative role of the LPN/LVN and RN, when developing a prioritized list of problem statements/nursing diagnoses, the two nurses use _____ to determine relationships among the data.

CRITICAL THINKING ACTIVITIES

1. You are caring for a patient with slow, shallow respirations due to anesthesia. Identify which interventions you would select for this problem and briefly explain why you selected each intervention. Also, for interventions that you rejected, give your rationale.

   a. Encourage use of incentive spirometer every 2 hours while awake.
   b. Encourage fluids (if not contraindicated).
   c. Monitor vital signs at least once per shift.
   d. Encourage ambulation as ordered.
   e. Assist to sit in the chair for meals.
   f. Splint the surgical incision for coughing.
   g. Encourage to stretch out time between doses of narcotic pain medication.

STEPS TOWARD BETTER COMMUNICATION

VOCABULARY BUILDING GLOSSARY

Term	Definition
base'line data	data for reference; the beginning data against which later information is measured
clue	a suggestion; added information or hints
cor'relate	make to match, compare points of several things
da'tabase (da' tah base)	basic information collected about the patient that is tabulated or recorded
dis'count	disregard, not pay attention to
enhance'	improve, make better, add to
entail'	includes or involves as a necessary inclusion
evalua'tion	process of judging
hi'erarchy (hi' er ark ee)	in order of importance or rank
in'put	information from someone about facts, feelings, or attitudes
implementa'tion	the carrying out of actions
men'tate	patient's capacity to think
on'going	in progress; continuing
pru'dent	wise or careful

COMPLETION

Directions: Fill in the blanks with the correct words from the Vocabulary Building Glossary to complete the statements.

1. The patient and family should have _____ on the goals of care and the treatment plan to increase compliance and success.

2. When items or concepts are placed in order according to their priority, they are in a(n) _____.

3. If you have a cold or cough, it is not _____ to work with patients with low resistance.

4. Don't _____ the statements the patient makes because it will give you some _____ as to how he is feeling.

5. Think of some ways you can _____ your patient's stay in the hospital.

6. Try to _____ the lab reports with what you observe with the patient.

7. Taking a good history will _____ getting adequate information from the patient.

CLINICAL ACTIVITIES

Asking for Assistance

Directions: Seek assistance when something is unclear or not understood.

1. If you feel awkward auscultating the heart and lungs, ask the instructor to demonstrate the skill on your patient by saying, "Would you please show me how to auscultate my patient's lungs (or heart) properly?"

2. If you are having difficulty hearing a patient's blood pressure accurately, ask for help by saying, "I'm not certain I'm getting my patient's blood pressure accurately. Could you help me?"

SHORT ANSWER

To assist patients with spiritual concerns, rather than saying, "Do you want...?", the patient might be more receptive if you would use a more polite form of question, such as "Would you like...?". Other polite phrases include "Might I...?", "May I...?", and "I would like to ... if that is all right with you."

Directions: In the spaces below, write polite phrases for asking a patient about reading to her, praying with her, sitting with her, calling a spiritual advisor, and calling friends. Example: "Would you like me to bring you something to read?"

1. _____

2. _____

3. _____

4. _____

5. _____

Writing Expected Outcomes

Directions: Write two expected outcomes for each of the following nursing diagnoses. Example: Patient will use PCA pump before pain becomes severe for 48 hours after surgery.

1. Pain due to surgical incision

   a. _____

   b. _____

2. Altered self-care ability due to paralysis of left side

   a. _____

   b. _____

3. Constipation due to side effects of medications

   a. _____

   b. _____

GRAMMAR POINTS

When taking a history, you need to be sure that you and the patient are talking about the same time period.

- When you are asking about medical history, you need to ask, "Have you had…*breathing problems…?*" (chronic conditions) or "Have you ever had…*a stroke…?*" (a one-time happening).

- If you are asking about current symptoms, you will need to ask, "Do you have…*vision or hearing problems…?*" (now).

If you do not pronounce the words carefully, or you are dealing with an older person with a hearing loss, or someone who is distracted or is a native speaker of another language, you may not receive the correct information.

Fluids, Electrolytes, Acid-Base Balance, and Intravenous Therapy

chapter

3

Answer Key: Review the related chapter to answer these questions. A complete answer key was provided to your instructor.

TABLE ACTIVITY

Edema Characteristics

Directions: Select the principle on the right that most accurately completes the statement on the left. (More than one principle may apply.)

1. Localized edema ___a, e___ .
2. Dependent edema ___b, c, d___ .

   a. occurs with inflammation
   b. is noted in feet, ankles, and lower legs
   c. is an effect of gravity
   d. is usually pitting
   e. is characterized by tight, shiny skin

MATCHING

Directions: Select the principle on the right that most accurately completes the statement on the left.

1. Maintaining normal composition and distribution of body fluids is essential to health because ___b___ .

2. The renin-angiotensin-aldosterone system causes renin ___d___ .

3. When there are differences in concentration of fluids in the various compartments ___a___ .

4. The substances in the body fluids can move in and out of capillaries and cell bodies because ___e___ .

5. A deficit of water in the extracellular compartment leads to cellular dehydration because ___c___ .

   a. osmotic pressure will move water from the area of lesser concentration of solutes to the area of greater concentration until the compartments are of equal concentration

   b. all the life processes of every cell of every organ take place in a fluid medium

   c. when a semipermeable membrane separates fluids of unequal concentration, molecules of water move from the less-concentrated to the more-concentrated solution

   d. to be released when there is decreased blood flow to the kidney

   e. diffusion provides a spontaneous mixing of molecules

COMPLETION

Directions: Fill in the blanks to complete these statements about fluid and electrolyte balance.

1. Whenever sodium is retained by the body and not excreted by the kidneys, ___water___ is also retained.

2. Normal transmission of nerve impulses and normal muscular activity, including that of the heart, require the presence of ___Calcium___.

3. A potassium deficit can cause cardiac ___arrest___.

4. When a patient becomes dehydrated from insufficient fluid intake, serum sodium levels ___rise___.

5. Four conditions that can lead to hypokalemia are improper use of ___diuretics___, as well as ___Vomiting___, ___diarrhea___, and continuous ___gastric suction___.

6. Examples of three foods high in potassium are ___Orange juice___, ___bananas___, and ___potatoes___.

7. Magnesium is important in ___Protein___ synthesis.

8. Good sources of magnesium include ___tuna, avocado, spinach & rolled oats___.

9. Phosphorus is essential for the formation of ___ATP___.

10. ___Phosphorus___ is also important as a(n) ___buffer___ to promote acid-base balance.

SHORT ANSWER

Fluids and Electrolytes

Directions: Fill in the blank or supply a short answer to complete the following statements about fluid balance and intake.

1. The average intake of liquids during a 24-hour period is ___2500___ mL.

2. A urinary output of less than ___30___ mL per hour indicates poor renal function.

3. List two treatments or nursing measures that can lead to water intoxication.
    a. ___Giving IV fluid too rapidly___
    b. ___Forcing fluids w/o noting output___

4. Name three nursing actions that can help relieve nausea and vomiting.
    a. ___Remove odors from room___
    b. ___Cool compress___
    c. ___antiemetic___

5. When a patient vomits, he loses water and which electrolytes? <u>Sodium, potassium,</u>
<u>magnesium + calcium</u>

6. To help in the assessment of fluid volume deficit related to diarrhea, list three observations the nurse should note and record.

   a. <u>Odor</u>
   b. <u>Color | Consistency</u>
   c. <u># of stools passed in 8 hours</u>

7. Name four nursing measures useful for treating fluid volume deficit related to diarrhea.

   a. <u>Provide fluids</u>
   b. <u>medication to slow diarrhea</u>
   c. <u>Restrict food | BRAT diet</u>
   d. <u>small sips of Gatorade</u>

8. Name two causes of fluid volume deficit in an older adult patient.

   a. <u>use of laxatives</u>
   b. <u>decreased thirst sensation</u>

9. List three nursing actions that should be included in the care plan of a patient with generalized edema.

   a. <u>daily weight</u>
   b. <u>measure input + output</u>
   c. <u>Restrict fluid intake if ordered</u>

10. List three common nursing problems for patients with problems of vomiting, diarrhea, or draining wounds.

    a. <u>fluid volume deficit</u>
    b. <u>Potential electrolyte imbalance</u>
    c. <u>Risk of infection due to impaired skin integrity</u>

SHORT ANSWER

Signs and Symptoms of Fluid and Electrolyte Imbalance

1. A 78-year-old patient is admitted with hyponatremia. What signs and symptoms of this problem would you expect to find in this patient?
   <u>Confusion, fatigue, lethargy, headache,</u>
   <u>anxiety, nausea, altered level of</u>
   <u>consciousness</u>

2. A patient with cardiac problems enters the hospital with diarrhea. He is hypokalemic. What signs and symptoms of hypokalemia are expected? Why is this condition so dangerous?

muscle weakness, abdominal pain, cardiac dysrhythmias, decreased reflexes, urinary retention. It's dangerous due to its potential for causing life-threatening cardiac dysrhythmias.

TABLE ACTIVITY

Fluid Deficits

Directions: Complete the following table comparing the three major conditions related to fluid deficits.

	Vomiting	Diarrhea	Draining Wounds
Clinical manifestations to be documented	nausea abdominal pain pallor cold/clammy skin	abdominal cramps general weakness frequent, watery bowel movements	shock pain infection dehydration
Possible causes	① pregnancy ② gi irritation from food, viruses, drugs/chemicals	local irritation of intestinal mucosa— infection or allergy	Burns fluid loss by drainage of wounds
Nursing interventions	quiet/cool environment offer small meals/cool drinks oral hygiene	physical/mental rest emotional support provide privacy	record intake/output monitor vitals emotional support
Medical management	antiemetic drugs antihistamines sedatives phenothiazine	replace fluids high-residue diet antispasmodics	analgesics fluid/electrolyte replacement

IDENTIFICATION

Intravenous Therapies

Directions: For each statement regarding intravenous therapy, indicate if it is true or false. If false, correct the sentence to make it a true statement.

___T___ 1. Older patients with heart problems are at increased risk for fluid overload.

___T___ 2. All equipment and fluids used for IV therapy must be sterile.

___F___ 3. One of the goals of care for a patient receiving IV fluids is to deliver the fluids as rapidly as possible.

___F___ 4. When adding a new bottle or bag of IV fluid for continuous infusion, clean technique is used.

___T___ 5. Standard precautions are used for discontinuing an IV catheter.

CALCULATIONS

Directions: Calculate the correct flow rates for the following orders and situations.

1. Ordered: 1000 mL D$_5$RL over 8 hours
    Administration set delivers 20 gtts/mL
    How many drops per minute should be administered? __42 gtts/min__

2. Ordered: 500 mL D$_{10}$W at 150 mL/hour
    Administration set delivers 20 gtts/mL
    How many drops per minute should be administered? __50 gtts/min__

3. Your patient had an IV count of 325 mL at the beginning of your shift. You infused two piggybacks during the shift; the first was 125 mL and the second was 50 mL. You hung a new 1000 mL bag of fluid at 1:00 PM. The IV count at the end of your shift was 800 mL.
    What was the total IV intake for the shift? __700 mL__

PRIORITY SETTING

You are assigned to care for the following patients:
    a. Ms. Toms, age 76, who has nausea, vomiting, and dehydration.
    b. Mr. Wilson, age 68, who had surgery and is receiving a transfusion of packed red cells.
    c. Mr. Whitts, age 36, who has pancreatitis and is receiving TPN.

1. After you receive report, which patient would you visit and check first? __b__

You have a nursing assistant assigned to help you with your patients. You need vital signs on all three patients at 8:00 AM.

2. Which patient would you assign to the nursing assistant for measuring vital signs? __~~a b~~ c__

3. You need to do an initial shift assessment on each of the three patients. Which one would you assess first? __a__

IDENTIFICATION

Blood Gas Analysis

Directions: Under each laboratory value given below, add ↓ if the value is below normal, ◊ if normal, and ↑ if above normal. Then decide whether the data set indicates metabolic acidosis, respiratory acidosis, metabolic alkalosis, or respiratory alkalosis. Also identify if the PaO_2 indicates normal oxygenation (N) or hypoxia (H). Normal oxygen levels should be 80–100 mm Hg.

Example: pH pCO_2 HCO_3 PaO_2

            7.32   44 mm Hg   21 mEq/L   82 mm Hg

              ↓   ◊   ↓   N

Indicates metabolic acidosis with normal oxygenation

1.   pH pCO_2 HCO_3 PaO_2

            7.33   50 mm Hg   26 mEq/L   60 mm Hg

    Indicates __respiratory acidosis__

2.   pH pCO_2 HCO_3 PaO_2

            7.48   32 mm Hg   25 mEq/L   90 mm Hg

    Indicates __respiratory alkalosis__

3.   pH pCO_2 HCO_3 PaO_2

            7.50   45 mm Hg   28 mEq/L   78 mm Hg

    Indicates __metabolic alkalosis__

REVIEW QUESTIONS FOR THE NCLEX® EXAMINATION

Directions: Choose the best answer(s) for the following questions.

1. General causes of edema are: *(Select all that apply.)*
   1. a loss of plasma protein.
   2. increased capillary circulation.
   3. increased lymphatic circulation.
   4. increase in capillary hydrostatic pressure.
   5. infusion of 4 L of normal saline.

2. The patient with hypokalemia shows signs of: *(Select all that apply.)*
   1. nausea.
   2. stupor.
   3. abdominal pain.
   4. cardiac dysrhythmias.
   5. paresthesias.

3. Safe administration of intravenous fluids includes:
    1. shaking the bag to mix the solution thoroughly.
    2. checking the infusion rate every 30–60 minutes.
    3. weighing the patient daily.
    4. checking electrolyte levels before hanging a new bag of IV solution.

4. The data indicating effectiveness of interventions for an older patient with a fluid volume deficit are: *(Select all that apply.)*
    1. weight gain of 2 pounds.
    2. successful infusion of 3000 mL of normal saline.
    3. patient can answer questions without confusion.
    4. moist mucous membranes in the mouth.
    5. drinking 8 ounces every 2 hours.

5. Nursing actions for a patient receiving intravenous fluids should include: *(Select all that apply.)*
    1. re-dress the IV insertion site each shift.
    2. stabilize the cannula in the vein to prevent trauma to the surrounding tissues.
    3. set the intravenous fluid to run at the prescribed rate of flow.
    4. speed up the flow rate of intravenous fluids when necessary to catch up on fluids that have not been administered at the prescribed rate.
    5. observe and record the patient's response to the administration of fluids.
    6. maintain strict asepsis when changing the intravenous tubing and bag.

6. A hypertonic solution would be used to:
    1. decrease the intravascular volume by pulling fluid into the interstitial space.
    2. maintain the normal tonicity of the blood.
    3. improve total body water distribution by moving fluid from the extracellular compartment to the intracellular compartment.
    4. pull fluid from the intracellular and interstitial spaces to the intravascular space.

7. Calculation: Find the correct number of drops per minute for the following order: 500 mL $D_5\frac{1}{2}NS$ IV q8h. Available: Microdrip tubing. _63 gtts / min_

8. Place an "X" on the diagram below where a central line would most likely be inserted for the administration of TPN or medications.

9. Metabolic acidosis is more likely to occur in a person who:
    1. is unable to metabolize carbohydrates normally or who ingests few or no carbohydrates.
    2. is unable to metabolize fats normally.
    3. suffers from kidney failure with excessive reabsorption of bicarbonate from the urine.
    4. has diarrhea with excessive loss of bicarbonates in the feces.

10. Nursing measures recommended to prevent central line infection include: *(Select all that apply.)*
    1. cleansing the insertion site with chlorhexidine solution for dressing changes.
    2. performing hand hygiene whenever changing fluids or performing dressing changes.
    3. daily review of the need for the central line.
    4. changing the dressing every 3 days.
    5. using barrier precautions when changing the dressing.

CRITICAL THINKING ACTIVITIES

Scenario: Intestinal Surgery

Your patient is a 68-year-old female who had intestinal surgery 2 days ago. She is NPO, has a nasogastric tube to suction, an intravenous line with $D_5\frac{1}{2}NS$ at 125 mL/hr. Physical assessment data includes: Alert and oriented but groggy, diaphoretic, fine crackles in the lower lobes of both lungs, moving all extremities, and complaining of abdominal pain and a dry mouth. Bowel sounds are hypoactive, no BM since surgery, and is voiding dark amber urine without difficulty. Urine sp. gr. is 1.030. NG output in last 2 hours is 200 mL of dark green secretions. Vital signs: T 101.2° F (38.4° C), P 92, BP 128/78. Intake last 24 hours: 2480 mL, output was 2010 mL. Laboratory values: K^+ 3.1 mEq/L, Na^+ 140 mEq/L, Cl^- 91 mEq/L.

1. What other assessment data should you acquire related to her fluid status?

    Skin turgor & condition of mucous membranes

2. Do the assessment findings indicate a fluid deficit or fluid excess problem? Explain using the assessment data.

    fluid volume deficit - urine is dark - specific gravity 1.030

3. What is her electrolyte status? Does she have any electrolyte abnormalities? If so, which one(s)? Give your rationale for your answers.

    Hypokalemic - potassium level 3.1 mEq
    Hypochloremic - chloride level 91 mEq/L

Scenario: Pneumonia

Your patient is a 76-year-old male who was just admitted with pneumonia. He is anorexic and has a temperature of 102.4° F (39.1° C), P 98, R 26 and shallow, BP 138/64. Pulse oximetry reading is 92% on room air. He is diaphoretic. Lung sounds reveal decreased breath sounds in bases with rhonchi in upper lobes. He is somewhat confused, which is not his normal status.

1. What assessments would you make regarding fluid and electrolyte status?

    Acid-base imbalance, hyponatremia from fever

2. What might be causing the patient's confusion?

    Fever - electrolyte imbalance causes confusion in elderly.

3. Would you expect that the patient would have an acid-base imbalance? If so, what would it probably be? *Respiratory acidosis – shallow breathing causing CO_2 build up.*

STEPS TOWARD BETTER COMMUNICATION

VOCABULARY BUILDING GLOSSARY

Term	Definition
syno'via (sin o' vee ah)	secreting membrane found in joints
a'queous (a' kwee us) hu'mor	transparent fluid between the lens of the eye and the cornea
paren'teral (pah ren' ter al)	by subcutaneous, intramuscular, intravenous, or method other than by mouth into the gastrointestinal tract
cru'cial (kru'shul)	of extreme importance
diaphore'sis (di ah for ee'sis)	excessive perspiration, a great deal of sweating
clam'my	cool and damp
sprue	disorder causing lack of nutrient absorption from the intestine
per'meable (per'mee a bul)	permitting passage of a substance (a property of membranes)
vis'cous (vis' kus)	thick, like honey (a property of fluids)

VOCABULARY EXERCISE

Table of prefixes to remember:

Prefix	Meaning	Examples
extra-	outside	extracellular
hyper-	more	hypertonic hyperglycemic
hypo-	less	hypotonic hypoglycemic
inter-	between, among	internal interstitial intervention
intra-	within	intracellular intravascular intravenous
iso-	same, equal	isotonic isometric
trans-	through, across	transcellular transfusion transport

COMPLETION

Directions: Fill in the blanks with the correct terms from the Vocabulary Building Glossary and the Vocabulary Exercise to complete the statements.

1. __Synovial__ fluid is located in the joints and acts as a lubricant for the joints.

2. Fluid balance is __Crucial__ to the well-being of an elderly person.

3. The patient with a high fever often experiences __diaphoresis__.

4. Normal saline intravenous solution is __isotonic__.

5. A 10% dextrose intravenous solution is __hypertonic__.

6. An intravenous infusion places fluid in the __intravascular__ space.

7. The patient who is experiencing shock has skin that feels __clammy__.

8. Enteral feeding solutions are more __viscous__ than intravenous solutions.

9. Patients who have __sprue__ often experience considerable diarrhea.

10. A membrane must be __permeable__ for diffusion to take place across it.

COMMUNICATION EXERCISE

Patient Teaching

A.   *Directions: A nurse is instructing a patient about intake and output. Note their interaction.*

Nurse: "Ms. T., the doctor wants us to measure everything you drink. This sheet will be here for you to write down the amount each time you drink something."

Ms. T.:   "How will I know how much I drank?"

Nurse: "See how this cup is marked with lines indicating the amount of fluid?"

Ms. T.:   "Oh, yes, I do see that now."

Nurse: "Now tell me what you will do."

Ms. T.:   "I need to look to see how much fluid is in the cup and then how much is left when I have had a drink. Do I subtract to determine the exact amount I drank?"

Nurse: "Yes, that's correct. If you have trouble, just call me and I'll help you. Let's try it now. The cup has 120 mL in it. Take a drink. Good. Now it has 60 mL left. So if we subtract 60 from 120, we find that you drank 60 mL. Let's write that down."

Ms. T.:   "It doesn't seem too complicated. Leave the paper and pencil next to the cup to remind me to write the amount down each time I drink, please."

Nurse: "Of course, Ms. T. Also, I need to measure your urine output. So whenever you use the toilet, be certain that the little white "hat" is sitting in it. Call me when you have finished and I will measure and record it. Try to drop any toilet paper into the toilet behind the hat so it doesn't alter the measurement."

Ms. T.:   "OK, I'll try."

B. *Directions: You have a patient who must take a diuretic because of fluid imbalance. What can you teach this patient about planning a diet that contains sufficient potassium? List at least five foods that are high in potassium.*

Explain that potassium rich foods such as avocado, bananas, dates, figs, + apricots. Also, potatoes, spinach + legumes provide potassium.

Care of Preoperative and Intraoperative Surgical Patients

chapter
4

Answer Key: Review the related chapter to answer these questions. A complete answer key was provided to your instructor.

COMPLETION

Preoperative Care

Directions: Fill in the blank with the correct word(s) to complete the sentences.

1. A technologic advance in surgery is use of a(n) _laperoscope_, as recovery for the patient is quicker.

2. The surgeon should be alerted if there is no _signed consent_ in the chart.

3. The elderly patient is more prone to fluid and electrolyte imbalances during and after surgery because they are more likely to have _impaired renal, hepatic, respiratory & cardiac function & chronic disease causing vulnerability to fluid/electrolyte imbalances_

4. Before surgery, it is important to know if the patient has any _allergies_ and if he is taking _any medications_.

5. Obese people are at higher risk with surgery because fat contains fewer blood vessels, causing _slower healing_ and a greater threat of _infection_.

6. Before surgery, it is imperative that _baseline vital signs_ are recorded on the chart for postoperative comparison.

7. Patients are encouraged to quit smoking before surgery because smoking has a negative effect on _wound healing_ and _pulmonary function_.

8. A patient who is allergic to _latex_ is at high risk of exposure during surgery.

9. Poorly controlled diabetes leads to postoperative complications such as _delayed healing_ and _infection_.

10. _Vitamin E_, _NSAIDs_, and _fish oil_ should be discontinued _7 to 14_ days before surgery.

PRIORITY SETTING

Directions: You have finished receiving report and are ready to begin patient care. You are assigned a preoperative surgery patient who is scheduled for surgery at 8:30 AM. How would you prioritize your actions? Number the actions listed below in the order (from 1 to 8) in which you would perform them.

6   a.   Complete the preoperative checklist.

1   b.   Check to see that the patient's signature is on the surgical consent form.

2   c.   Check that all diagnostic test results are back and determine if there are any abnormal lab values.

3   d.   Have the patient shower, if possible.

4   e.   Remind the patient to remain NPO and not to swallow any fluids or food.

5   f.   Have the patient remove any metal hairpins and jewelry and all underclothes, leaving on only a clean hospital gown.

7   g.   Start the presurgical nurse's notes in the chart, which will be finished when the transport person comes for the patient.

8   h.   Explain to the family where the surgical waiting room is and how to get there.

MATCHING

Surgical Risk Factors and Their Effects on Recovery

Mr. J. is admitted to the same-day surgery unit for repair of an inguinal hernia. He is 48 years old, has diabetes mellitus for which he takes insulin, is 140 pounds overweight, and smokes one and a half packs of cigarettes a day. He has smoked since age 15 and has chronic bronchitis with a productive cough.

Directions: Match each of Mr. J.'s surgical risk factors with the effect it can have on his recovery from surgery. (Note that there may be more than one effect for each risk factor.)

1.   **d, g**   Diabetes mellitus

2.   **b, f, h, i**   Smoking and chronic bronchitis

3.   **a, c, e**   Obesity

a.   Slower healing and risk of infection because adipose tissue has fewer blood vessels

b.   Decreased lung expansion due to chronic lung disease

c.   Decreased lung expansion due to upward pressure of enlarged abdomen against thorax

d.   Wide variations in blood glucose levels

e.   Potential for wound dehiscence because of added stress on sutures

f.   Accumulations of secretions in air passages

g.   Infection related to less phagocytic action against microorganisms

h.   Reduced level of functional hemoglobin

i.   Abnormal clot formation and obstruction of blood vessels

COMPLETION

Directions: Fill in the blank with the correct word(s) to complete the statements.

1. The function of the _____liver_____ is important in the surgical patient because this is where anesthetic agents are metabolized.

2. The ___Circulating___ nurse is responsible for opening sterile supplies during surgery.

3. Surgery is a risk for the elderly patient because ___thrombus___ formation is greater for the older the patient.

4. In addition to physiologic preparation, most surgical patients have a need for _emotional_ _psychosocial_ support.

5. As the patient leaves for surgery, family members should be informed about which three things?

   a. ___Where they can wait___
   b. ___When they will be able to see the patient___
   c. ___How long the surgery will take___

6. When a patient asks why he can't have anything to eat or drink for 8 hours prior to surgery, how should the nurse respond?

   ___Anesthesia depresses gag reflex + sometimes causes nausea. This makes the patient susceptible to aspiration___

APPLICATION OF THE NURSING PROCESS

Scenario: Ms. Sutton, age 38, is to undergo a simple mastectomy for early breast cancer. She will have general anesthesia. She has recently remarried and is concerned about her husband's feelings regarding her surgery.

1. List the patient problem statements that would be appropriate for Ms. Sutton in the preoperative period.

   ___Anxiety due to surgery + husband's possible reaction to surgery outcome. Grief over loss of breast Disrupted sleep due to anticipation of surgery.___

2. State an outcome objective for each of the above nursing diagnoses. ___Patient will manage anxiety with relaxation exercises. Patient will express concerns to husband about his feelings about the loss of her breast.___

3. List interventions that you would perform when the transport person comes to take Ms. Sutton to surgery.

   Both check the patient's ID bracelet with the medical record. Check for jewelry. Help transfer the patient to the stretcher + cover the patient. Complete the documentation note + Check the preoperative checklist is complete. Remind patient that the surgeon will verify + mark the surgical site prior to surgery.

4. How would you evaluate the preoperative care given to Ms. Sutton? Evaluate whether the interventions on the care plan were completed + if they were effective. Verify the patient discussed her concerns with her husband. Ask if her anxiety has lessened.

SHORT ANSWER

Intraoperative Care

Directions: Provide a brief answer to each question.

1. Describe autologous blood collection and reinfusion. Blood is withdrawn from the patient at a blood bank prior to surgery. It is stored + prepared for reinfusion should the patient require it.

2. What are the advantages of regional anesthesia? Less expensive + less dangerous

3. List four procedures for which local anesthesia is used.
   a. tissue biopsy
   b. Cyst excision
   c. pacemaker insertion
   d. Vascular access device insertion

4. Name three measures used to prevent the possibility of surgical infection in the operating suite.
   a. positive air pressure to prevent airborne entry of microorganisms
   b. Room temperature is kept low to discourage microbial growth
   c. Surgical asepsis is practiced by OR personnel

5. Identify the various measures used to prevent "wrong patient, wrong site" surgery from occurring.

The procedure is verified by the surgeon + preoperative nurse. The patient's ID bracelet is verified that it matches the medical record. The site is marked + verified by the patient. Before surgery begins a "time out" occurs + final verification occurs.

6. No matter what type of anesthesia is used, the goals of anesthesia should be kept in mind. They are:

   a. to prevent pain

   b. to achieve adequate muscle relaxation

   c. to calm fear, ease anxiety + induce forgetfulness of experience

7. Potential complications of surgery include the following. Describe an intervention to monitor and/or prevent their occurrence.

   a. Infection: Ensure sterile technique is maintained during surgery + preparing skin preparation prior to surgery

   b. Fluid volume imbalance: maintain fluid infusion at ordered rate; monitor urine output if catheter is inserted

   c. Hypothermia/hyperthermia: Monitor patient's temperature during surgery. Warming blanket as needed

   d. Injury: Pad all bony prominences when patient is positioned on the operating room table. Secure patient with safety straps.

REVIEW QUESTIONS FOR THE NCLEX® EXAMINATION

Directions: Choose the best answer(s) for the following questions.

1. Measures to prepare a patient psychologically for surgery include:
   1. making certain that the spouse is in favor of the surgery.
   2. teaching the patient to use the incentive spirometer before surgery.
   3. showing the patient the area that will be prepped and where the incision will be.
   4. allaying fears by teaching what will happen before, during, and after surgery.

2. The patient who has liver disease is at increased risk from surgery because: *(Select all that apply.)*
   1. good liver function is needed to metabolize drugs and anesthetics.
   2. the liver helps cleanse the blood of microorganisms.
   3. blood pressure swings are likely when liver function is poor.
   4. clotting times may be affected, causing the patient to bleed excessively.
   5. the liver stores extra blood that can be released if the patient becomes hypovolemic.

3. Skin preparation is performed before surgery to: *(Select all that apply.)*
   1. provide a better visual field for the surgeon.
   2. sterilize the skin.
   3. help prevent wound contamination. ⭕
   4. facilitate postoperative dressing changes.
   5. reduce the number of microorganisms at the surgical site. ⭕

4. The patient is scheduled for an exploratory laparotomy for an abdominal mass. The preoperative laboratory results are listed below. Which test finding would you report to the surgeon?
   1. CBC: Hgb 14.5 g, RBC 5.1
   2. WBC: 8600
   3. UA: sp. gr. 10.25, glucose negative, ketones negative, WBCs 57 per low-power field, casts 10 ⭕
   4. Blood glucose: 85 mg/dL

5. Advantages of general inhalant anesthesia include: *(Select all that apply.)*
   1. no nausea or vomiting occurs postoperatively.
   2. the patient is unaware of pain or discomfort. ⭕
   3. deep muscle relaxation is achieved. ⭕
   4. the patient recovers a few minutes after surgery.
   5. the patient is not awake during surgery. ⭕
   6. the patient can eat immediately after surgery.

6. Functions of the scrub nurse include: *(Select all that apply.)*
   1. assisting with ties of surgical team's gowns.
   2. preparing the instrument table. ⭕
   3. labeling and handling surgical specimens. ⭕
   4. assisting with transfer of the patient to the operating table.
   5. handing instruments and supplies to the OR team during surgery. ⭕
   6. maintaining sterility within the sterile operating field during surgery. ⭕

7. Procedural sedation is used for many surgeries. It consists of:
   1. a nerve block combined with oral sedation.
   2. local or regional anesthesia and IV sedation. ⭕
   3. inhalation of short-acting anesthetic.
   4. intravenous anesthesia and sedation.

CRITICAL THINKING ACTIVITIES

Scenario: Ms. Holt is scheduled for a colectomy for diverticulosis after many episodes of diverticulitis. She has been feeling much better since she finished the antibiotics for the last episode. You have the preoperative checklist in hand and are preparing her for surgery. She tells you that she has decided she doesn't want the surgery after all because she is feeling so much better.

1. What do you do? Describe the specific steps you would take in this situation. Verify the patient is positive she doesn't want the surgery. Inform the charge nurse + request the surgeon by informed. Stop preoperative procedures.

2. How would you document this event in her medical record? Document your actions in the medical record after noting patient's statement about not proceeding with surgery. Note the time the surgeon was notified + by whom.

STEPS TOWARD BETTER COMMUNICATION

VOCABULARY BUILDING GLOSSARY

Term	Definition
laparoscopic (lap a ro skop' ik)	seen or performed though a laparoscope, an instrument for direct visualization into the peritoneal body cavity
invasive (in vay' siv)	involving a puncture or incision of the skin
hemodilution (hee' mo di loo' shun)	increase of the fluid content of the blood, which decreases its concentration
coercion (co er' shun)	using force or threats to make a person do something

COMPLETION

Directions: Fill in the blanks with the correct words from the Vocabulary Building Glossary to complete the statements.

1. Administering too much intravenous fluid may cause ___hemodilution___.

2. Telling a patient that she will surely die without the surgery would be ___coercion___ to get the patient to sign the surgical consent form.

3. Even laparoscopic surgery is ___invasive___.

4. Gallbladder surgery is usually a(n) ___laparoscopic___ procedure these days.

GRAMMAR POINTS

Verb Forms—Future Tense

The nurse prepares the patient for surgery by performing preoperative teaching. Instructions to the patient are given using the future tense, such as "You will...", "You should...", or "The nurse is going to...". For the following set of orders, write out the instruction or explanation you would give to the patient as part of the preoperative teaching.

1. NPO after midnight: ___No eating or drinking anything after midnight.___

2. Report at 0600 to outpatient surgery unit: ___You need to be at the outpatient surgery desk at 6:00 Am.___

3. Surgical prep: ___Your skin will be cleansed with an antimicrobial solution in the operating room.___

4. Temazepam (Restoril) 30 mg PO hs: ___A sleeping pill is ordered for you at bedtime.___

Directions: Other instructions you would give to the patient might include the following. Fill in the blanks with the proper verb forms.

5. "The nurse _____will help_____ you to cough and deep-breathe every 2 hours."

6. "Turning _____is_____ required every 2 hours after surgery."

7. "You will need _____to ask_____ for pain medication and should do so before the pain becomes severe."

8. "Your valuable belongings _____will be_____ locked up in the business office or given to your husband."

9. "You _____will remove_____ your necklace prior to surgery."

10. "The side rails _____will be_____ raised after you have been given your preoperative medications."

CULTURAL POINTS

1. What special items might you need to think about if you are preparing an older patient for surgery?

   Hearing aid, dentures, glasses
   Cane /walker
   Prosthesis

2. What information would you give him or her about the items? Write out how you would state that information.

   Give location of where the item will be stored.
   Your hearing aid will be in the top drawer
   of the bedside table. I've notated the
   chart as well.

Care of Postoperative Surgical Patients

chapter

5

Answer Key: Review the related chapter to answer these questions. A complete answer key was provided to your instructor.

TABLE ACTIVITY

Anesthesia Implications

Directions: Complete the following table comparing the nursing implications of various types of anesthesia.

Type of Anesthesia	Postoperative Nursing Implications
Inhalation (general anesthesia)	① monitor for respiratory & circulatory difficulties ② Reduced need for narcotics after surgery as effects of inhaled anesthetic persists after pt regained consciousness
Intravenous drugs (procedural sedation)	① monitor airway & vital signs ② monitor level of consciousness & ability to respond to verbal commands
Regional or topical	① observe for depression of respirations & lowered blood pressure ② Patient remains conscious, fewer respiratory difficulties & cardiovascular complications occur

SHORT ANSWER

PACU Care

Directions: Provide the answers to the following questions in the blank spaces provided.

1. The correct way to open the airway of a patient who is still unconscious after surgery with general anesthesia is to:

   Jaw-thrust maneuver; place fingers behind the angle of the jaw & lift the jaw forward

2. Oxygen is administered in the PACU to the patient who has undergone general anesthesia for two reasons, which are:

    a. _to eliminate anesthetic gases_

    b. _to help meet increased metabolic demand for oxygen caused by surgery_

3. Discharge criteria from the PACU is based on a scoring system that includes assessment of:
    Circulation, respiration, skin color, activity, consciousness
    & oxygen saturation level

Postoperative Care

Directions: Answer the following questions in the spaces provided.

1. General anesthesia causes some atelectasis. The nurse must encourage deep-breathing and coughing to reexpand the lung alveoli because:
    If any area of the lung remains atelectatic for more than 72
    hours, hypostatic pneumonia from retained secretions is likely to occur

2. List five nursing responsibilities regarding the care of active surgical drains.

    a. _Monitor frequently to be sure it is open & draining_

    b. _Use strict aseptic technique when handling the drain & changing dressings_

    c. _Measure the amount, note characteristics of drainage_

    d. _Assess skin around drain_

    e. _Maintain suction by periodically compressing device_

3. Signs that circulation is adequate distal to the surgical site are: _Pulses are present, skin_
    is warm to the touch; no undue swelling

4. If there is no written order for dressing changes, what should be done? _Reinforce the dressing_
    as needed. & report abnormal drainage

5. What should be recorded on the patient's chart when a dressing is changed and drainage has occurred?
    Amount, color, odor, viscosity & clots

6. What signs and symptoms indicate an infected surgical wound? _Pain, redness, swelling_
    & hardness / fever

7. What is the correct procedure for the immediate care of a patient who experiences wound dehiscence with evisceration?
    Patient supine — cover wound & intentinal contents
    with sterile towels or moistened with saline dressings.
    Notify surgeon immediately

COMPLETION

Directions: Fill in the blanks to complete the statements.

1. Besides checking the rate of respirations, it is important to check both the _____quality_____
    _____ and ___depth of respiration_____.

2. Besides medicating for pain, measures to promote comfort in the immediate postoperative period include providing __warmth_____ and medicating as needed for ____nausea_____.

3. The four initial classic signs of shock resulting from hypovolemia due to hemorrhage are
    ___thirst_____, ___blurred vision_____, ___restlessness_____, and
    ___blurred vision____.

4. In addition to those above, describe other physical changes that occur with the progression of shock.
    a. Pulse: ___increases – bounding at first then thready____
    b. Blood pressure: ___falls_____
    c. Respirations: ___rapid_____
    d. Skin: ___cold & clammy, pale; cyanosis of lips & nail beds occurs late__
    e. Level of consciousness: ___decreases until comatose_____

5. Another complication to which the elderly patient is more susceptible is overhydration. Signs that would make the nurse suspect overhydration include:
    ___Crackles in lungs; shortness of breath, confusion_____

6. A postoperative patient is complaining of shortness of breath and chest pain. He is very anxious and has a cough, rapid pulse, and rapid respirations. These could indicate the complication of:
    ___Pulmonary embolus or myocardial infarction_____

APPLICATION OF THE NURSING PROCESS

Scenario: Mr. Honda, age 73, has undergone a colectomy. He did well through surgery and in the recovery room. He has an IV with D$_5$NS hanging, an NG tube set to low suction, and a urinary catheter. He has a history of arthritis and chronic bronchitis. He is usually an "active senior," playing golf several times each week and tending his garden. He is breathing shallowly when you assess him and is complaining of pain at 7 out of 10 on the pain scale.

1. Choose the top four patient problems that would appropriate for Mr. Honda during this postoperative period.
    a. ___Altered breathing pattern_____
    b. ___Pain, acute_____
    c. ___Altered skin integrity_____
    d. ___Potential infection_____

2.   Write at least one expected outcome for each of the above problem statements.

   a. Patient will have no signs of wound infection at discharge

   b. Patient's incision will remain clean, dry & intact

   c. Patient's pain will be controlled to under a level of 5

   d. Patient's oxygen saturation ↑ 95%.

3.   What nursing interventions should be included on the plan of care to monitor for pulmonary problems?

Monitor patient's temperature, pulse & respirations. Auscultate breath sounds & monitor oxygen saturation level every 4 hours.

4.   What adjunct measures could you use along with pain medication to treat this patient's pain?

Encourage patient to try relaxation, deep breathing, imagery. Encourage patient to keep room noise to a minimum & be sure room is tidy.

5.   What measures would you institute to promote good oxygenation and circulation? Instruct on using incentive spirometer encouraging every 2 hours. Have patient sit up & encourage patient to cough

6.   What evaluation criteria would tell you that the patient is breathing effectively? Chest expansion adequate & equal bilaterally. No sign of Dyspnea & Oxygen Saturation level between 95 & 100.

7.   What evaluation criteria would tell you that the patient's pain is adequately controlled? If patient rates pain under a level of 5 & decreases with pain medication

PRIORITY SETTING

You are assigned to care for Mr. Johnson, who has just returned from surgery for colon resection. You receive report from the PACU nurse and settle the patient in the bed. Number the actions listed below in the order (from 1 to 12) in which you would perform them.

<u>2</u>   a. Inspect the surgical dressing.

<u>3</u>   b. Check all tubes and drains for patency.

<u>1</u>   c. Take vital signs.

<u>6</u>   d. Adjust the IV drip rate to the ordered flow rate.

<u>8</u>   e. Inquire about the patient's pain level.

<u>9</u>   f. Ask the patient to take four deep breaths.

<u>4</u>   g. Hook the NG tube to the suction.

<u>12</u>   h. Document the postoperative assessment.

<u>5</u>   i. Verify that the correct IV solution is hanging.

<u>10</u>   j. Provide an additional warmed blanket.

<u>11</u>   k. Allow the family to visit.

<u>7</u>   l. Auscultate the heart and lungs.

REVIEW QUESTIONS FOR THE NCLEX® EXAMINATION

Directions: Choose the best answer(s) for the following questions.

1. Measures to prevent thrombophlebitis in a postoperative patient who has had an abdominal incision are: *(Select all that apply.)*
   1. PCA use for pain.
   2. application of sequential compression devices on the legs.
   3. early ambulation with sessions three times a day.
   4. promote sufficient hydration via oral and IV fluid.
   5. encouraging leg exercises at least every 2 hours while awake.

2. The patient *most* likely to have pulmonary complications after surgery is the one who has had a(n):
   1. appendectomy.
   2. hysterectomy.
   3. tonsillectomy.
   4. colectomy.

3. Adynamic ileus can occur after anesthesia and abdominal surgery. Signs and symptoms found on assessment include:
   1. high-pitched, frequent bowel sounds in all four quadrants.
   2. diarrhea, cramping, and high-pitched bowel sounds.
   3. absence of bowel sounds in upper quadrants.
   4. abdominal distention, pain, no passage of feces or flatus, and no bowel sounds.

4. Coughing after surgery is evaluated not only by the amount of airflow produced by the cough but also by:
   1. the loudness of the sound made.
   2. the number of coughs produced at one time.
   3. the degree of inspiration prior to the cough.
   4. whether secretions are moved up and out of the bronchial tree.

5. Mastectomy surgery may cause psychological problems. The nurse should assess for signs of ineffective coping such as:
   1. excessive pain.
   2. withdrawn behavior.
   3. constant complaining.
   4. demanding behavior.

6. A sign of wound infection is:
   1. serous drainage.
   2. purulent drainage.
   3. pink granular tissue at edges of wound.
   4. reddish-yellow wound drainage.

7. The plan of care for the immediate postoperative period should include which safety measure?
   1. Keeping an emesis basin within the patient's reach
   2. Positioning the patient on their side until they are alert enough to prevent aspiration
   3. Talking to the patient and reorienting them frequently
   4. Covering the patient with warmed blankets to decrease chilling

8. Safety measures for the postoperative patient include: *(Select all that apply.)*
   1. cautioning the patient not to get out of bed without assistance while receiving narcotic analgesics.
   2. answering the patient's call light promptly.
   3. assessing the patient for bladder distention every 8 hours.
   4. monitoring fluid intake and output closely.
   5. assessing urine output every 2 hours.
   6. assessing vital sign trends.

9. The order reads: Infuse D$_5$RL 1000 mL over 6 hours. The IV tubing delivers 10 drops per mL. The drop rate should be _____ gtts/minute. *(Fill in the blank.)*
   1. 21
   2. 28
   3. 31
   4. 26

10. When assisting the patient to arise from the bed postoperatively, you would have them *first*:
    1. push up from the bed with the elbows.
    2. turn toward the side of the bed from which they are going to exit.
    3. bend the knees and plant the feet flat on the mattress.
    4. grab the top side rail and push up to a sitting position.

CRITICAL THINKING ACTIVITY

Scenario: Mr. H. has just returned to his room from the PACU. He has had a colectomy performed. He is receiving IV fluids and antibiotics.

1. On the second postoperative day, he has decreased breath sounds and some dyspnea. He is not coughing much. What complication of surgery might he be experiencing?

   Atelectasis & retained secretions

2. He has an NG tube attached to suction and is NPO. The last shift assessment found that he is tachycardic, has decreased urine output, poor skin turgor, and his blood pressure has dropped 20 points. What would you suspect is the problem?

   Dehydration

3. Mr. H. improves and is ready for discharge. He will continue oral antibiotics at home. What instructions should he be given?

    Diet, medication schedule, activity, wound care,
    respiratory care, next appointment

STEPS TOWARD BETTER COMMUNICATION

VOCABULARY BUILDING GLOSSARY

Term	Definition
allay' (ah lay')	to calm, to place at rest
induce' (in doos')	to bring on by outside means
grog'gy	unsteady or shaky with an unclear mind
numb (num)	lack of sensation; no feeling
kink'ed (kinkt)	bent sharply so as to block the flow inside
malaise' (mah layz')	general feeling of bodily discomfort

COMPLETION

Directions: Fill in the blanks with the correct words from the Vocabulary Building Glossary to complete the statements.

1. Ms. P. is awake from anesthesia but is still very _groggy_.

2. The nurse must carefully check each tube and drain after turning a patient to be certain that no tube is _kinked_.

3. After spinal anesthesia, the patient's legs are _numb_ for a few hours.

4. Mr. R.'s wound was healing nicely but he is suffering from _malaise_.

5. Certain drugs can sometimes _induce_ anaphylactic shock.

GRAMMAR POINTS

As a nurse, you will be giving postoperative discharge instructions to your patients. Some instructions are about things the patient *should* do (ought or are strongly advised to do); others are about things that they *should not* do. Certain things *must* be done (are necessary to do, cannot be avoided) to prevent complications; other things *must not* be done or they may interfere with recovery. Insert the correct instruction before each statement.

You should   You should not   You must   You must not

1. _You should_ walk for 5–10 minutes three times a day.

2. _You must_ inspect the incision for signs of redness or drainage every day.

3. _You should not_ scratch the incision if it starts to itch.

4. _You must not_ lift anything heavier than 5 pounds for at least 4 weeks.

5. _You should_ call the health care provider if your temperature rises to 100.2° F (38.0° C).

COMMUNICATION EXERCISE

Dialogue Example

Joan, an LVN, is getting Mr. Cox out of bed to sit in the chair for the second time since his surgery yesterday. Note how Joan interacts with Mr. Cox.

Joan:	"Mr. Cox, it is time to get you up to sit in the chair for about 20 minutes now. I'll help you sit on the side of the bed and put on your robe."
Mr. Cox:	"Do I have to get up now? I just finished breakfast."
Joan:	"Yes, your doctor left orders for you to be up in the chair after breakfast."
Mr. Cox:	"You won't leave me there too long, will you?"
Joan:	"No, I'll be back in about 20 minutes to help you back into bed."
Mr. Cox:	"OK."
Joan:	"Place your left hand on the side rail and turn toward me." (She raises the head of the bed slightly and helps Mr. Cox to turn on his side and swing his feet over the side of the bed into a sitting position. She helps him put his arms into his robe while he is seated.)
Mr. Cox:	"Whee, I feel just a little dizzy."
Joan:	"Just sit here for a moment until the dizziness passes."
Mr. Cox:	"OK. I feel better now."
Joan:	"Let me put your slippers on your feet and then I'll help you to stand up. Place your hands on my shoulders and stand on the count of three." (Joan helps Mr. Cox to stand by supporting him while he rises.)
Mr. Cox:	"I made it."
Joan:	"That was very good. Now we'll walk over to the chair and turn so that you are ready to sit down."
Mr. Cox:	"I don't want to miss the seat when I sit down."
Joan:	"Move back so the chair is touching the back of your legs. Place your right hand on the arm of the chair and slowly lower yourself into the chair." (Mr. Cox does this successfully.) "That was great. Would you like a blanket over your legs to keep you warm?"
Mr. Cox:	"No, I'm warm enough. That wasn't as hard as it was yesterday. Thank you."
Joan:	"OK. It is 9:10 now, so I'll be back at 9:30."

Infection Prevention and Control

Answer Key: Review the related chapter to answer these questions. A complete answer key was provided to your instructor.

COMPLETION

Directions: Fill in the blanks to complete the statements.

1. All streptococci and staphylococci are gram-____*positive*____ organisms.

2. A large factor in the contraction of disease is the status of the patient's ____*immune system*____.

3. Insufficient hand hygiene by medical staff and other people in contact with patients is a major cause of ~~~~ *health care- associated* infections.

4. Chlamydia is typically transmitted via ____*sexual*____ contact.

5. Pathogens are transmitted by three routes: ____*airborne*____, ____*contact*____, and ____*droplet*____.

6. Viruses are of three types: ____*latent*____, ____*active*____, or ____*oncogenic*____.

7. Ebola is a(n) ____*active*____ virus that is extremely ____*lethal*____.

8. Caring for a patient with Ebola virus requires strict precautions including a(n) ____*buddy*____ to assist when donning and doffing personal protective equipment (PPE).

SHORT ANSWER

Causes and Symptoms of Infection

Scenario: You are caring for patients on a general medical-surgical unit. Currently, there are several postoperative patients; therefore, you are vigilant for signs and symptoms of infection in these patients. You also have an elderly patient who is fairly immobile so you are aware of the need to assess them for signs of pneumonia.

Directions: Provide the answers to the following questions.

1. List four specific signs and symptoms that suggest presence of a respiratory infection such as pneumonia.

   a. _Cough_

   b. _Fever_

   c. _Malaise_

   d. _Increased respiratory rate_

2. What are five local signs and symptoms of inflammation?

   a. _Heat_

   b. _Redness_

   c. _Swelling_

   d. _Pain_

   e. _Loss of function_

3. Identify seven signs and symptoms of systemic or generalized infection.

   a. _Fever_

   b. _Headache_

   c. _Chills_

   d. _Malaise_

   e. _Loss of appetite_

   f. _Diaphoresis_

   g. _Muscle ache_

Nursing Interventions for Patients with Infections

Directions: Provide the answers to the following questions.

1. List three nursing interventions that can be used to reduce high fevers.

   a. _Increase fluid intake_

   b. _Control environmental temperature_

   c. _Provide tepid baths_

2. What are three teaching points to help patients avoid spreading respiratory infections to others?

   a. _Cover mouth when coughing_

   b. _Dispose of used tissues in trash_

   c. _Hand hygiene_

3. List five things that you should do to help prevent health care–associated infections.

a. _Hand hygiene_

b. _If patient has C Diff healthcare workers need to use soap_

c. _Do not place soiled items on floor_

d. _Inform housekeeping about C Diff_

e. _Hand hygiene before + after any direct patient contact_

TABLE ACTIVITY

Directions: Complete the following table by supplying appropriate information in each column. Some of the blocks have been filled in for you.

Category-Specific Isolation Expanded Precautions (Transmission Based)

Isolation Category	Private Room	Masks	Gowns	Gloves	Common Diseases Placed into Isolation Category
Airborne Infection Isolation	Always; door to room must be kept closed at all times	N-95 respiratory	No, unless draining wounds	No - unless draining wounds	Pulmonary or laryngeal tuberculosis, or draining tuberculous skin lesions; smallpox; viral hemorrhagic fever; severe acute respiratory syndrome (SARS); measles; varicella, disseminated zoster
Contact Precautions	Preferred cohorting of patients with same type of infection	Situation dependent	Always - if patients cohorted staff must perform hand hygiene + change PPE	Always; if patients are cohorted, staff must perform hand hygiene and change PPE *between* patients	MRSA VRE ESBL + MDRO infections
Droplet Precautions	Preferred cohorting of patients with same type of infection	Wear a surgical mask when entering room; patient should wear mask during transport and observe cough etiquette	not usually	When helping with cough-inducing procedures	Pertussis Influenza Rubella Pneumonia
Ebola Precautions (Requires "buddy" to assist donning/ doffing PPE.)	Mandatory	Cover hair Full-face shield must wear N-95 respiratory mask	Change into hospital-issued scrubs or disposable scrubs, then don impervious cover gown and hood that covers all of the neck and chest. If activities performed in the patient's room are likely to dislodge cuff or gown, secure cuff with Coban or tape.	Don first pair before donning impervious shoe/ leg cover, don cover gown. Second pair is donned after face mask, hair cover, and hood are donned.	Airborne, Contact precautions with "buddy" observing all aspects of care provided to ensure no exposure

PRIORITY SETTING

Scenario: You are caring for a patient who was admitted for a leg infection. She needs IV antibiotic medication. She is unsure but she believes that it will be the first time that she will receive this medication.

Directions: Prioritize the steps below for safe administration.

_____ a. Check the order and know why the patient is to receive an antimicrobial drug.

_____ b. Check that the dosage of the antimicrobial drug is appropriate for the patient.

_____ c. Verify allergies with the patient before administering an antimicrobial drug.

_____ d. Obtain cultures prior to administering the antimicrobial agent.

_____ e. Check to see if serum drug levels or cultures have been ordered.

_____ f. Monitor patient for signs of allergic reaction, such as rash, hives, itching, drug fever, swelling of the mucous membranes, difficulty breathing, or anaphylaxis.

SHORT ANSWER

Sepsis

Scenario: You are working in an extended-care facility. Mr. Fayed is an elderly patient who is generally alert, cheerful, and conversant. Today, you immediately notice a marked change in his behavior and he appears very ill. You are aware that he has had some urinary symptoms (i.e., frequency and urgency) over the past 2 days.

Directions: Answer the following questions about sepsis.

1. List four signs and symptoms of sepsis.

   a. _____

   b. _____

   c. _____

   d. _____

2. How might these symptoms differ in an elderly person? _____

   _____

   _____

APPLICATION OF THE NURSING PROCESS

Care of the Patient at Risk for Infection

Directions: Write a short-term and a long-term goal and 4–6 interventions and an example of an evaluation statement for the short-term goal.

Mr. Jackson is a 76-year-old patient residing in an extended-care facility. He has chronic poor circulation to his lower extremities; the skin just above the ankles has a brownish discoloration and is very leathery. He complains of itching and frequently scratches his legs; there are some very faint scratch-type marks above the ankles.

Problem Statement/Nursing Diagnosis: Potential for infection related to poor circulation and skin ulceration

Goals/Expected Outcomes	Nursing Interventions	Evaluation

REVIEW QUESTIONS FOR THE NCLEX® EXAMINATION

Directions: Choose the correct answer(s) for the following questions.

1. When a nurse assesses the patient for signs of local infection, which sign(s) or symptom(s) would indicate a local infection? *(Select all that apply.)*
   1. Redness of skin and adjacent tissues
   2. Swelling at the site and surrounding tissues
   3. Pain at the site and surrounding tissues
   4. Limited function of the involved part
   5. Decreased peripheral pulses

2. The patient requires Transmission-Based Precautions because of a draining wound positive for methicillin-resistant *Staphylococcus aureus* (MRSA). The patient must go to the radiology department for diagnostic testing. What should the nurse do?
   1. Call the health care provider and ask if the testing is really needed.
   2. Reschedule the test for after the MRSA is resolved.
   3. Put a mask on the patient just prior to transport.
   4. Communicate with the radiology department regarding the presence of MRSA.

3. A patient has a staphylococcal infection that developed in an abdominal wound. The dressing must be changed once each shift. The patient is underweight, suffering from malnutrition, and has a fever. Which nursing action(s) is/are essential? *(Select all that apply.)*
   1. Assess bowel and urine elimination regularly.
   2. Monitor temperature and promptly report abnormal readings.
   3. Encourage the patient to eat well-balanced, nutritious meals.
   4. Strictly adhere to precautions to avoid spreading infection.
   5. Plan active exercise to promote mobility.

4. A medication likely to be prescribed to combat a fungal infection is:
   1. acetaminophen (Tylenol).
   2. trimethoprim-sulfamethoxazole (Septra).
   3. ketoconazole (Nizoral).
   4. penicillin V (Pen-Vee K).

5. A patient has a hacking cough, a runny nose, and painful swallowing because of a sore throat. He is diagnosed with a streptococcal infection of the throat. The nurse should use gloves for which type of activity?
    1. Taking a history from the patient
    2. Obtaining a throat swab for a culture and sensitivity test
    3. Delivering the throat culture tube to the lab
    4. Reviewing the culture results with the patient

6. Which patient(s) is/are most likely to have depression of the immune system? A patient who: *(Select all that apply.)*
    1. takes antibiotics for a urinary tract infection
    2. drinks alcohol excessively
    3. has chronic renal failure
    4. has been on corticosteroids for a long time
    5. is overweight for height
    6. is employed in a long-term care facility

7. To help a patient recover from a throat infection, what should he be advised to do?
    1. Continue his normal workout routine but to get plenty of rest at night.
    2. Drink 8 ounces of liquid every hour while he is awake.
    3. When the sore throat stops, discontinue prescribed medications.
    4. Take an antipyretic with meals or a snack.

8. The patient comes to the clinic for a chief complaint of burning with urination and urinary urgency. Based on her complaints, what additional assessment data would be most appropriate to obtain *first*?
    1. Assess her genitalia for signs of inflammation.
    2. Check her chart for a history of kidney problems.
    3. Check her temperature to assess for a fever.
    4. Ask her about drug and food allergies.

9. When assessing a patient for an infection, the nurse suspects infection when the white blood cell count is:
    1. 4500 mm^3.
    2. 6500 mm^3.
    3. 3000 mm^3.
    4. 13,200 mm^3.

10. The nurse observes a new nursing assistant using a mask, a gown, foot covers, and gloves for every patient she is assigned to. What should the nurse do *first*?
    1. Check the assignment sheet to see what kinds of patients the assistant is assigned to.
    2. Ask the charge nurse to intervene because the assistant is wasting supplies.
    3. Assess the assistant's understanding of Standard and Transmission-Based Precautions.
    4. Allow her to continue to work because her actions prevent health care–associated infection.

11. Alcohol-based hand sanitizer is frequently adequate; however, when caring for patients with infections, which types of pathogens require strict soap-and-water hand hygiene? *(Select all that apply.)*
    1. *Clostridium difficile*
    2. *Staphylococcus aureus*
    3. *Candida albicans*
    4. *Pseudomonas aeruginosa*
    5. *Klebsiella pneumoniae*

12. Which action(s) would the nurse take to reduce the risk of health care–associated infections for patients who are at risk? *(Select all that apply.)*
    1. Position the patient in a supine position for comfort.
    2. Offer and assist with frequent oral hygiene.
    3. Obtain an order for indwelling catheter for incontinent patients.
    4. Encourage patients to cough and deep-breathe.
    5. Be protective of skin when moving and repositioning the older adult.
    6. Use strict aseptic technique for any invasive procedure.

13. The patient is being treated for a skin infection. The nurse sees an order for metronidazole (Flagyl). What should the nurse do *first*?
    1. Give the medication as ordered and observe for side effects.
    2. Review the nursing implications for the drug.
    3. Ask another nurse if this drug is appropriate for the patient.
    4. Check laboratory results to verify presence of an anaerobic infection.

14. The order is to give an older adult 350 mg of liquid preparation of cephalexin (Keflex) every 6 hours. On hand is cephalexin 250 mg/5 mL oral suspension. How many milliliters (mL) should be given for each dose? _5.4_ *(Fill in the blank.)*

15. The health care provider orders 600 mg of acetaminophen. The pharmacy delivers a 3-ounce bottle of acetaminophen 325 mg/10.15 mL. How many mL should be given? _18.7_

CRITICAL THINKING ACTIVITIES

Scenario A: You observe that a new nursing assistant has a cough and runny nose. She is assigned to care for a patient under protective precautions. You realize that she may be unfamiliar with this type of isolation, or that she may not know how to deal with the situation.

1. What should you do? _____

    _____

    _____

Scenario B: You see a laboratory technician drawing blood from a patient. He is not wearing gloves, stating, "I don't need gloves." He appears to be competent and is quickly able to draw the blood without apparent contact with body fluids.

1. Explore how you would handle this situation. _____

    _____

    _____

    _____

    _____

STEPS TOWARD BETTER COMMUNICATION

VOCABULARY BUILDING GLOSSARY

*Directions: The following words from Chapter 6 have the long **a** sound, as in* name. *Perhaps you can find others.*

Term	Definition
surveil'lance (ser vay'lenz)	continuous watching for something
malaise' (mah layz')	feeling of illness
-phage (fahj)	eating, swallowing
mac'rophage (mak' row fahj)	large phagocytic cell
phagocyto'sis (fag ow sytow' sis)	surrounding of microorganism by phagocytes
asep'tic	free from bacteria
asep'sis	method to prevent infection, keep bacteria-free

PRONUNCIATION SKILLS

*The long **a** sound can be spelled in a number of ways.*

Spelling	Examples
a	latent, anal, patient, dangerous, table, dilation, incubation
a–e	invade, isolate, palpate, dilate, lactate, incubate, drape, -phage, make, mistake (silent "e" at end)
ai	brain, pain, malaise, daily, wait, straight
ay	day, say, stay, May
ea	great, break, steak
ei	vein, weigh, nucleic, eight
ey	they, obey

MATCHING

Directions: Match the following terms with their correct definitions.

1. _____ Asepsis
2. _____ Malaise
3. _____ Exudate
4. _____ Purulent
5. _____ Surveillance

a. General feeling of illness, not well
b. Containing pus
c. Watching for
d. Keeping free from bacteria
e. Discharge composed of tissue, fluid, and dead cells

PRONUNCIATION SKILLS

*Directions: In the following sentences, underline the letters in the words that have the long **a** sound.*

1. Draping the patient on the table before a procedure protects the patient's privacy and modesty. It helps to maintain aseptic conditions.

2. Ms. Clay has fever and malaise and her wound has green exudate.

3. Ms. James is not having any pain but she has gained more than eighteen pounds in weight.

COMMUNICATION EXERCISES

Directions: Write out what you would say for the following situations.

1. Ms. Compton had a laparoscopic hysterectomy yesterday and has been found to have an abscess (boil) in the axilla. The abscess has been drained. How would you explain the importance of hand hygiene and using clean towels and washcloths to bathe when she goes home?

    _____

    _____

    _____

    _____

    _____

    _____

2. You have a patient with a large infected wound on his shin. How would you explain to him how infection is spread and the precautions that must be taken in caring for him and changing his dressings?

    _____

    _____

    _____

    _____

    _____

    _____

    _____

    _____

Care of Patients with Pain

Answer Key: Review the related chapter to answer these questions. A complete answer key was provided to your instructor.

TABLE ACTIVITY

Common Terms to Help Patients Describe Their Pain

Directions: Fill in the table with some common terms to help your patient describe pain.

Degree of pain (from least to most severe)	
Quality of pain	
Frequency of pain	

COMPLETION

Directions: Fill in the blanks to complete the statements.

1. The body produces _____, which can attach to pain receptors and block the pain sensation.

2. Sinus infection pain reflected in the upper molars is termed _____ pain.

3. Rest _____ pain tolerance and improves response to analgesia.

4. One "rule" to keep in mind is that massage should *not* be used on areas _____.

5. A dressing change or an uncomfortable procedure can be made less painful if you ask the patient questions and _____ his attention during the procedure.

6. Repositioning is an important measure in _____ pain, especially in the elderly.

7. Examples of narcotic analgesics are _____, _____, and

    _____.

8. A measure of the effectiveness of control of chronic pain is how well the patient can accomplish

    _____.

SHORT ANSWER

Pain and Pain Management

Directions: Read the scenario and answer the questions that follow.

Scenario: You have been asked to assist the nurse manager to develop an in-service for the nursing staff about pain and pain management. He has asked you to collect some relevant information that can be reviewed with the staff and to make a handout that compares acute and chronic pain.

1. What are five facts that dispel false perceptions about pain?

    a. _____
        _____

    b. _____

    c. _____
        _____

    d. _____
        _____

    e. _____
        _____

2. List four nonphysical factors that affect pain tolerance.

    a. _____

    b. _____

    c. _____

    d. _____

3. List at least six nonpharmacologic approaches that can be used as adjuncts to medication.

    a. _____

    b. _____

    c. _____

    d. _____

    e. _____

    f. _____

4. Briefly explain how imagery and meditation can assist with pain control._____

    _____

TABLE ACTIVITY

Acute Versus Chronic Pain

Directions: Fill in the table to compare features of acute and chronic pain.

Pain	Acute	Chronic
Duration		
Prognosis for relief		
Cause		
Psychosocial effects		
Effect of therapy		

APPLICATION OF THE NURSING PROCESS

Caring for a Patient with Acute Pain

Directions: Provide the answer to the following scenarios.

Mr. Takanali sustained injuries in a tour bus accident and was transferred 2 days ago from the ICU to the general medical-surgical unit. He has a broken arm, rib fractures, and soft tissue trauma on both legs. Mr. Takanali has a difficult time verbalizing his pain to the nursing staff and frequently declines medication. He is quiet and withdrawn and often appears very uncomfortable.

1. List at least six physiologic clues that upon assessment might indicate Mr. Takanali is experiencing pain.

    a. _____

    b. _____

    c. _____

    d. _____

    e. _____

    f. _____

2. List at least five behaviors you might observe that indicate that Mr. Takanali may be having pain.

   a. _____

   b. _____

   c. _____

   d. _____

   e. _____

3. You are reinforcing teaching points to help Mr. Takanali understand pain management. *(Select all that apply.)*
   a. Medication is more effective if taken before pain is too severe.
   b. Taking medication regularly helps control the pain.
   c. Pain actually interferes with wound healing.
   d. Addiction to narcotics happens in usually less than 1% of patients.
   e. Pain tolerance does not vary greatly from one person to the next.

4. List five areas that should be covered in documentation about pain and measures taken for the treatment of pain.

   a. _____

   b. _____

   c. _____

   d. _____

   e. _____

PRIORITY SETTING

Directions: Read the scenarios and prioritize tasks and patients' needs appropriately.

Scenario A: You are caring for Mr. Pulido. He sustained a broken ankle with severe soft tissue swelling and many abrasions in a motorcycle accident. He was admitted and has an external fixation procedure for the ankle fracture. He received IV morphine before the procedure, procedural sedation, and a nerve block for the fixation. He is receiving morphine by PCA pump. Prioritize the following nursing responsibilities related to giving analgesic medications. Ibuprofen 800 mg is ordered as needed every 6 hours for his many abrasions and muscle pain.

_____   a. Verify PCA pump settings with order.

_____   b. Reinforce teaching about medications.

_____   c. Use nonpharmacologic measures such as elevation or ice packs.

_____   d. Report to the health care provider when measures are not effective.

_____   e. Assess the patient's pain.

_____   f. Check the medication record for last dose of ibuprofen.

Scenario B: You are caring for several patients on a busy medical-surgical unit. While you are aware that all patients expect and deserve to receive timely and adequate relief of their pain, you also recognize the need to organize and prioritize your actions. Based on your knowledge of pain and pathophysiology, prioritize the order in which you will attend to the analgesic needs of these patients.

_____ a. Mr. Johnson is postoperative for a hernia repair. He complains of pain 8/10 in the lower abdominal area.

_____ b. Ms. Quick reports pain in the left neck and jaw that radiates down to the back.

_____ c. Mr. Ben-David reports severe pain that started 10 minutes ago, in the area distal to his lower extremity cast.

_____ d. Mr. Ramous is a diabetic who has continuous neuropathic pain in his lower legs.

REVIEW QUESTIONS FOR THE NCLEX® EXAMINATION

Directions: Choose the best answer(s) for the following questions.

1. The patient is experiencing pain in a limb after amputation. What type of pain is this patient experiencing?
   1. Chronic pain
   2. Phantom pain
   3. Referred pain
   4. Nociceptive pain

2. The nurse understands that the choice of a pain scale to use for a patient depends on the:
   1. pain scales available on the unit.
   2. age and physical and cognitive ability of the patient.
   3. nurse's preference for a pain scale.
   4. World Health Organization's recommendation.

3. When teaching about the side effects of opioid pain medication, you would tell the patient to take measures to prevent:
   1. dizziness.
   2. drowsiness.
   3. constipation.
   4. urinary retention.

4. Gabapentin (Neurontin) is given to relieve which type of pain?
   1. Acute pain
   2. Chronic pain
   3. Neuropathic pain
   4. Nociceptive pain

5. A patient is undergoing rehabilitative therapy. When would be the *best* time to give analgesic medication?
   1. Give PRN medications every 4–6 hours.
   2. Give early in the morning before performing activities of daily living.
   3. Give on a schedule to minimize pain during therapy sessions.
   4. Give whenever the pain is greater than 4/10.

6. The patient is unable to verbalize pain. Which patient behavior is the best indicator that pain medication is successfully addressing the patient's pain?
   1. Patient sleeps unless aroused by nurse.
   2. Patient watches TV without grimacing.
   3. Patient actively participates in physical therapy.
   4. Patient smiles at friends and family when they visit.

7. The nurse gives the patient a 4-mg IV dose of morphine at 10:00 AM. When should the nurse next evaluate the effectiveness of the pain control medication?
   1. 10:30 AM
   2. 11:00 AM
   3. 11:30 AM
   4. 12:30 PM

8. When evaluating the effectiveness of pain medication, in addition to assessing physical body language, the nurse should rely on:
   1. the length of time between requests for pain medication.
   2. how sedated the patient becomes after receiving the medication.
   3. whether the patient experiences nausea from the medication.
   4. what the patient says about his pain relief.

9. Packs or compresses for heat therapy are usually left in place for:
   1. 1 hour.
   2. 30 minutes.
   3. 10 minutes.
   4. 20 minutes.

10. Intramuscular analgesic injections are not recommended for the elderly because:
    1. kidney function is decreased and the drug is excreted more slowly.
    2. circulation is sluggish and the medication is not picked up quickly.
    3. skin and tissue are more fragile and bruising is likely.
    4. muscle and fat tissue are diminished, which may affect bioavailability.

CRITICAL THINKING ACTIVITIES

Scenario: Ms. Cole, age 74, is admitted to the hospital for a laparoscopic cholecystectomy. She has a history of chronic gallbladder disease with episodes of pain, nausea, and vomiting. During her initial assessment upon admission, you learn that Ms. Cole has had rheumatoid arthritis of the knees and hips for about 15 years.

1. Which statement most accurately applies to Ms. Cole's problem of arthritis pain?
   a. If she does not mention having pain due to her arthritis, it is because she has gotten used to it over the years and it no longer bothers her much.
   b. Unless some degeneration of the joints is shown by x-rays, there is little reason to believe that a person has pain with arthritis.
   c. The use of moist heat in the morning upon arising can diminish pain with movement.
   d. Ibuprofen, a nonnarcotic analgesic, and hot packs applied to her knees help relieve Ms. Cole's pain at home and could be continued in the hospital.

2. If Ms. Cole states that she often feels pain under her right shoulder blade when her gallbladder "acts up," you can assume that Ms. Cole:
   a. probably also has an undiagnosed heart condition.
   b. is feeling referred pain.
   c. is confused about where her pain really is.
   d. is pretending to have pain that does not really exist.

3. The admitting health care provider has not ordered anything for relief of Ms. Cole's arthritic pain. In this circumstance, the best nursing action would be to:
   a. explain to Ms. Cole that whatever she receives for pain after surgery will probably relieve the pain she has in her knees and hips.
   b. ignore the omission of orders because Ms. Cole's arthritic pain is not as important as her gallbladder disorder.
   c. ask Ms. Cole what measures she uses at home for relief of her arthritic pain, record the information, institute nursing measures, and ask her provider to order the analgesic she uses.
   d. tell Ms. Cole nothing can be done about her painful joints because her provider did not write an order for any relief measures.

4. On the evening after her surgery, Ms. Cole has a long visit with her daughter. During that time, you look in on Ms. Cole and she seems to be comfortable and happy. After her daughter leaves, Ms. Cole asks for something for pain. Ms. Cole's behavior probably indicates that:
   a. she does not have as much real pain as she says she has.
   b. she is afraid to complain in her daughter's presence.
   c. her daughter brought some medication from home to relieve her mother's pain.
   d. her daughter's visit effectively distracted Ms. Cole and diverted her attention from her pain.

STEPS TOWARD BETTER COMMUNICATION

VOCABULARY BUILDING GLOSSARY

Term	Definition
com pounds'	(verb) increases or adds to; makes worse
creep'ing	moving slowly and with difficulty
frail	having delicate health; weak; easily breakable
grim'ace	tense facial expression indicating pain
im'agery	mental pictures
indic'ative	suggesting; pointing out; revealing
place'bo	a substance given during a controlled study as medication that contains no actual medication
keep a "stiff upper lip"	bear something without an outward show of emotion or body change (slang); to endure without complaint
tol'erance	point in drug therapy where the drug no longer works

COMPLETION

Directions: Fill in the blanks with the correct words from the Vocabulary Building Glossary to complete the statements.

1. The use of _____ helps patients relax and take a short "mental vacation."

2. The patient was experiencing back pain and was _____ across the room to the bathroom.

3. When the nurse turned the patient onto his left side, his _____ indicated that he was experiencing pain.

4. Fatigue _____ the problem of pain and makes it more difficult to cope with.

5. The 88-year-old lady had lost 7 pounds and appeared very _____.

6. Some patients respond well to a(n) _____ in place of a narcotic analgesic.

7. Mr. Thomas presented a(n) _____, not even flinching when the doctor bent his knee after surgery.

8. When a patient frequently complains of pain much sooner than usual after a dose of pain medication, either something is making the pain worse or the patient is developing _____ to the pain medication.

9. When a pain medication is no longer effective for the patient, it is _____ of the need for a change in the medication order.

MATCHING

Directions: Match the abbreviations with their correct terms.

1. _____ OTC
2. _____ PCA
3. _____ TENS

   a. Transcutaneous electrical nerve stimulation
   b. Over-the-counter
   c. Patient-controlled analgesia

TERMINOLOGY

Evaluating Pain

Directions: Rank (from 1 to 9) the following words for degrees of pain from the least to the worst.

_____ Moderate

_____ Minimal

_____ Extremely severe

_____ Exquisite

_____ Mild

_____ Very severe

_____ Absent

_____ Fairly severe

_____ Severe

MATCHING

Directions: Match the terms indicating the quality of pain on the right with the correct category headings on the left. (Each category will have more than one term.)

1. _____ Heat
2. _____ Knife
3. _____ Stretching
4. _____ Vibrating
5. _____ Pressure

a. Burning
b. Pulsating
c. Dull
d. Twisting
e. Tearing
f. Throbbing
g. Biting
h. Searing
i. Stabbing
j. Crushing
k. Tingling
l. Pulling
m. Sharp

COMMUNICATION EXERCISES

Directions: Read the following scenarios and answer the related questions.

1. Your patient's ordered medication is not controlling the pain for more than 1 hour. You need to call the health care provider and ask for the order to be changed. Write out what you would say during the phone call. (Remember you will need to know the current vital signs.)

   _____

   _____

   _____

   _____

2. Your patient has received IV morphine for pain. A half hour later, you notice that the patient's respirations have dropped to 10 per minute. You must notify the charge nurse of the patient's condition. Write out how you would tell the charge nurse this information.

   _____

   _____

   _____

   _____

Care of Patients with Cancer

Answer Key: Review the related chapter to answer these questions. A complete answer key was provided to your instructor.

COMPLETION

Directions: Fill in the blanks to complete the statements.

1. Malignant cells grow in a(n) _____ manner compared to normal cells.

2. An abnormal replication of cells is called a(n) _____.

3. Malignant growths are divided into four main types: _____, arising from mesenchymal tissue; _____, originating from the epithelial tissue; _____ and _____, cancers of the blood-forming system; and _____, which is malignancy of the pigment cells of the skin.

4. TNM staging system identifies cancers by how much the malignancy has spread and includes three basic parts: *T* for _____, *N* for _____, and *M* for _____.

5. _____, _____, air and water pollution, and certain _____ found in food packaging are all considered to be carcinogens.

6. There are three traditional modes of therapy for malignancies: _____, _____, and _____.

7. Many antineoplastic drugs are _____, which can cause tissue damage and severe local injury if they escape from the vein into which they are administered.

8. Suppression of the _____ is the major reason that doses of chemotherapy must be limited.

9. A patient undergoing radiation therapy must wear_____ and _____ when outdoors.

10. Radiation therapy of the abdomen or newer targeted therapies often produce _____, which can lead to dehydration if not treated.

11. The health care provider orders Roxanol 20 mg PO q4h for pain. The pharmacy delivers a 90-mL bottle of Roxanol 10 mg/mL. How many mL should be given? _____

MATCHING

Risk Factors for Cancer

Directions: Match the word on the right with the correct definition on the left.

1. _____   Diet heavy in pickled or salted foods
2. _____   Frequent sex in early teens
3. _____   Early menarche; late menopause
4. _____   Estrogen therapy
5. _____   Over age 65; African American
6. _____   Heavy smoker; asbestos exposure
7. _____   Use of smokeless tobacco

a.   Stomach
b.   Prostate
c.   Uterine and endometrial
d.   Breast
e.   Uterus and cervix
f.   Lung
g.   Mouth

SHORT ANSWER

Interventions for the Side Effects of Chemotherapy

Directions: Read the clinical scenario and answer the questions that follow.

Scenario: You are caring for a patient who is receiving chemotherapy. List at least five nursing activities (assessments or interventions) to include in the care plan of the patient experiencing the common problems related to cancer or the toxic side effects of chemotherapy.

1.   Common problem: fatigue

a.   _____

b.   _____

c.   _____

d.   _____

e.   _____

2.   Toxic effect: thrombocytopenia

a.   _____

b.   _____

c.   _____

d.   _____

e.   _____

3.   Toxic effect: mucositis

a.   _____

b.   _____

c.   _____

d.   _____

e.   _____

4. Toxic effect: immunosuppression

a. _____

b. _____

c. _____

d. _____

e. _____

APPLICATION OF THE NURSING PROCESS

Caring for a Patient with Non-Hodgkin Lymphoma

Directions: Provide the answer to the following questions.

Scenario: Ms. Junic is diagnosed with non-Hodgkin lymphoma. She is receiving combination chemotherapy and radiation. She is trying to be brave and "not bother the nurses or worry her family," but you walk in and find that she is crying. She admits to nausea, vomiting, and diarrhea, but she states, "I know that is just part of the therapy, so I am trying to deal with it."

1. List at least four things to assess related to Ms. Junic's vomiting and diarrhea.

a. _____

_____

b. _____

_____

c. _____

_____

d. _____

_____

2. Which nursing problem is a priority for Ms. Junic?
a. Potential for altered nutrition due to nausea, vomiting, and diarrhea
b. Diarrhea due to effects of cancer treatment
c. Insufficient knowledge due to drugs and side effects
d. Limited coping ability due to side effects of treatment

3. List six nonpharmacologic interventions for nausea.

a. _____

b. _____

c. _____

d. _____

e. _____

f. _____

4. List at least five online resources that a cancer patient and his or her family might use to help them cope with the problems associated with malignancy.

a. _____

b. _____

c. _____

d. _____

e. _____

5. Which statement by Ms. Junic indicates that she understands how to deal with the side effects of chemotherapy?
    a. "All drugs, including chemotherapy drugs, have side effects."
    b. "I should report side effects; they could be an adverse response to therapy."
    c. "After I learn to recognize the side effects, I can cope independently."
    d. "A few side effects are okay as long as they don't interfere with activities of daily living."

PRIORITY SETTING

Directions: Read the following scenario and prioritize as appropriate.

Scenario: You are assigned to care for five patients on an oncology unit. You have just received report from the night shift nurse. Prioritize the order in which you will attend to the needs of these patients.

_____   a. Ms. Hobbs needs her AM dose of Megace.

_____   b. Ms. Hiroshi needs assistance with eating breakfast.

_____   c. Mr. Lopez' laboratory report shows a platelet count of $10,000/mm^3$.

_____   d. Mr. Nehru is asking for a PRN pain medication.

_____   e. Ms. Jaiswal wants information about cancer support groups.

REVIEW QUESTIONS FOR THE NCLEX® EXAMINATION

Directions: Choose the best answer(s) for the following questions.

1. There are many risk factors for different cancers, but there are some commonalities that are risks for all cancers. Some facts about all cancers are: *(Select all that apply.)*
    1. all cancers are genetic.
    2. although cancer can strike at any age, older people are more susceptible.
    3. cancer can develop from viruses.
    4. nutritional factors can account for up to 30% of cancers.
    5. using a cell phone causes cancer.

2. Having an intrinsic risk factor for cancer means a person: *(Select all that apply.)*
    1. has a risk factor which is "built in" and cannot be altered, such as age, sex, or racial group.
    2. has a risk factor which is modifiable, such as weight, diet, or sleeping habits.
    3. carries a gene that could develop into cancer.
    4. maintains a lifestyle conducive to catching a cancer virus.
    5. Uses a tanning bed and is at increased risk for skin cancer.

3. There are several steps that may be taken as a cancer preventive measure. Some of these are: *(Select all that apply.)*
    1. lose weight.
    2. limit salted, smoked foods intake.
    3. reduce coffee consumption.
    4. avoid indoor activities when it is warm and sunny outside.
    5. limit alcohol consumption.

4. The nurse directs the nursing assistant in safety measures to be used while caring for a patient undergoing radiation therapy with a sealed implant. Which would be appropriate to include?
    1. Use ordinary Standard Precautions; nothing else is required.
    2. Limit total time in patient's room to 60 minutes/8-hour shift.
    3. Wear a radiation detection badge to detect the amount of radiation exposure.
    4. Wear a lead apron to decrease exposure to radiation.

5. When providing care for a patient undergoing internal radiation, you would:
    1. wear a lead apron when at the bedside.
    2. quickly and efficiently provide hands-on care.
    3. stay out of the patient's room as much as possible.
    4. ask a family member to feed the patient.

6. When evaluating the patient's response to chemotherapy, which assessment finding is the greatest immediate concern?
    1. Constipation and straining
    2. Bleeding after brushing teeth
    3. Alopecia or change in hair color
    4. Fatigue and irritability

7. The patient is newly diagnosed with cancer and faces enormous stress. Which response by the nurse would be the most useful in helping the patient cope?
    1. "The health care provider will give you all the information you need to know."
    2. "Tell me what the health care provider told you and maybe I can help to clarify things."
    3. "Try to read or watch television. Just keep your mind busy."
    4. "Don't worry about chemotherapy. My aunt had it and she did just fine."

8. When assessing for the side effect of bone marrow depression from chemotherapy, the nurse would: *(Select all that apply.)*
    1. check the CBC lab results.
    2. assess for easy bruising.
    3. assess for signs of infection.
    4. check for hearing loss.

9. Alopecia resulting from chemotherapy is:
    1. temporary.
    2. irreversible.
    3. treatable.
    4. preventable.

10. Which statement by the family indicates an understanding of palliative care?
    1. "We want him to be comfortable, so oral medications are preferred."
    2. "We should encourage water and other nourishment as much as possible."
    3. "He'll feel short of breath and we'll hear the 'death rattle'."
    4. "He'll continue with his cancer treatments if they don't cause side effects."

11. The patient is having diarrhea secondary to radiation therapy of the pelvic area. Which statement by the patient indicates a need for additional teaching about the diarrhea?
    1. "I will cleanse the rectal area and apply petroleum jelly."
    2. "I will report an increase in the number and frequency of bowel movements."
    3. "I will avoid eating foods such as bananas and cheese."
    4. "I may need to have my electrolytes checked if the diarrhea is severe."

12. *Promoters* are substances that:
    1. help prevent cancer cells from invading other cells.
    2. cause cancer cells to grow faster.
    3. help cancer cells metastasize to other areas.
    4. enhance the effect of chemotherapy drugs.

CRITICAL THINKING ACTIVITIES

Scenario: Mr. Long is scheduled to begin receiving external radiation therapy to his chin and neck for cancer of the mandible.

1. Which are correct teaching points to share with Mr. Long about his therapy? *(Select all that apply.)*
    a. Local skin irritation may not appear immediately but may appear later.
    b. The treatment will be delivered in divided doses over many days.
    c. He must avoid contact with others to prevent exposing them to radiation.
    d. Written instructions are provided to help manage the expected side effects.
    e. Skin damage will be permanent, but the area will be very small.

2. Which side effect is most likely to occur as a result of radiation to the neck?
    a. Thrombocytopenia
    b. Loss of taste
    c. Alopecia
    d. Leukopenia

3. Choose measures that would be included in the care plan for Mr. Long. *(Select all that apply.)*
    a. Increase fluid intake
    b. Artificial saliva to be used as needed
    c. Minimal brushing of teeth to reduce irritation
    d. Avoid spicy food and alcohol
    e. Limit protein intake

4. To minimize damage to the skin exposed to radiation, Mr. Long should be instructed to:
    a. wear a tight-fitting scarf around his neck to protect it from sunlight.
    b. wash the skin gently with mild soap, tepid water, and a soft washcloth.
    c. avoid applying any lotions or powders unless prescribed by the health care provider.
    d. examine the condition of his skin weekly and report any blistering.

5. Mr. Long becomes unusually angry and demanding after his third treatment. You recognize that:
    a. he had a bad experience with the radiation therapy team.
    b. anger is one of the normal stages of the grieving process.
    c. the health care provider should be notified to prescribe an anxiolytic drug.
    d. confusion and personality changes are side effects of therapy.

6. In helping Mr. Long deal with his anger, choose the most therapeutic response.
    a. "Everything will be okay, Mr. Long. Let me sit with you for a while."
    b. "You don't seem like your usual self. Tell me what happened."
    c. "Those treatments are really tiring. Just rest for a while."
    d. "I can see that you are upset. Why are you acting this way?"

STEPS TOWARD BETTER COMMUNICATION

VOCABULARY BUILDING GLOSSARY

Term	Definition
ad′juvant	serving to help or assist; used in addition to (another treatment)
be′nign	not malignant; gentle or kind
carcin′ogen	substance that tends to produce a cancer
depletes′	uses up; seriously decreases the supply
immunocom′petent	able to develop immunity
in si′tu	contained within the original site
intrin′sic	naturally belonging to or within something
malig′nant	uncontrolled growth that is harmful and may cause death
metas′tasis	spread of cancer cells to other parts of the body
oc′cult	hidden; not readily detectable
transforma′tion	change in nature, character, or appearance
ves′icant	agent that causes severe irritation and can cause blisters

WORD ATTACK SKILLS

Combining Forms: Prefixes

adeno-	gland
carcino-	cancer
melano-	black
fibro-	fiber; refers to connective tissue
leio-	smooth muscle
leuko-	white blood cell; white
lipo-	fat; lipid
lympho-	lymphocyte (clear tissue fluid)
osteo-	bone
radio-	radiant energy waves such as in radiation therapy

Combining Forms: Suffix

-oma	tumor

Word Families

metas′tasis	(noun) invasive spread of tumor cells
metas′tasize	(verb) to spread throughout the body
metasta′tic	(adjective) capable of spreading throughout the body
carcino′ma	(noun) malignant tumor of epithelial tissue
carcin′ogen	(noun) agent that may cause cancer
carcinogen′ic	(adjective) capable of causing cancer

PRONUNCIATION SKILLS

Directions: Look at the accent mark on each of the following words and practice their pronunciations.

mes en chy' mal (*ch* sounds like "k")

ma lig' nant

per i to ne' al

car cin o gen' ic (car sin o jen ik)

mi cro scop' ic ally (*ically* sounds like "ikly")

prog no' sis

car cin no' ma (kar sin no ma)

car cin' o gens (kar sin o jens)

de oxy ribo nu cle' ic (dee oxy rybow noo klay ic)

COMPLETION

Directions: Fill in the blanks with the correct words from the Vocabulary Building Glossary to complete the statements.

1. _____ is the movement of cancer cells from the original site to other areas of the body.

2. A tumor whose cells reproduce in an uncontrolled, nonstructured pattern is called a(n) _____ tumor.

3. If a malignant tumor occurs in the gastrointestinal tract, the only early symptom may be _____ bleeding.

4. When certain body cells are exposed to a(n) _____ repeatedly over time, the cells may undergo malignant changes.

5. When chemotherapy or radiation is effective on a solid tumor, the cells in the tumor undergo a(n) _____ and the tumor shrinks or stops growing.

6. A brain tumor may be _____ and still be life-threatening.

7. The excessive malignant growth of a tumor places a strain on the body and _____ nutritional stores.

8. The use of tamoxifen is a(n) _____ therapy added to surgery, radiation, and/or chemotherapy for breast cancer.

9. A normal, healthy body has the _____ ability to fight and kill beginning cancer cells.

10. Poor nutrition, exposure to toxic substances, chronic illness, and long periods of excessive stress make the body less _____ and may contribute to the growth of cancer.

11. When found _____, cervical cancer has a very good cure rate.

12. Breast cancer and many other types of cancer tend to _____ to other parts of the body if not caught and treated early.

Types of Tissues

Directions: From what type of tissue does each of the following tumors arise?

1. Adenocarcinoma: _____

2. Leiomyoma: _____

3. Lymphoma: _____

4. Melanoma: _____

5. Osteosarcoma: _____

6. Fibroma: _____

COMMUNICATION EXERCISE

Mr. Tomm, age 72, has metastatic prostate cancer. He is to undergo radiation therapy. Practice what you would say in the remainder of the dialogue.

Nurse: "Good morning, Mr. Tomm. How do you feel this morning?"

Mr. Tomm: "Pretty good, I guess. I woke up a lot last night."

Nurse: "Were you worrying about this morning's radiation treatment?"

Mr. Tomm: "I am a bit anxious, yes."

(Continue with statements by both the nurse and Mr. Tomm.)

Chronic Illness and Rehabilitation

chapter

9

Answer Key: Review the related chapter to answer these questions. A complete answer key was provided to your instructor.

SHORT ANSWER

Chronic Illness and Immobility

1. List five chronic diseases or conditions that require extra care or rehabilitation.

   a. _____

   b. _____

   c. _____

   d. _____

   e. _____

2. List four goals of care in a long-term care facility.

   a. _____

   b. _____

   c. _____

   d. _____

3. Patients with a chronic illness often feel they will never become healthy, happy, or strong again. The nurse must help these patients improve their _____.

4. The patient must develop new _____ mechanisms in order to effectively deal with the changes the illness or situation has brought.

5. Restorative programs focus on _____ and _____.

6. Prevention actions for rehabilitation continue until _____
   _____.

7. Early effects of immobility include: _____
   _____
   _____
   _____

8. The elderly are more susceptible to the complications of immobility. It is especially important to monitor an elderly immobile patient for signs of:

a. _____

b. _____

c. _____

d. _____

e. _____

TABLE ACTIVITY

Directions: Complete the following table with the measures used to prevent complications within the particular body system.

Body System	Measures to Prevent Complications
Musculoskeletal	
Gastrointestinal	
Cardiovascular	
Neurologic	
Renal/urinary	
Respiratory	
Integumentary	

COMPLETION

Directions: Fill in the blanks to complete the statements.

1. When working with a rehabilitation patient, the nurse must recognize that the patient is the
    _____ of the team.

2. The rehabilitation team often consists of the health care provider, nurse, vocational counselor,
    and the _____, _____, _____,
    _____, and _____ therapists.

3. The basis of the philosophy of rehabilitation nursing is recognition of _____
    _____.

4. Safety restraints may only be used if they _____ or are needed for
    _____.

5. The first step in the prevention of falls is recognition of which _____
    _____.

6. The second step in the prevention of falls is recognition of _____
    _____ that could precipitate a fall.

7. Encourage elderly residents of long-term care facilities to _____ to pick up some-
    thing and _____ to dry the feet to help prevent dizziness or loss of balance and a
    fall.

8. Older patients are at greatly increased risk for complications of _____.

9. To help relieve or prevent venous stasis in the immobile patient, encourage _____
    _____ every 2 hours.

10. Sensory deficits such as impaired _____ or _____ may add to
    a patient's confusion and anxiety at night.

11. Patients who are taking diuretics must be constantly monitored for _____
    _____, which might cause confusion.

12. A major psychosocial issue for the greatly immobilized patient is _____
    _____ due to inability to socialize.

13. The goal of home care is to keep the patient _____ and enable him or her to
    _____.

14. In the long-term care facility, the core caregivers are _____ and they should be
    treated respectfully.

REVIEW QUESTIONS FOR THE NCLEX® EXAMINATION

Directions: Choose the best answer(s) for the following questions.

1. A patient who has suffered burns over 35% of the body has a nursing diagnosis of Altered skin integrity. The best expected outcome for this patient would be:
   1. patient will regain mobility within 3 months.
   2. patient's skin will heal with grafting as needed within 3 months.
   3. patient's pain will be well-controlled within 1 week.
   4. patient will consume enough calories for tissue regeneration.

2. Within the long-term care environment, the LPN/LVN usually functions in the capacity of:
   1. supervisor of the facility.
   2. admission nurse with Medicare paperwork duties.
   3. basic caregiver.
   4. charge nurse guiding the care team.

3. A priority of the National Patient Safety Goals and the Joint Commission for patients in long-term care include:
   1. provide meals of the quality of restaurant food.
   2. make care safer by reducing harm caused in the delivery of care.
   3. concentrate on improving mental health.
   4. make sure all patients have advance directives.

4. Restorative care programs are beneficial in preventing falls. A restorative program focuses on:
   1. restoring skin integrity.
   2. muscle strengthening.
   3. maintaining functionality.
   4. disability prevention.

5. When working with a rehabilitation patient, the nurse recognizes that: *(Select all that apply.)*
   1. fall prevention is a high priority.
   2. those with chronic physical conditions are more likely to experience mental illness.
   3. the Joint Commission has yet to develop National Patient Safety Goals.
   4. patients should never be restrained.
   5. elderly patients usually heal rapidly.

6. An appropriate expected outcome for the nursing diagnosis of Altered physical mobility for the patient who is right-handed and who has right-sided hemiparesis from a stroke is:
   1. bedrest will be maintained at all times.
   2. patient will begin crutch walking within 4 weeks.
   3. patient will comb hair and brush teeth by the end of 4 weeks.
   4. patient will show no signs of infection at time of discharge.

7. When assigning a task to an unlicensed assistive person (UAP), as the charge nurse, you must:
   1. be sure it is acceptable to the patient for the UAP to perform the task.
   2. ask the UAP if he or she knows how to perform the task.
   3. be certain that competence in performing the task has been documented for the UAP.
   4. test the UAP for competence.

8. Patients who have physical restraints must be assessed for body alignment visually:
   1. every shift.
   2. daily.
   3. every 30 minutes.
   4. by someone who is in attendance around the clock.

9. Physical and chemical restraints may be ordered and applied only when the patient:
    1. pulls the tubes out repeatedly.
    2. refuses to stay where he belongs.
    3. keeps interrupting the activities of others.
    4. is a danger to himself or others.

10. When working with a confused patient on dressing, it is best to gain cooperation by:
    1. providing a variety of choices of what to do when.
    2. limiting choices and the need to make decisions.
    3. decreasing sensory input as much as possible.
    4. keeping the patient engaged in activities during the day.

CRITICAL THINKING ACTIVITIES

Scenario A: Mr. Timmons, age 22, was in a motorcycle accident. He fractured his left leg and cervical spine (nondisplaced) and sustained a head injury. He is in the rehabilitation institute for rehabilitative care. He is in halo traction, has a leg brace, and is alert, but has some cognitive problems such as aphasia and memory loss.

1. What services would you expect to be included in Mr. Timmons' care?

2. What specific interventions should be on his interdisciplinary care plan related to his skin?

3. What measures would be on the plan to preserve and promote mobility?

Scenario B: Ms. O'Rourke, age 78, has limited vision and is suffering from sundowning. She gets confused at night and sometimes feels she must leave the facility.

1. What do you think would be the overall goals for this patient?

2. What therapies would have the highest priority?

3. What physical concerns should be addressed within her care plan?

STEPS TOWARD BETTER COMMUNICATION

VOCABULARY BUILDING GLOSSARY

Term	Definition
ascertain' (as er tayn')	(verb) make certain or sure
co'ping (ko'ping)	(verb) dealing with difficulties and problems and attempting to overcome them; managing difficulties
op'ti'mal	ideal; the highest; the best, as in *the best treatment*
peo'ple skills	social abilities that help a person get along well with other people
sub'op'ti'mal	less than ideal
sundowning	(noun) when a person becomes confused as the sun goes down

COMPLETION

Directions: Fill in the blanks with the correct words from the Vocabulary Building Glossary to complete the statements.

1. The nurse and social worker work with the patient to improve his _____ skills.

2. Mr. Jones exhibited _____ by becoming very agitated during the evening shift.

3. Sometimes the nurse must _____ what is preventing the patient from making progress toward his goals.

4. Mr. Otong achieved a(n) _____ recovery from his stroke, as he can walk quite well.

5. To work well on a rehabilitation team, the nurse must develop very good _____.

6. Ms. Krause has not regained use of her arm after her stroke and her recovery is considered

   _____.

PRONUNCIATION SKILLS

The consonant blend **th** in English is difficult for many people, especially since it has two different sounds. To make the **th** sound, such as in "**th**ank you" and "**th**ree," put your tongue between your front teeth and blow out air between your tongue and top teeth; slide your tongue back, scraping the top of your tongue against your upper teeth. Practice. Practice the following words:

arthritis	thanks
bath	thigh
birthday	thin
breath	thirst
month	three
mouth	thumb
teeth	Thursday

To make the voiced <u>th</u> sound, such as in "<u>th</u>ere" and "<u>th</u>ey," make the **th** sound but use your voice; try not to slide your tongue backwards—let it vibrate against your upper teeth. Compare the following:

Noun	Verb
bath	ba<u>the</u>
teeth	tee<u>the</u>
breath	brea<u>the</u>

Notice that the silent **e** makes the preceding vowel sounds long. Practice the following words having voiced <u>th</u> sounds:

ba<u>the</u>	<u>th</u>ere
brea<u>the</u>	<u>th</u>ese
o<u>th</u>er	<u>th</u>ey
<u>th</u>an	<u>th</u>is
<u>th</u>at	<u>th</u>ose
<u>th</u>e	toge<u>th</u>er

COMMUNICATION EXERCISES

1. Read the following communication. Circle every "th" sound, and put a line under every *voiced* <u>th</u> sound.

    The therapist will come to see you on Thursday. We will come together. I hope your arthritis is better by then. Take your bath and brush your teeth before we come. These are the breathing exercises that you need to practice. They will help you feel better. Thanks for being such a good sport.

2. You are working in a long-term care facility. Write out what you would say when you ask another nurse to cover your assigned patients while you are at lunch.

    _____

    _____

    _____

    _____

    _____

    _____

Student Name_____ Date_____

The Immune and Lymphatic Systems

Answer Key: Review the related chapter to answer these questions. A complete answer key was provided to your instructor.

COMPLETION

Review of Anatomy and Physiology

Directions: Fill in the blanks to complete the statements.

1. _____ patches help defend against ingested pathogens.

2. _____ are immunoglobulins that identify and neutralize foreign objects.

3. The _____ is the first barrier encountered by pathogens.

4. The neutrophils and macrophages of the hematologic system assist the immune system by _____ when an antigen is encountered.

5. When the body produces an immune response to a "self" cell or tissue, this causes a(n) _____ disorder.

LABELING

Anatomy of the Organs of the Immune System

Directions: Label the following structures on the diagram of the body.

tonsils
thoracic duct
thymus gland
inguinal lymph nodes
spleen
bone marrow
right lymphatic duct
axillary lymph nodes

Caring for a Patient with an Immune Disorder

Directions: Read the clinical scenario and answer the questions that follow.

Scenario: You are caring for Mr. Carson. He has an immunodeficiency condition. The health care provider orders Transmission-Based Isolation Precautions (protective). Mr. Carson appears very apprehensive when you first meet him and he tells you that he is not sure why he is isolated, what to expect, or what he should be doing to help himself.

1. Explain the purpose of isolation to Mr. Carson:_____

    _____ .

2. Share three goals of nursing care with Mr. Carson to help him understand the plan of care.

    a. _____

    b. _____

    c. _____

3. Describe some of the psychological implications for patients who have isolation precautions. _____

    _____

    _____

    _____

    _____

    _____

4. Name three important teaching points for Mr. Carson to help him understand things he can do to prevent infection after being discharged from the hospital.

    a. _____

    b. _____

    c. _____

PRIORITY SETTING

Directions: Read the scenario and prioritize as appropriate.

Scenario: You are preparing to do a physical assessment on Mr. Hitachi. He reports having some generalized fatigue and intermittent tenderness in "my neck, just underneath my ears." He was referred to the clinic for an immunologic workup. Prioritize the order of the elements below that are part of the physical assessment.

_____   a. Inspect the skin for color, turgor, texture, and presence of lesions.

_____   b. Palpate lymph nodes in the neck to identify enlargement or tenderness.

_____   c. Take vital signs, noting if there is an increase in temperature or pulse rate.

_____   d. Auscultate lung fields and assess work of breathing.

_____   e. Inspect extremities for edema.

_____   f. Analyze lab results such as CBC, C-reactive protein, and antibody screening tests.

APPLICATION OF THE NURSING PROCESS

Caring for a Patient with an Allergic Reaction

Directions: Provide the answer to the following questions.

Scenario: Ms. Cohan comes to the clinic for a rash after eating strawberries several days ago. She also reports, "This has never happened to me before and this really itches! Is this going to happen to me again?"

1. While you are examining Ms. Cohan's skin, what assessments and observations are you making?

   _____

   _____

   _____

2. Write a patient-centered goal for the following problem: altered skin integrity due to irritation and scratching.

   _____

3. List five interventions to use for Ms. Cohan's potential for impaired skin integrity.

   a. _____

   b. _____

   c. _____

   d. _____

   e. _____

   f. _____

4. Which statement(s) indicate(s) that Ms. Cohan has understood the patient education regarding allergy testing? *(Select all that apply.)*
   a. A scratch test may be done by dropping extracts of allergens into scratches made on the skin.
   b. Intradermal injection of allergens will cause an anaphylactic reaction.
   c. Patches containing allergens can reduce fruit allergies.
   d. Inflammation and itching identify those allergens that provoke the immune system.
   e. Allergy testing is not necessary, because her immune reaction was typical for strawberry allergy.

REVIEW QUESTIONS FOR THE NCLEX® EXAMINATION

Directions: Choose the best answer(s) for the following questions.

1. What is necessary for a humoral immune response to occur?
   1. Detection of the absence of a foreign agent when it leaves body cells
   2. Exacerbation of the process of inflammation
   3. Inhibition of phagocytosis and the membrane-attack complex
   4. Presence of a particular antibody that responds to an antigen

2. Having a case of chickenpox provides a person with which type of immunity?
   1. Passive artificial immunity
   2. Active naturally acquired immunity
   3. Active artificially acquired immunity
   4. Natural (innate) immunity

3. The patient sustains trauma to the right lower extremity. To reduce the pain and edema associated with the inflammatory response, which action would the nurse perform *first*?
    1. Obtain an order for an antiinflammatory medication.
    2. Assess the distal pulses and sensation to touch.
    3. Elevate the right lower extremity.
    4. Immobilize the leg with a splint.

4. What is the purpose of giving "booster doses" of an immunizing agent, such as tetanus toxoid?
    1. Provides an immediate supply of antibody when a person is in danger of contracting the disease
    2. Provides active immunity for a short period until any danger of the person developing the disease has passed
    3. Stimulates the memory of plasma cells and thereby stimulates synthesis of greater quantities of antibody
    4. Boosts the synthesis of antibodies by sensitizing the immune cells for the first time

5. The health care provider has ordered an annual influenza vaccination and a tetanus booster for an elderly patient living in a long-term care facility. The patient refuses to cooperate. What is the best response?
    1. "I'll be really quick and gentle, because I know you don't like shots."
    2. "It's okay to refuse. We can wait and talk to your provider about this."
    3. "Everyone in the facility is getting the vaccines, including all the staff."
    4. "I'd like to understand your point of view, so let's talk about your decision."

6. The patient has a fever. Which task(s) would be appropriate to assign to the nursing assistant? *(Select all that apply.)*
    1. Help the patient remove excess clothing.
    2. Ask the patient about fever and chills.
    3. Obtain an antipyretic from the medication room.
    4. Take the temperature with a temporal artery thermometer.
    5. Talk to the patient about over-the-counter fever reducers.
    6. Get the patient a cold drink.

7. The nurse is reviewing a patient's laboratory values. Which laboratory value indicates that the patient is having the desired response to antibiotic therapy?
    1. White blood cell count of 8500/mm³
    2. Red blood cell count of 5.4 million/mm³
    3. Platelet count of 150,000/mm³
    4. Culture results show sensitivity to antibiotic

8. A nursing student is assisting the nurse to perform cooling measures for a patient with a high fever. The nurse would intervene if the student took which action?
    1. Removed excess blankets from the patient
    2. Obtained a basin of cold water for sponging
    3. Offered the patient cool oral fluids
    4. Checked the health care provider's order for an antipyretic

9. Your patient has had blood drawn to measure the level of several immunoglobulins. What is the most important factor to consider when interpreting the results?
    1. The type of disorder that is being investigated
    2. Presenting signs and symptoms
    3. Age of the patient
    4. Other existing health problems

10. The nurse is working in a clinic that provides immunization service to the community. Which action would the nurse take to address possible adverse hypersensitivity reactions to immunizing agents? *(Select all that apply.)*
    1. Advocate that all patients should have scratch testing prior to immunization.
    2. Administer vaccines only if patients have previously been immunized.
    3. Ask all patients about history of allergies and allergic reactions prior to immunization.
    4. Ensure the emergency equipment and rescue medications are easily accessible.
    5. Advise all patients to remain in the clinic for 20 minutes after receiving an injection.

CRITICAL THINKING ACTIVITIES

Scenario: You are working with a new nursing assistant and you have asked her to carefully monitor vital signs for a patient with a fever. She appears eager and willing to help you.

1. What specific directions should you give to the nursing assistant about this task? _____

_____

_____

_____

_____

_____

STEPS TOWARD BETTER COMMUNICATION

VOCABULARY BUILDING GLOSSARY

Term	Definition
bad'ger	harass, annoy, or pester, bother frequently
con sti tu' tion	a person's overall health or disposition (also structure or organization); general body strength
im mu no glob' ulin	protein that functions as an antibody
jog	nudge as a reminder (also run at a slower pace)
mi' grate	move around
neu' tral ize	make safe or to reduce the effect
pre dis pose'	to be inclined toward, to have a tendency toward
sur veil' lance (ser va'lenz)	watch regularly or monitor

COMPLETION

Directions: Fill in the blanks with the correct words from the Vocabulary Building Glossary to complete the statements.

1. There are five classes of _____ (Ig): IgA, IgD, IgE, IgG, and IgM.

2. Antivenoms that contain antibodies may _____ snake venom.

3. Living in close proximity to others (i.e., homeless shelters, long-term care facilities) may

   _____ an individual to infectious disease.

4. Advise your patient that although he may have a naturally strong _____, adequate

   nutrition, immunizations, and healthy lifestyle habits will help to prevent immune disorders.

5. The Centers for Disease Control perform _____ for infectious disease, such as West

   Nile virus.

6. When supervising nursing assistants, give instructions and feedback about performance, but do not

   _____ them about minor mistakes.

7. Cancer cells can _____ to different locations in the body.

8. Taking a review course will help to _____ your memory before you take the test for

   licensure.

WORD ATTACK SKILLS

Prefixes and Suffixes

A *prefix* is attached to the beginning of a word or a word root to change the meaning. A vowel is used when needed to connect the prefix to the word.

a-, an-	no, not, without, absence of
anti-	against, opposing
auto-	self, by itself
hyper-	excessive, more than normal; higher than needed
hypo-	decreased, less than normal; lower than needed
immun/o-	provide immunity
in-	not; (or into)
lymph/o-	lymph, lymphatic
lys/o-	destruction

A *suffix* is attached to the end of a word or root to change the meaning or the way the word is used.

-cyte	cell
-penia	deficiency of
-genic	produced by

COMPLETION

Directions: Complete the sentences with the correct prefix or suffix.

1. If sterile technique is not used for Foley catheter insertion, the patient may develop an iatro-_____

   infection.

2. Lupus erythematosus is an example of a(n) _____ -immune disorder.

3. In a person with a normally functioning immune system, the presence of an antigen in the body will cause formation of a(n) _____ -body.

4. Patients with neutro-_____ are very susceptible to infection.

Word Families

Actor	Action	Process	Result
pro tec′ tor	pro tect′	pro tec′ tion	
med′ ia tor	me d′ iate	me dia′ tion	
re ac′ tor	re act′	re ac′ tion	
al′ ler gen			al′ ler gy

Singular and Plural Forms

Singular

serum
diagnosis
phenomenon
criterion

Plural

sera
diagnoses
phenomena
criteria

PRONUNCIATION SKILLS

The following words have the long **e** sound (underlined), as in the word "he." Notice the sound can be written with e, ee, ea, ei, i, or y.

me ′di ate
di ag no′ses
pro ce ′dure
re′ nal
se cre′ tions
tech nique′
fe′ver
deep breath′ing
de crease′ / in crease′

*Directions: Underline the letters in the words that make the long **e** sound.*

1. Please use standard precautions for handling body secretions.

2. Her fever has increased but she is breathing deeply.

3. Does he know the procedure for keeping the needles clean?

GRAMMAR POINTS

Active Versus Passive

Immunizations can be active or passive, and the English language can be active or passive, too. In acquired immunity, a person can either actively produce his own antibody or passively receive antibodies that have been produced by another person or animal. In English, when the subject of a sentence or clause does the action, the sentence or clause is called *active*.

Examples: *The housekeeper cleans the room.*
                 A nurse takes vital signs several times a day.
                 People produce their own antibodies.

The housekeeper, the nurse, and people do the action, so these are active sentences.

Passive sentences or clauses are used when it is not known who does the action or it is less important who or what does the action.

Examples: *The bed is made.*
                 Vital signs are taken in the morning and evening.

The bed and vital signs do no action (some other agent does it), so these are passive sentences.

Scientific writing often uses the passive form because there may not be an actor, or there may be no action, only a state of being. However, it is preferable to use active voice whenever possible.

Examples: *Allergies are divided into three major groups.*
                 Antibodies are found in the serum of blood.

Who or what divides or finds is not important.

If the agent of the action must be included, a "by" or "through" phrase is usually used to tell who or what does the acting.

Examples: *Temperatures and blood pressures are taken <u>by a nurse</u>.*
                 The bed is made <u>by the housekeeping staff</u>.
                 Antibodies are produced <u>by the plasma cells</u>.
                 Trends can been seen <u>by taking vital signs</u> on a regular schedule.
                 Vaccination became accepted <u>through the efforts of Edward Jenner</u>.
                 AIDS is caused <u>by transmission of HIV</u>.
                 Edema is characterized <u>by tight, shiny skin</u>.

The action is not done by the subjects of these passive sentences, but rather by the nouns in the underlined phrases.

A *passive verb* is formed by using the verb "to be" in any form (am/is/are, was/were, have/has been, will/would be, and so on) followed by a past participle. The *past participle* of a regular verb is its *-ed* form, such as *divided, prepared,* and *used.* Other past participles are irregular, such as *found, taken, seen, made,* and *known.*

Care of Patients with Immune and Lymphatic Disorders

Answer Key: Review the related chapter to answer these questions. A complete answer key was provided to your instructor.

TERMINOLOGY

Directions: Match the term on the left with the correct definition, function, or statement on the right.

1. _____ Disseminated
2. _____ Lymphedema
3. _____ Sentinel infections
4. _____ Anaphylaxis
5. _____ Urticaria
6. _____ Barrier protection
7. _____ Autoimmune disorder
8. _____ T helper cells
9. _____ ART
10. _____ Coccidioidomycosis

a. Extreme allergic reaction that is life-threatening
b. Hives
c. Fungus found in soil
d. Widespread
e. Large amounts of fluid accumulate, causing swelling
f. Antiretroviral therapy
g. T cells that have the protein CD4 on their surface
h. Opportunistic infection that indicates immunosuppression
i. Latex, polyurethane, or deproteinized latex condoms
j. Immune system reacting against the body's own cells

TABLE ACTIVITY

Directions: In the table below, list the effects that could occur with exposure to different allergens.

Four Broad Categories of Allergens

Category	Method of Exposure	Triggers	Effects
Contactants	Direct contact with mucosa/skin/tissue	Dust, wool fabrics, detergents, soaps, lotions, cosmetics, plants such as poison ivy, dyes, metals in jewelry, latex	
Ingestants	Swallowed	Food: citrus fruits, tomatoes, strawberries, cow's milk, wheat, eggs, dairy products, seafood, chocolate, nuts, monosodium glutamate (MSG), other preservatives, and artificial food coloring Drugs: aspirin, barbiturates, anticonvulsants, antimicrobials, but any drug may cause an allergic reaction	
Inhalants	Entry through nose or mouth	Dust, molds, pollen, fragrances, animal dander, insect feces, and some chemicals	
Injectables	Via needle; i.e., hypodermic, intramuscular, intravenous Animal or snake bites, insect stings	Medications, vaccines, animal saliva, snake or insect venoms	

APPLICATION OF THE NURSING PROCESS

Disorders of Inappropriate Immune Response

Directions: Read the scenario and write brief answers for the following questions.

Scenario: Juanita Ramos suspects that she may have allergies to environmental allergens. She reports runny nose, sneezing, and watery eyes that seem to be unassociated with a fever or cold.

1. Identify five factors that should be assessed in collecting data and taking a history from Ms. Ramos.

   a. _____

   _____

   b. _____

   _____

c. _____

_____

d. _____

_____

e. _____

_____

2. List four types of drugs that are used to alleviate systemic reactions to allergens.

a. _____

b. _____

c. _____

d. _____

3. The health care provider suggests that she initially try an over-the-counter medication. List four common side effects of medication such as diphenhydramine (Benadryl).

a. _____

b. _____

c. _____

d. _____

4. List six suggestions that will help Ms. Ramos control environmental allergens.

a. _____

b. _____

c. _____

d. _____

e. _____

f. _____

PRIORITY SETTING

Directions: Read the scenario and prioritize nursing actions as appropriate.

Scenario: You are working in a smaller clinic and you hear one of the X-ray technicians calling for help. The patient is having an anaphylactic reaction to IV contrast dye and the radiologist asks you to help. The patient has a patent IV line and the emergency equipment is in the room. Prioritize these five measures used to treat anaphylaxis.

_____ a. Provide psychological support.

_____ b. Administer oxygen.

_____ c. Establish a patent airway.

_____ d. Administer antihistamine (diphenhydramine hydrochloride [Benadryl]).

_____ e. Administer aqueous epinephrine.

COMPLETION

Directions: Fill in the blank(s) to complete the following sentences.

1. HIV is a(n) _____ that integrates itself into the genetic material of the host cell.

2. An unsafe practice is to be the _____ partner in anal or vaginal intercourse without using some form of _____ such as a latex condom.

3. In HIV-infected individuals, _____ usually manifest as white patches on the surface of the tongue and buccal mucosa.

SHORT ANSWER

HIV/AIDS

You are working in an HIV/AIDS clinic that provides testing, information, referrals, and outpatient care. The clinic also takes an active role in the community to provide health information seminars and a resource for families.

Directions: Write brief answers for the following questions.

1. List at least five of the initial symptoms of AIDS.

   a. _____

   b. _____

   c. _____

   d. _____

   e. _____

2. Identify four modes of transmission for HIV.

   a. _____

   b. _____

   c. _____

   d. _____

3. Identify at least four teaching points for people who are HIV positive.

   a. _____

   _____

   b. _____

   _____

   c. _____

   _____

d. _____

_____

REVIEW QUESTIONS FOR THE NCLEX® EXAMINATION

Directions: Choose the best answer(s) for the following questions.

1. Opportunistic infections occur when:
   1. the body is weakened or the immune system is suppressed.
   2. heavy exposure to tuberculosis occurs.
   3. another infection is already present in the body.
   4. antiviral therapy has affected the immune system.

2. Which statement by an elderly patient indicates a need for additional patient teaching about risk for HIV?
   1. "I may have to remind my health care provider to ask about sexual health."
   2. "There is a decline in functioning of the immune system for elderly people."
   3. "Condoms are not needed because pregnancy is not an issue."
   4. "Skin and mucous membranes are more fragile in the elderly person."

3. A patient is diagnosed with herpes zoster. What is the drug of choice for herpes?
   1. Cidofovir (Vistide)
   2. Foscavir (Foscarnet)
   3. Valganciclovir (Valcyte)
   4. Acyclovir (Zovirax)

4. The patient comes to the clinic for a physical examination and HIV testing. He tells the nurse that he thinks he may have been recently exposed to HIV. Which assessment item(s) should be included at this point? *(Select all that apply.)*
   1. Sexual history
   2. IV drug use
   3. Current medications
   4. Vital signs
   5. Presence of anasarca
   6. Change of mental status

5. The health care provider orders several diagnostic tests including an HIV test for a patient. What is appropriate information to give to the patient?
   1. He can use an FDA-approved home test for HIV which is adequate and confidential.
   2. He will first have a nucleic acid test (NAT).
   3. He will have a rapid HIV antibody test as the initial screening for HIV.
   4. He must fast after midnight and return in the early AM for specimen collection.

6. The nurse hears in report that a patient with AIDS also has thrush. What intervention would the nurse plan to use during the shift?
   1. Restock the supplies for contact isolation.
   2. Ensure that the patient has a patent IV for antibiotics.
   3. Check to make sure there is an order for folic acid.
   4. Offer the patient ice pops or chilled applesauce.

7. Which group of drugs commonly tends to cause allergies in many people?
   1. Antihypertensives, diuretics, and antiarrhythmics
   2. Aspirin, barbiturates, anticonvulsants, and antibiotics
   3. Vitamin and mineral supplements and electrolyte replacements
   4. Antibiotics, antianginals, sedatives, and antipsychotics

8. Which problems are related to the use of antihistamines in aging males?
   1. Hesitancy and urinary retention
   2. Orthostatic hypotension and dizziness
   3. Angina and cardiac dysrhythmias
   4. Depression and general malaise

9. A patient was recently diagnosed with systemic lupus erythematosus. Which sign(s) and symptom(s) would the nurse expect to find documented in this patient's medical record? *(Select all that apply.)*
   1. Painful or swollen joints
   2. Red rash usually on the face
   3. Fatigue and weakness
   4. Nausea, vomiting, and diarrhea
   5. Unexplained fever
   6. Sensitivity to the sun

10. Which medications are likely to be prescribed for a patient with systemic lupus erythematosus?
    1. NSAIDs and prednisone
    2. Doxorubicin (Adriamycin) and vincristine (Oncovin)
    3. Isoniazid (INH) and rifampin (Rifadin)
    4. Lamivudine (Combivir) and ethambutol (Myambutol)

11. The nurse is giving skin care instructions to a patient with systemic lupus erythematosus. Which set of instructions is appropriate?
    1. Use alcohol-based skin care products for the antibacterial action.
    2. Avoid use of cosmetics, moisturizers, and soaps.
    3. Wear long pants, a long-sleeved shirt, and a hat when in the sun.
    4. Apply over-the-counter hydrocortisone cream as needed.

12. The health care provider recommends that a patient be scheduled for a diagnostic test to detect presence of Reed-Sternberg cells in the tissues to rule out lymphatic cancer. Which diagnostic test will detect these cells?
    1. Computed tomography
    2. Biopsy of the lymph nodes
    3. Biopsy of the bone marrow
    4. Positron emission tomography

13. The patient begins to cry. "I am really scared. Am I going to die of cancer? Why is this happening to me?" What is the best response?
    1. "Let me get your wife and the two of you can have some privacy."
    2. "You should not be using your energy to worry right now. You should wait until the health care provider verifies the diagnosis."
    3. "I'd be scared too. My aunt had cancer and I know just how you feel."
    4. "I can tell you're scared and I don't know why this is happening, but we are here to give you support and information."

14. The patient asks the nurse to explain some of the differences between Hodgkin and non-Hodgkin. What information about Hodgkin is correct?
    1. It is more widespread through the lymphatic tissues.
    2. It is less widespread through the lymphatic tissues.
    3. It identified as B cell and T cell lymphoma.
    4. It has a lower survival rate and a worse prognosis.

CRITICAL THINKING ACTIVITIES

Scenario A: You are working in walk-in clinic. The health care provider orders an antibiotic injection for a patient. You give the medication as ordered. Almost immediately after receiving the medication, the patient tells you, "I feel kind of funny. Maybe a little short of breath. Is that normal?"

1. What should you do? _____

   _____

   _____

   _____

   _____

   _____

   _____

2. List four signs and symptoms that may indicate an anaphylactic reaction.

   a. _____

   b. _____

   c. _____

   d. _____

Scenario B: You are taking a patient history on a young woman who admits to having sex with several young men whom she knows and describes as "good friends." The woman states that, "I'm pretty sure that none of us have HIV."

1. What kinds of questions should you ask?

2. What would you recommend regarding testing for HIV?

3. If this young woman declines a screening test for HIV, what are your responsibilities?

Scenario C: The health care provider orders IV hydration for a patient postmedication administration. The current maintenance IV is infusing at 125 mL/hour per pump. The order is to increase the IV fluid to 200 mL/hour x 3 hours then resume previously ordered rate. It is now 8:00 AM.

1. What volume should the patient have received at the end of 3 hours? _____.

2. At 8:00 AM, you should set the pump to deliver how many mL/hour? _____.

3. At 11:00 AM, you should reset the pump to deliver how many mL/hour? _____.

STEPS TOWARD BETTER COMMUNICATION

VOCABULARY BUILDING GLOSSARY

Term	Definition
gay	homosexual (male or female)
iatrogenic	a side effect caused by medical treatment
immunosuppression	inhibit the normal immune system response
myth (mith)	traditional belief or ancient story
relapse	reappearance of cancer cells; also a return to a former state
remission	disease is under control
syndrome	group of symptoms associated with a condition

PRONUNCIATION AND MEANING

When you encounter long medical words, try breaking them down into smaller parts. This will help you with their meanings.

Example: antiretroviral = anti (against) + retro (backward) + viral (relating to a virus)

It will also help you to pronounce the words correctly.

Examples:

anaphylaxis	(ă-nă-fă-LĂK-sĭs)
cryptococcosis	krip' tow kok o' sis
cytomegalovirus	si' tow meg' ah low vi' rus
disseminate	di sim' in ate
environment	(ĕn-VĪ-rŏn-mĕnt)
erythema	(ĕr-ĭ-THĒ-mă)
immunosuppression	im' you no sa pre' shun
insufficiency	(ĭn-să-FĬSH-ăn-sē)
lymphedema	(lĭm-fĕ-DĒ-mă)

COMPLETION

Directions: Fill in the blanks with the correct words from the Vocabulary Building Glossary to complete the statements.

1. After the patient completed treatment for cancer, there was a(n) _____ of symptoms.

2. The patient's prolonged usage of steroids resulted in _____ effects.

3. Goodpasture's _____ affects lungs and the kidneys.

4. _____ can be therapeutic for transplant patients.

5. There have been many cases of AIDS transmitted from partner to partner among the

    _____ population in this country.

6. The belief that elderly adults are unlikely to contract AIDS is a(n) _____ .

7. The patient with lymphoma who had been successfully treated developed symptoms again during a(n)

    _____ .

TERMINOLOGY

Directions: Name the organ or structure to which each condition below is related. (Hint: each word contains a part that means a specific organ or structure.)

1. Retinitis: _____

2. Meningitis: _____

3. Encephalopathy: _____

4. Nephrotoxicity: _____

5. Mucocutaneous: _____

6. Neuralgia: _____

7. Neutropenia: _____

MATCHING

Directions: Match the acronym (abbreviated term) on the left with what it stands for (meaning) on the right.

1.	_____	ART	a. Personal protective equipment
2.	_____	CDC	b. Nucleoside reverse transcriptase inhibitor
3.	_____	HSV	c. Opportunistic infection
4.	_____	NRTI	d. Enzyme-linked immunospecific assay
5.	_____	MAC	e. Antiretroviral therapy
6.	_____	PPE	f. Herpes simplex virus
7.	_____	OI	g. Centers for Disease Control
8.	_____	ELISA	h. *Mycobacterium avium* complex

WORD ATTACK SKILLS

In this chapter, you learned how the immune system protects the body and how failure of the immune system manifests as different types of disease and disorders. *Immuno-* is a combining form that is frequently used in this chapter.

Directions: Below are several terms that begin with "immuno-." Can you remember other words from Chapter 11 that also used the combining form "immuno-"?

immunodeficiency (ĭm-ū-nō-dĕ-FĬSH-ĕn-sē)

immunocompromised (ĭm-ū-nō-KŎM-pro-mīzd)

immunocompetence (ĭm-ū-nō-KŎM-pĕ-tĕns)

immunotherapy (ĭm-ū-nō-THĔR-ă-pē)

_____

_____

_____

_____

_____

_____

_____

Student Name_____ Date_____

The Respiratory System

chapter
12

Answer Key: Review the related chapter to answer these questions. A complete answer key was provided to your instructor.

REVIEW OF ANATOMY AND PHYSIOLOGY

Terminology

Directions: Match the term on the left with the correct statement, function, or definition on the right.

1. _____ Bronchioles
2. _____ Pleural cavity
3. _____ Cilia
4. _____ Compliance
5. _____ Cough reflex
6. _____ Ventilation
7. _____ Oxyhemoglobin
8. _____ Inspiration and expiration
9. _____ Elastance
10. _____ Total lung capacity

a. Movement of air in and out of the lungs
b. Carry air to alveoli
c. Hairlike projections that trap and help expel inhaled foreign particles
d. Elasticity of the lungs
e. Carries majority of the oxygen to the cells of the body
f. When depressed, secretions are retained and pneumonia may occur
g. Pressure within is less than that of outside atmosphere
h. Controlled by movement of diaphragm and muscles in chest wall
i. Extent to which lungs can return to their original position after being stretched
j. Amount of air or gas lung can hold at end of maximal inspiration

Completion

Directions: Fill in the blank(s) to complete the following sentences.

1. _____ decreases surface tension on the alveolar wall, allowing it to _____ more easily with _____ and preventing alveolar collapse upon _____.

2. Two conditions that can interfere with oxygen and carbon dioxide exchange are _____ surfactant and interstitial _____.

3. Respiratory gases are carried mostly in the bloodstream by the _____.

4. A large percentage of carbon dioxide is transported in the blood plasma in the form of _____ ions.

5. Carbon dioxide combines with _____ within the red blood cell, forming _____.

SHORT ANSWER

Age-Related Changes Affecting the Respiratory System

Directions: Provide a short answer to the following questions.

1. Why are the elderly more susceptible to respiratory infections?_____

_____

2. Why is the potential for aspiration greater in the elderly person? _____

_____

_____

3. What is the significance to the respiratory system of the 50% decrease in total body water after age 70?

_____

_____

4. What alveolar changes affect respiration in the elderly person?_____

_____

_____

5. How could osteoporosis impact respiratory function?_____

_____

_____

TERMINOLOGY

Assessment

Directions: Match the terms on the left with the statements on the right that best describe them. (There may be more than one answer for each.)

1. _____ Assessment of mouth and pharynx

2. _____ Indirect laryngoscopy

3. _____ Thoracentesis

4. _____ Capnography

5. _____ Throat culture

a. Simple removal of polyps can be done during this procedure.
b. Endoscope is passed to visualize interior of larynx.
c. Patient is NPO until gag reflex returns.
d. Uses a nasal cannula, skin sensor, or endotracheal tube attachment.
e. Usually performed to confirm infection with streptococcus.
f. To remove pleural fluid, instill medication, or obtain fluid for diagnostic studies.
g. Examiner uses warm laryngeal mirror, head mirror, and light source.
h. Examiner uses tongue blade and light source.
i. Biopsy can be taken during examination.
j. Food and liquids withheld 6–8 hours before procedure.

SHORT ANSWER

Directions: Provide a short answer to the following questions.

1. Why is obtaining a history of smoking and alcohol intake pertinent to a respiratory assessment?

   _____

   _____

2. What can skin color tell you that is pertinent to a respiratory assessment? _____

   _____

   _____

3. What is the best position in which to place the patient for lung auscultation?_____

   _____

   _____

PRIORITY SETTING

Directions: Indicate the order of priority in which you would perform actions for the following scenario.

Scenario: You are performing a physical assessment of the respiratory system.

_____   a. Instruct the patient to breathe deeply and slowly through the mouth.

_____   b. Observe the head and look for facial puffiness over the sinus area.

_____   c. Note the posture and the way abdominal muscles are used.

_____   d. Note skin color.

_____   e. Move your stethoscope to compare one side of the chest to the other.

_____   f. Place the diaphragm of the stethoscope against the skin with moderate pressure.

REVIEW QUESTIONS FOR THE NCLEX® EXAMINATION

Directions: Choose the best answer(s) for the following questions.

1. Evaluation of the effectiveness of deep-breathing and coughing is best done by:
   1. auscultating the lungs bilaterally both before and after.
   2. assessing the color and amount of secretions produced.
   3. observing the respiratory rate and quality afterward.
   4. asking the patient whether he is breathing easier.

2. When performing a respiratory assessment, which action(s) should be performed? *(Select all that apply.)*
   1. Inquire about exposure to respiratory inhalants.
   2. Obtain a throat culture and a sputum specimen.
   3. Auscultate the lungs bilaterally.
   4. Assess the patient's knowledge of respiratory disease.
   5. Assess color of mucous membranes.
   6. Assess the rate and quality of respirations.
   7. Check for use of accessory muscles.
   8. Look for signs of anxiety or restlessness.

3. The patient has chest congestion and the nurse instructs him to increase fluid intake. What is the best rationale for this intervention?
   1. Fluids help to decrease the cough reflex.
   2. Coughing may cause dehydration.
   3. Fluid helps to thin secretions.
   4. Congestion increases the chance for sepsis.

4. The nurse notes in the medical record that the patient has orthopnea. Which intervention would the nurse use to address this condition?
   1. Offer the patient extra pillows.
   2. Assist the patient to turn every 2 hours.
   3. Obtain an order for continuous oxygen.
   4. Monitor the patient after mild exertion.

5. The nurse is assessing the oxygenation status of the patient. Which are the best indicators of oxygenation?
   1. Respiratory rate, lung sounds, skin color
   2. Arterial blood gases (ABGs), lung sounds, SpO_2
   3. Skin color, ABGs, chest X-ray
   4. SpO_2, ABGs, skin color

6. Which position is best for the patient undergoing a thoracentesis?
   1. Sitting up, leaning forward on an overbed table
   2. Side-lying, affected side up, head slightly raised
   3. Side-lying, affected side down, head flat
   4. High Fowler position

7. An elderly patient with a severe respiratory infection is seen in the emergency department. The health care provider orders an IV of $D_5\frac{1}{2}NS$ 1000 mL over 12 hours. The IV tubing delivers 10 drops per mL. At what drip rate should this IV be administered? _____ 30 10 gtts/min

8. Indicate on the diagram where you would place the stethoscope to begin the respiratory assessment.

9. When a patient is scheduled for a lung ventilation and perfusion scan, what patient teaching is pertinent?
    1. The test will be done using CT technology.
    2. Radioactive agents will be inhaled and injected IV.
    3. The test can be done at the patient's bedside.
    4. The machine doing the imaging is loud and ear protection will be provided.

10. The patient has just returned from having a bronchoscopy. The nurse would intervene if the nursing student performs which action?
    1. Takes the patient's vital signs.
    2. Obtains food and fluids for the patient.
    3. Raises the head of the bed to 30 degrees.
    4. Auscultates the lung fields.

11. The nurse is caring for a patient with emphysema. What is the most essential point in administering oxygen to this patient?
    1. Instructing the patient to call for assistance as needed.
    2. Initiating continuous pulse oximetry monitoring.
    3. Frequently checking the skin underneath the cannula.
    4. Ensuring that oxygen flow is set at the correct rate.

12. Which instruction set should the nurse give to the patient to obtain a good sputum specimen?
    1. Perform mouth care just before giving the specimen.
    2. No fasting or other special preparation is required.
    3. The specimen should be obtained in the morning before eating.
    4. Cough deeply and spit the specimen into a clean container.

13. A patient with a long history of smoking and emphysema has a nursing diagnosis of Inadequate health management related to the inability to stop smoking. Which outcome statement is the best? The patient will:
    1. list three health reasons to stop smoking.
    2. receive smoking cessation information.
    3. explain how smoking became a habit.
    4. verbalize two strategies to stop smoking.

14. A postoperative patient has increased CO_2 levels. What is the best intervention by the nurse?
    1. Have the patient cough and turn.
    2. Have the patient take several deep breaths and use the incentive spirometer.
    3. Listen to the patient's lung sounds and check the surgical dressing.
    4. Ambulate the patient and make sure she is hydrated.

15. The nurse is preparing to give a patient an influenza vaccination. Which patient statement is the biggest concern?
    1. "I am afraid of needles; could I have the inhaled form?"
    2. "I recently stopped smoking and I seem to be coughing a lot."
    3. "I have a lot of allergic reactions to many common foods."
    4. "I have a history of chronic congestive heart failure."

CRITICAL THINKING ACTIVITIES

1. Describe particular ways you would adjust your teaching for an elderly patient who needs to be taught to use an incentive spirometer and cough effectively.

2.   Within your extended family, determine the risk factors for respiratory disorders.

STEPS TOWARD BETTER COMMUNICATION

VOCABULARY BUILDING GLOSSARY

Term	Definition
malaise'	(noun) general feeling of bodily discomfort
refrain'	(verb) to avoid doing something
dysphag'ia (dis fa' jee ah)	(noun) difficulty swallowing
hypocapnia	deficiency of carbon dioxide in the blood
hypercapnia	excess of carbon dioxide in the blood
surfactant	an agent that reduces fluid surface tension
naris (*plural* nares)	nostril
adventitious (ad ven ti' shus)	accidental, occasional; abnormal, outside of the usual place
apneusis (ap nu' sis)	long inspiration unrelieved by expiration

COMPLETION

Directions: Fill in the blanks with the correct words from the Vocabulary Building Glossary to complete the statements.

1.   Bronchitis is usually evident upon auscultation of the lungs because _____ sounds are present.

2.   The elderly patient seemed to have a general feeling of _____.

3.   A(n) _____ is used to make soaps more effective, as well as being found naturally in the body.

4.   Please _____ from smoking near the entryway.

MATCHING

Directions: Match the combining form or abbreviation on the left with its meaning on the right.

1.   _____   -itis
2.   _____   -oscopy
3.   _____   MRI
4.   _____   CT

a.   Magnetic resonance imaging
b.   Computed tomography
c.   Inflammation
d.   Process of visually examining

TERMINOLOGY

Directions: Identify the correct term for each definition.

1. Examination of the larynx: _____

2. Sinuses next to the nose: _____

3. Abnormal lung sounds: _____

4. Oxygen-deficient: _____

5. Difficulty breathing: _____

PRONUNCIATION

Directions: Practice saying these words with a partner.

1. "l" as the initial sound: (Curl the tip of your tongue and place it against the back of your front teeth. Air will flow around the sides of your tongue.)

laryngi'tis	le'sions	lung
larynx	lined	

2. "l" as the final sound:

cell	na'sal	tonsil
fron'tal	or'al	vo'cal
muco'sal	skull	

COMMUNICATION EXERCISE

1. With a partner, practice an explanation to an elderly person of the steps she should take to avoid contracting an upper respiratory infection (immunization, staying out of crowds, prompt treatment of any symptoms, avoid children with coughs and colds, maintain adequate rest and nutrition, good handwashing).

2. Switch roles and explain to a grade school–age child how to avoid catching and spreading respiratory diseases (covering coughs—cough into elbow, disposing of tissues, handwashing—sing the ABC song 2–3 times to expand alveoli, don't go to school or parties when you are sick or contagious, stay away from crowded places).

3. You do not speak your patient's language. What resources are available for you to complete the above exercise in the clinical setting?

Care of Patients with Disorders of the Upper Respiratory System

chapter

13

Answer Key: Review the related chapter to answer these questions. A complete answer key was provided to your instructor.

SHORT ANSWER

Directions: Provide a short answer for the following questions.

1. List three common symptoms of sinusitis.

   a. _____

   b. _____

   c. _____

2. Explain what life-threatening complication is possible with epiglottitis and other inflammatory upper airway disorders.

   _____

3. Why is strep screening done when tonsillitis is identified? _____

   _____

APPLICATION OF THE NURSING PROCESS

Upper Respiratory Disorders

Directions: Provide a short answer for the following questions.

1. Write one expected outcome for each of the following nursing diagnoses.

   a. Altered communication ability related to inability to speak due to tracheostomy _____

   _____

   b. Risk for aspiration related to impaired swallowing_____

   _____

   c. Altered airway clearance related to physical changes in airway (tracheostomy) _____

   _____

2. List two nursing interventions for each of the following nursing diagnoses for a patient who has obstructive sleep apnea.

   a. Altered breathing pattern while sleeping: _____

   _____

   b. Sleep deprivation: _____

   _____

COMPLETION

Directions: Fill in the blanks to complete the statements.

1. A nursing intervention to help promote drainage in the patient with acute sinusitis is _____

   _____.

2. Warning signs of cancer of the larynx include _____

   _____.

3. When cleaning the tracheostomy site and tube, the nurse must be careful not to allow _____

   _____.

4. The nurse's chief concern for the postoperative tonsillectomy patient is _____.

5. One way to detect postoperative bleeding in the tonsillectomy patient is to observe for frequent

   _____.

6. When suctioning a tracheostomy, the nurse must use _____ technique.

7. If a radical neck dissection must be performed, a(n) _____ is performed at the

   same time.

PRIORITY SETTING

1. You are assigned the following patients:
   - M.S., a preoperative patient scheduled for radical neck dissection surgery at 10:00 AM
   - O.T., a postoperative tonsillectomy (adult) patient being admitted as an inpatient due to excessive bleeding
   - M.R., a postlaryngectomy patient with a tracheostomy who is first-day postoperative

Directions: Indicate the order of priority in which you would do the following: (Use 1, 2, 3.)

_____   Provide preoperative care for M.S., including the preoperative checklist.

_____   Assess O.T.'s status.

_____   Assess M.R.'s status.

2. Which patient should be your first priority? _____. Give rationale.
   a. The patient with the tracheostomy who is having considerable difficulty breathing.
   b. The postoperative patient just arriving on the unit from surgery.
   c. The radical neck dissection patient who is complaining of considerable pain.

REVIEW QUESTIONS FOR THE NCLEX® EXAMINATION

Directions: Select the best answer(s) or fill in the blank with the correct word(s) for the following questions.

1. The priority assessment for any patient with any problems of the upper airway is:
    1. anxiety and pain.
    2. adequacy of oxygenation.
    3. presence and thickness of nasal and oral secretions.
    4. signs of dyspnea.

2. A patient comes to the emergency department with a nosebleed. Which is the first action the nurse should initiate?
    1. Applying ice to the back of the neck.
    2. Having the patient tip the head way back, hyperextending the neck.
    3. Packing the nose with gauze.
    4. Applying pressure to the nose with the thumb and forefinger.

3. When drugs are prescribed for treatment of rhinitis and sinusitis, which type(s) of drugs would be included? *(Select all that apply.)*
    1. Decongestants
    2. Bronchodilators
    3. Antihistamines
    4. Antitussives
    5. Antipyretics
    6. Mucolytics

4. Which statement regarding rhinitis and the elderly patient is true?
    1. Complementary and alternative therapies are ineffective in the older adult.
    2. Antihistamines and decongestants should be used with caution.
    3. Antipyretics and antibiotics are not used because of risk of allergic reactions.
    4. Viral rhinitis is self-limiting and comfort measures are not necessary.

5. The patient with acute pharyngitis has a nursing diagnosis of Discomfort and pain related to inflammation. Which intervention would the nurse use for this diagnosis?
    1. Advise to use warm saline gargles.
    2. Obtain a throat culture.
    3. Monitor the patient's temperature.
    4. Assess the potential for aspiration.

6. The patient reports a long history of smoking and now complains of hoarseness and a lump-like feeling in the throat. Which question is the most relevant to collect data about possible signs of throat cancer?
    1. Are you coughing up green or gray sputum?
    2. Do you experience any wheezing after exercise?
    3. Does the lump in your throat disappear when you swallow?
    4. Have you had hoarseness for more than 3 weeks?

7. The patient is being discharged after undergoing a rhinoplasty for a nasal fracture. Which discharge instruction would the nurse question?
    1. Use a humidifier at home to decrease mucosal dryness.
    2. Take ibuprofen every 6 hours for pain.
    3. Apply a cool compress over the nose and face.
    4. Use a stool softener as needed to avoid straining.

8. In the immediate postoperative period after a tonsillectomy, what is the highest priority?
   1. Pain control
   2. Adequate hydration
   3. Prevention of aspiration
   4. Treatment of nausea

9. A patient undergoing sinus surgery has a preoperative piggyback of cefazolin (Ancef) ordered, with 500 mg of the drug dissolved in 50 mL of IV solution. The powdered drug was mixed with 10 mL of sterile water before it was added to the IV solution. The drug is ordered to be administered over 20 minutes. The IV tubing delivers 10 drops per mL. The IV should run at ____32____ drops per minute.

10. What assessments should be done for patient with a new tracheostomy? *(Select all that apply.)*
    1. Cuff inflation
    2. Lung sounds before and after suctioning
    3. Redness or swelling of tonsils
    4. Hoarseness when speaking
    5. Condition of insertion site
    6. Work of breathing

11. The nurse is caring for patients who have been diagnosed with laryngeal cancer. Which patient is likely to have the best outcome after medical treatment?
    1. An elderly man with a long history of smoking and difficulty swallowing
    2. A middle-aged man who reports having persistent hoarseness
    3. A young man who complains of pain in the region of the Adam's apple
    4. An elderly woman who reports weakness and difficulty breathing

12. A man eating in a restaurant suddenly stands up and grasps his throat with his hands. What is the priority action?
    1. Call 911 and stay with the man.
    2. Direct the man to cough forcefully.
    3. Start cardiopulmonary resuscitation.
    4. Initiate abdominal thrusts.

13. The nurse observes that a patient is having severe respiratory distress. Which action should be delegated to the nursing assistant?
    1. Calling the health care provider
    2. Staying with the patient
    3. Obtaining an Ambu bag
    4. Setting up suction equipment

14. A patient with a new tracheostomy has a nursing diagnosis of Altered airway clearance. What is the most likely etiology of this problem?
    1. Improper suctioning technique
    2. Failure of the tracheostomy tube
    3. Inadequate oral hygiene
    4. Inability to cough up secretions and mucus

15. A patient's wife reports that her husband frequently snores. Which question would the nurse ask to identify another symptom of obstructive sleep apnea?
    1. "Does he wake suddenly at night?"
    2. "Does he have shortness of breath on waking?"
    3. "Does he complain of a sore throat in the evening?"
    4. "Does he go to bed early or late in the evening?"

CRITICAL THINKING ACTIVITIES

Scenario: A 76-year-old male patient possibly has laryngeal cancer. He is to undergo diagnostic testing and if cancer is diagnosed, he will have a laryngectomy.

1. What diagnostic tests would most likely be done for this patient?

2. If the patient has a laryngectomy and a tracheostomy, how would you provide a means of communication?

3. What criteria would you use to determine when the patient's tracheostomy needs suctioning?

4. What are the two most important principles to be observed when suctioning?

STEPS TOWARD BETTER COMMUNICATION

VOCABULARY BUILDING GLOSSARY

Term	Pronunciation	Definition
diligent	dil' ah jent	(adj.) hardworking, dedicated at all times
vigilant	vij' ah lent	(adj.) watchful, alert to danger
prevalent	prev' ah lent	(adj.) commonly occurring, widespread
susceptible	sus cep' ti ble	(adj.) easily affected by something—physical or emotional
patent	pa' tent	(adj.) open

COMPLETION

Directions: Fill in the blanks with the correct words from the Vocabulary Building Glossary to complete the statements.

1. Immediate postoperative care of a tonsillectomy patient focuses on maintaining a(n)

    _____ airway and observing for hemorrhage.

2. To prevent a respiratory infection in a tracheostomy patient, the nurse must be _____

    with hand hygiene before suctioning.

3. The elderly are very _____ to upper respiratory infections.

4. When a patient suffers from dysphagia, the nurse must be _____ for signs of aspiration when the patient is eating or drinking.

5. The belief that immunizations are important for children is _____ in Western culture.

SHORT ANSWER

Directions: Write the word to match the definition.

1. Nosebleed: _____

2. Removal of the adenoids: _____

3. Inflammation of the sinuses: _____

IDIOMATIC USAGES

Idioms are phrases used in everyday speech that do not translate literally from one language or culture to another. Below are some common English language idioms.

"Catching" a cold means getting a viral infection.

"Stuffier" means becoming more congested.

"Dull" can mean mentally slow, as well as referring to a soft, toneless sound. The opposite would be "sharp, clear" for all of these meanings.

A "magic slate" is a board covered with wax and a plastic sheet on top that can be written on with a stylus. The words show, but are erased when the sheet is lifted so that it can be reused.

PRONUNCIATION

In English, the consonant sound **"l"** is found at the beginning, middle, or end of words. It is made by putting the tip of the tongue against the back of the top front teeth with the lips open a little. The tongue lies in the bottom of the mouth and the air comes out on both sides. The voice is used.

Directions: Practice saying these words with a partner.

1. "l" as the middle sound:

air-filled	irregular'ity	physiol'ogy
al'lergy	malig'nant	plaque
car'tilage	max'illary	pol'yps
cil'ia	mobil'ity	re'flex
cold	mus'cle	swal'lowed
eld'erly	olfact'ory	swell'ing
epiglot'tis	pa'late	til'ted
flu	pal'lor	ulcera'tion
glot'tis	pal'pate	
inflamma'tion	par'ticles	

2. "l" is silent:

calm	half	talk
could	should	would

SPELLING AND PRONUNCIATION SKILLS

ph = f

When the letters **"ph"** occur in the same syllable in English, they are pronounced like **"f."** They may occur at the beginning, middle, or end of words. The sound is made by touching the top teeth with the bottom lip. Air is blown out between the lip and the teeth.

Directions: Practice saying the following words.

dysphagia	esophageal	facial	frontal
esophagus	pharynx	lymph	

Care of Patients with Disorders of the Lower Respiratory System

chapter

14

Answer Key: Review the related chapter to answer these questions. A complete answer key was provided to your instructor.

REVIEW OF ANATOMY AND PHYSIOLOGY

Terminology

Directions: Match the term on the left with its best description on the right.

1. _____ Diffusion
2. _____ Tidal volume
3. _____ Vital capacity
4. _____ Resistance
5. _____ Perfusion
6. _____ Surfactant
7. _____ Ventilation

a. Movement of air from outside body to alveoli and back to the outside
b. Amount of gas in air one can exhale after maximal inhalation
c. Amount of gas either inhaled or exhaled with each breath
d. Chiefly determined by radius or caliber of airway
e. Prevents collapse of lung by stabilizing alveoli and decreasing capillary pressure
f. Passage of fluid through vessels of an organ
g. Takes place between gas in alveolar space and blood in capillaries of lung

APPLICATION OF THE NURSING PROCESS

Directions: List specific nursing actions that could be planned for a patient.

1. List four points to include in the assessment of a patient with a cough.

   a. _____

   b. _____

   c. _____

   d. _____

2. Name four interventions that can help prevent pneumonia.

   a. _____

   b. _____

   c. _____

   d. _____

Directions: Provide a nursing action to address the problem.

3. Data: "My husband coughs as hard as he can, but he just can't get the phlegm up from his lungs."

    Nursing action: _____

4. Data: "It seems that I have to come to the hospital at least twice a year for an infection in my lungs. I suppose there is nothing I can do about it now that I have chronic bronchitis and emphysema."

    Nursing action: _____

5. Data: "I get short of breath just trying to take a bath and brush my teeth. Here at the hospital, there is someone wanting to do something to me every time I turn around. I wish I could get some rest."

    Nursing action: _____

MATCHING

Directions: Match the symptoms with the disease. (Choose all that apply.)

_____ 1. Rhinitis (common cold)   a. Pain in the chest
                                                   b. Cough
_____ 2. Influenza   c. Muscle aches
                                                   d. Headache
_____ 3. Pneumonia   e. Fever
                                                   f. Nasal congestion
                                                   g. Chills
                                                   h. GI symptoms

SHORT ANSWER

1. List four signs or symptoms to note during data collection when caring for a patient with a lower respiratory disorder. *Example: Sits leaning forward with shoulders elevated.*

    a. _____

    b. _____

    c. _____

    d. _____

2. Name three reasons that health care workers are routinely screened for tuberculosis.

    a. _____

    b. _____

    c. _____

3. List five disorders that can be caused or triggered by smoking.

   a. _____

   b. _____

   c. _____

   d. _____

   e. _____

COMPLETION

Directions: Fill in the blanks to complete the statements.

1. _____ is an extensive inflammation of the lung with either consolidation of the lung tissue as it fills with exudate or interstitial inflammation and edema.

2. _____ occurs when the fluid within the pleural cavity becomes infected and the exudate becomes thick and purulent.

3. The most common fungal lung infections are _____ and

   _____.

4. The fatigue that is often present in patients with respiratory disease is usually caused by a deficit in the _____ supply to the tissues.

5. Excessively high concentrations of inhaled oxygen can bring about collapse of the alveoli because of an interruption in production of _____, which stabilizes the alveoli.

PRIORITY SETTING

Directions: It is 7:15 AM. Your patients have the following needs. In what order would you try to meet them? Number in order of priority. Discuss your answers with a classmate and state your rationale.

_____ a. A patient who had a thoracotomy is complaining of pain in spite of using his PCA pump.

_____ b. A patient vomited and needs a clean gown and sheets.

_____ c. A patient with pneumonia did not get his breakfast tray and is asking for it.

_____ d. A nursing assistant has just told you that a patient is febrile.

_____ e. A patient with a tracheostomy needs suctioning.

REVIEW QUESTIONS FOR THE NCLEX® EXAMINATION

Directions: Select the best answer(s) or fill in the blank with the answer for the following questions.

1. Safety factors for administering oxygen to the patient with chronic obstructive pulmonary disease (COPD) include:
   1. auscultating the lungs when the patient coughs.
   2. carefully titrating oxygen delivery.
   3. placing the patient in a recumbent position.
   4. filling the humidifier with warm tap water.

2. A nursing intervention that can *best* help prevent atelectasis in the patient with compromised lung function is to:
   1. encourage at least 3000 mL of fluid intake per day.
   2. assist with all activities of daily living (ADLs) to prevent excess fatigue.
   3. have the patient turn, cough, and deep-breathe at least every 2 hours.
   4. administer an expectorant to help clear airways.

3. Patients with chronic respiratory diseases can benefit from teaching that includes: *(Select all that apply.)*
   1. when and how to use pursed-lip breathing.
   2. dress warmly when leaving the house.
   3. verify safety of over-the-counter medications with health care provider.
   4. avoid crowds during flu season.
   5. food and hydration recommendations.
   6. use antihistamines to clear up congestion.

4. The nurse is assessing the patient for early stage emphysema. What sign would the nurse look for?
   1. Dyspnea
   2. Pale skin color
   3. Yellow, tenacious sputum
   4. Rapid, pounding pulse

5. The nurse is assessing the patient with a chest tube placed 3 days ago for a pneumothorax. Which finding indicates that there may be a problem with the apparatus?
   1. There is bloody drainage in the collection chamber.
   2. There is continuous bubbling in the water seal chamber.
   3. There is rigorous bubbling in the suction chamber.
   4. The water level fluctuates in the water seal chamber with breathing.

6. The nursing diagnosis for a patient with tuberculosis is Nonadherence with medication therapy. However, the etiology of the problem is unclear. What is the priority nursing action?
   1. Suggest that the patient wear a mask until the problem is resolved.
   2. Notify the public health department to follow up on exposed family and friends.
   3. Assess the patient's understanding of the therapy and treatment plan.
   4. Engage the family to remind the patient to take the scheduled doses.

7. Your pneumonia patient is encouraged to increase his fluid intake. He had 340 mL at breakfast, 60 mL with pills, 280 mL midmorning, 410 mL with lunch, and 240 mL midafternoon. How much more fluid does he need to reach the goal of 3000 mL for the day? _____1750_____

8. When administering respiratory medications to a patient, which medication should be administered *last*?
   1. Albuterol (Proventil)
   2. Montelukast (Singulair)
   3. Robitussin cough syrup
   4. Advair Diskus

9. The laboratory results for arterial blood gas analysis show that the patient has respiratory alkalosis. Before calling the health care provider, what additional assessment information is the most relevant?
   1. Current setting of the supplemental oxygen
   2. Pulse oximetry reading on room air
   3. Respiratory rate and breathing pattern
   4. Patient's subjective feeling of dyspnea

10. What is a major intervention to prevent further lung damage in the patient with chronic respiratory disease?
    1. Institute a plan to balance rest and activity.
    2. Convince the patient to quit smoking.
    3. Teach proper breathing techniques.
    4. Teach ways to maintain optimal health.

11. There is an order for a pneumonectomy patient to "avoid turning onto unoperated side." What is the best rationale for this order?
    1. Tension on the bronchial stump could occur.
    2. Position would cause kinking of the chest tubes.
    3. Patient could have increased chest excursion.
    4. The stomach and intestines will cause distention.

12. The nurse is checking the oxygen delivery system at the beginning of the shift. What is included in the assessment of the system and equipment? *(Select all that apply.)*
    1. Check to make sure that the oxygen flow rate is less than 3 L/min.
    2. Observe the tubing for kinks or blockage.
    3. Make sure that the tubing and connections are not touching the floor.
    4. Verify that the flow rate is set according to the health care provider's order.
    5. Make sure that the oxygen source or tank is not combustible.

13. Which nutritional suggestion would the nurse give to a COPD patient?
    1. Restrict fluids to prevent fluid overload and possible pulmonary edema.
    2. Perform mild exercise just before eating to stimulate appetite.
    3. Eat three regular meals a day, but limit protein intake.
    4. Cook when feeling most energetic and freeze extra portions.

14. A postoperative patient suddenly and unexpectedly becomes very anxious and complains of dyspnea. What is the priority nursing action?
    1. Encourage expression of feelings.
    2. Assess for other symptoms.
    3. Notify the RN or MD.
    4. Tell the patient to calm down.

15. The nurse is caring for a trauma patient and notes that with inhalation, a portion of the chest is drawn inward and with exhalation, the portion expands outward. What is the significance of this observation?
    1. This is a normal and expected pattern of chest movement.
    2. The patient is having excessive pain that is interfering with respiration.
    3. Several ribs are fractured and the patient should be turned onto the affected side.
    4. This pattern is associated with a pneumothorax or hemothorax.

CRITICAL THINKING ACTIVITIES

A patient who had been living in Southeast Asia for the past 2 years has just been diagnosed with tuberculosis. He is complaining of night sweats, fatigue, and weight loss. He has a cough.

1. Therapy for tuberculosis consists of several medications. What medications would you expect to be prescribed? What teaching points are especially important for this patient?

2. At what point will this patient no longer be considered contagious?

3. In what population of the United States is the incidence of tuberculosis the highest? Why?

STEPS TOWARD BETTER COMMUNICATION

VOCABULARY BUILDING GLOSSARY

Term	Definition
re′coil	to move back quickly; to return with force to an original position
flar′ing	getting wider; extending outward at the edges or tips
pursed (purst)	rounded, gathered together (as when lips are ready to blow out a candle or to whistle)
com′bustion (kŏm bust′ shŭn)	burning or fire
suscep′tible (su sep′ ti bel)	likely or probably will be affected; at risk of; prone to catch sickness
aggres′sive care	vigorous, strong, frequent care that follows all guidelines
cor′relate	link together two or more things; fit together into a pattern (e.g., *correlate* the symptoms with the disease)
ag′gravate	to cause to increase; to make worse
paradox′ical (par ah dok′ si kel)	something that looks contradictory but is true; two things that are working opposite of usual; contrary to what is normal or expected
hall′mark	sign, criteria; standard signal or feature of some condition
fluc′tuate	to change, vary up and down
cal′ibrate	to measure exactly, usually with markings
occlud′ed	blocked
emerging	rising or coming up

PRONUNCIATION OF DIFFICULT TERMS

Directions: Practice pronouncing the following words:

Term	Pronunciation	Definition
kyphosis	ki fo′ sis	abnormal outward curvature of the spine; hunchback
scoliosis	sko lee o′ sis	S-type curvature of the spine
empyema	em pie ee′ ma	accumulation of pus in a body cavity
hemoptysis	he mop′ ti sis	coughing and spitting of red, frothy blood
hematemesis	hem ah tem′ e sis	vomiting of blood

COMPLETION

Directions: Fill in the blanks with the correct words from the Vocabulary Building Glossary to complete the statements.

1. Learning to breathe with _____ lips helps decrease dyspnea for the patient with emphysema.

2. People with chronic respiratory disease are more _____ to respiratory infections than the general public.

3. When a chest tube is functioning properly, the fluid in the water seal chamber will _____ with each breath.

4. Oxygen is *not* explosive; however, oxygen does support _____.

5. When several ribs are fractured, _____ chest motion will be observed.

6. When respiratory distress is occurring, the nurse may observe _____ of the patient's nostrils.

7. A(n) _____ of acute respiratory distress syndrome (ARDS) is respiratory failure.

8. The Centers for Disease Control monitor _____ infectious diseases, such as SARS.

9. When turning a patient who is attached to a ventilator, the nurse must be careful to check that the ventilator tubing is not _____.

10. Patients with severe _____ or _____ of the spine often have restrictive lung disease.

WORD ATTACK SKILLS

Directions: Look at the word elements defined below and then break the listed words into their word parts using vertical lines. Write the meaning of each word as in the example below:

anti/venom   *an agent that counteracts the effect of a poison from snake or insect bite*

-oid: resembling

-megal/o: enlargement

-osis: condition

anti-:   against

1. Cytomegalovirus: _____

2. Immunocompromised:_____

3. Immunosuppressive: _____

4. Antiinfective: _____

5. Coccidioidomycosis:_____

COMMUNICATION EXERCISE

Directions: Here is an example of what you would say to teach a patient ways to prevent the spread of a respiratory infection.

"You can help prevent the spread of your respiratory infection by good hand hygiene. Use hand sanitizer or wash your hands frequently with soap and warm water. Cover your mouth with a tissue or your elbow when you cough or sneeze. Throw away used tissues immediately and perform hand hygiene. Be careful not to touch objects after coughing or sneezing before you cleanse your hands. Try to sit and stand several feet away from other people while your nose is running and you are coughing and sneezing. Stay out of crowded places."

Directions: With a peer, practice performing a respiratory assessment.

Take and record the respiratory history. Document your physical assessment findings. Ask your instructor to review your documentation of the assessment.

The Hematologic System

chapter

15

Answer Key: Review the related chapter to answer these questions. A complete answer key was provided to your instructor.

REVIEW OF ANATOMY AND PHYSIOLOGY

Completion

Directions: Fill in the blanks to complete the statements.

1. The type of blood cell responsible for the transport of oxygen is the _____.

2. Erythropoiesis must continue throughout life because the average life span of a red blood cell (RBC) is _____.

3. An infection in the body stimulates the production of _____, resulting in _____.

4. The normal adult range of white blood cells (WBCs) is 4500 to $11,000/mm^3$ with a life span of _____.

5. The major function of thrombocytes is to promote _____.

6. Bone marrow activity decreases by about _____ percent as years advance, making the older person more _____.

7. The storage and release of blood and the removal of old blood cells are major functions of the _____ and _____.

8. Basophils release _____ in response to allergens.

COMPLETION

Age-Related Changes Affecting the Hematologic System

Directions: Complete each of the following statements.

1. A problem that might be caused by the decrease in plasma volume after age 60 is: _____

_____

_____

2. The elderly are at greater risk for infection because _____

    _____.

3. People younger than age 60 are less likely to have clotting problems than older adults because there is

    _____.

4. Changes in blood coagulation make the elderly person more at risk for _____

    _____.

SHORT ANSWER

Causes and Prevention of Hematologic Disorders

Directions: Provide a short answer for each of the following questions.

1. Inherited disorders that interfere with normal blood function are:

    a. _____

    b. _____

    c. _____

2. These groups have tendencies for which hematologic problems?

    a. African Americans: _____

    b. Scandinavian descent:_____

    c. Middle-Easterners: _____

3. Complete the statements for drugs that can cause particular blood dyscrasias (abnormalities):

    a. Procainamide may cause:_____

    b. Furosemide may cause:_____

    c. Quinidine may cause: _____

    d. Oral contraceptives may cause:_____

4. Nutritional deficiencies that may interfere with erythropoiesis are: _____

    _____

5. Lifestyle factors that can help prevent anemia are: _____

    _____

    _____

6. Excessive blood loss can be prevented by: _____

    _____

7. Two ways to help prevent blood dyscrasias are:

    a. _____

    _____

    b. _____

    _____

SHORT ANSWER

Assessment and Diagnostics

Directions: Briefly answer the following.

1. List the five kinds of data that should be obtained during history-taking for assessment of a patient with a blood disorder.

    a. _____

    b. _____

    c. _____

    d. _____

    e. _____

2. State the possible cause or condition usually associated with each of the following (*example: Tarry stools: intestinal bleeding*).

    a. Jaundice: _____

    b. Bruises and petechiae: _____

    c. Polycythemia: _____

    d. Sore, bleeding gums: _____

    e. Smoky brownish urine: _____

    f. Swollen and painful joints: _____

    g. Weakness and intolerance to physical activity: _____

    h. Irritability, dizziness, and difficulty concentrating: _____

3. Inquiring about occupation and hobbies is important to a hematologic history because: _____

    _____

    _____

4. If during assessment, a patient's urine is noted to be a brown tea color, it could indicate that _____

    _____ is occurring.

5. Two nursing responsibilities for obtaining a urine specimen for monoclonal protein testing are:

    a. _____

    b. _____

6. When blood collection is performed, nursing responsibilities are to:

    a. _____

    b. _____

    c. _____

7. On the blood count differential, allergy may be indicated by the presence of _____
_____.

8. A d-Dimer blood test is useful for diagnosing _____.

PRIORITY SETTING

Directions: You have been asked to obtain a blood sample for a CBC from a patient in the ambulatory clinic. Number the following tasks in the order in which you would perform them. Consider that a task may be performed more than once. (See Skill 16-1 on Evolve.)

_____   a. Obtain the needed supplies.

_____   b. Place the label on the specimen tube.

_____   c. Don latex gloves.

_____   d. Write the information on the specimen label.

_____   e. Send the specimen to the laboratory.

_____   f. Perform the venipuncture.

_____   g. Cover the wound.

_____   h. Identify the patient using two identifiers.

_____   i. Remove the gloves.

_____   j. Fill out the laboratory requisition slip.

_____   k. Stop bleeding at the site.

_____   l. Perform hand hygiene.

_____   m. Explain to the patient what you are going to do.

REVIEW QUESTIONS FOR THE NCLEX® EXAMINATION

Directions: Choose or supply the best answer(s) for the following questions.

1. The main functions of blood are to: *(Select all that apply.)*
    1. transport nutrients to the cells and waste products away from the cells.
    2. assist in regulating fluid volume.
    3. assist in regulating body temperature.
    4. manufacture protein.
    5. regulate pH and acid-base balance.

2. Erythropoiesis cannot occur normally if: *(Select all that apply.)*
   1. bone marrow activity is suppressed.
   2. there is a lack of vitamin K.
   3. there are insufficient amino acids available.
   4. the diet does not include sufficient green and yellow vegetables.
   5. vitamin E is insufficient.
   6. linoleic acid is not present.

3. The normal range for platelets in adults is _____ /mm³.

4. The functions of plasma proteins are to: *(Select all that apply.)*
   1. combat arthritis.
   2. prevent fluid from leaking out into the tissue space.
   3. assist in the formation of blood clots.
   4. assist with skeletal mobility.
   5. combine with drugs and lipids to transport them throughout the body.

5. When gathering assessment data, you would: *(Place the choices in proper sequence.)*

   _____ 1. inspect the skin for abnormal color.

   _____ 2. inquire about family hereditary diseases.

   _____ 3. check scleral and conjunctival color.

   _____ 4. inquire about headaches or palpitations.

   _____ 5. inquire about ease of bleeding.

   _____ 6. measure vital signs.

   _____ 7. check for swollen or painful joints.

   _____ 8. check condition of fingernails and hair.

6. Yellowed skin or sclera and conjunctiva may occur from: *(Select all that apply.)*
   1. anemic state.
   2. excess bilirubin in the blood.
   3. inadequate platelet function.
   4. hemolysis.
   5. excess consumption of carrots.

7. A sign of spleen enlargement is:
   1. feeling of fullness in upper left abdomen.
   2. complaints of stomach pain from pressure.
   3. decreased erythrocyte count.
   4. an upper left quadrant lump felt upon palpation.

8. When a patient is anorexic, things that may interfere with eating are:
   1. providing socialization during meals.
   2. odors in the room.
   3. serving small frequent meals and snacks.
   4. providing mouth care before each meal.

9. People who have a blood abnormality may be prone to bleeding problems and _____

   _____ .

10. When a patient has a prolonged clotting time, after drawing blood, you should:
    1. apply pressure for 2 full minutes.
    2. have the patient apply pressure to the site until the bleeding stops.
    3. apply pressure for 5–10 minutes.
    4. use a styptic pencil to stop the bleeding.

11. Activity intolerance and fatigue occur with some hematologic disorders because:
    1. too many blood cells make blood thicker and circulation sluggish.
    2. a deficiency of hemoglobin decreases the oxygen-carrying capacity of the blood.
    3. oxygen molecules will not attach to faulty erythrocytes and can't reach the cells.
    4. oxygen cannot diffuse through alveolar membrane thickened by abnormal cells.

12. The patient with a blood abnormality is at higher risk for infection. Therefore, the nurse should make which intervention a priority?
    1. Treat pain immediately.
    2. Correct nutritional deficiencies.
    3. Use aseptic technique.
    4. Prevent undue fatigue.

CRITICAL THINKING ACTIVITIES

1. If you came upon an auto accident, stopped to help, and found someone on the ground spurting blood from the upper thigh, what would you do first? After that, what would you do?

2. You have been assigned to a recent postoperative patient who has just had a thoracotomy. You know that postoperative hemorrhage is always a potential complication. What would you specifically assess to assure yourself as best you can that a postoperative hemorrhage is not occurring?

STEPS TOWARD BETTER COMMUNICATION

VOCABULARY BUILDING GLOSSARY

Term	Definition
ag'gregate	(verb) bring separate parts together in a group, to combine
brought on	caused to occur, induced by, emerged from
clot	a thickened mass of liquid, especially of blood
perni'cious (per nish' us)	having a very harmful effect
pleth'ora	red complexion caused by excessive blood

COMPLETION

Directions: Fill in the blanks with the correct words from the Vocabulary Building Glossary to complete the statements.

1. When a cut occurs and a blood vessel is damaged, platelets _____ as part of the clotting process.

2. _____ anemia is caused by an inability of the body to absorb vitamin B_{12} from the intestinal tract.

3. Fibrinogen is another factor in addition to platelets that work to form a blood _____.

4. Patients suffering from polycythemia vera often display _____.

5. Lymphedema may be _____ by the lymph node extraction that accompanies a radical or modified mastectomy.

PRONUNCIATION

Directions: With a peer, practice pronouncing the following words. Use each word in an appropriate sentence.

Term	Pronunciation	Definition
dyscra'sia	dis kray' zee ah	imbalance in the elements of something
erythropoi'etin	a rith' ro poy' e tin	hormone that stimulates red blood cell production
erythropoie'sis	a rith' ro poi ee' sis	red blood cell production
fatigue'd	fa teeg' d	very tired, completely weary, exhausted
parenterally	pah ren' ter ah lee	by a route other than the digestive tract
pete'chia	pa tee' ki a	round, red spot
splenomeg'aly	splen' o meg' a lee	enlargement of the spleen
throm'bocytope'nia	throm' bo si to pee' ne ah	decrease in the number of platelets

MATCHING

Directions: Match the prefix or suffix on the left with its correct meaning on the right.

1. _____ -cyte
2. _____ -chrom
3. _____ -phils
4. _____ a-
5. _____ normo-
6. _____ gran-
7. _____ neo-
8. _____ mono-
9. _____ macro-
10. _____ leuko-
11. _____ erythro-

a. Have affinity for
b. Normal, usual
c. Negative prefix (not or without)
d. White
e. Cell
f. Large, long
g. Color
h. Sole, one
i. Grain, particle
j. New, young
k. Red

SHORT ANSWER

Directions: Write the meaning of each word, referring to the word elements in the exercise above. Use your dictionary as needed.

1. Macrophage: _____

2. Monochrome: _____

3. Leukocytosis: _____

4. Erythropoietin: _____

5. Granulocyte: _____

6. Neutrophil: _____

7. Agranulocyte: _____

8. Normochromic: _____

Care of Patients with Hematologic Disorders

chapter
16

Answer Key: Review the related chapter to answer these questions. A complete answer key was provided to your instructor.

COMPLETION

Hematologic Disorders

Directions: Fill in the blanks to complete the statements.

1. Anemia occurs because there is/are not enough _____ or _____.

2. Treatment of pernicious anemia consists of _____.

3. The primary difficulty caused by anemia is failure to meet the _____

   _____.

4. Sickle cell disease is present in about _____% of African Americans. Other groups are also affected, including _____,_____,_____, and _____.

5. When both parents have sickle cell trait, the chances of their children having sickle cell disease rise to

   _____%.

6. The symptoms suffered during a sickling crisis are the result of _____

   _____.

7. Leukemia is a cancer and the cause is _____.

8. Leukemia patients receiving chemotherapy should avoid eating _____.

9. There is a hereditary link for _____ leukemia.

10. Patients who are anemic and receiving iron therapy should increase their intake of vitamin C because it

    helps _____.

11. A patient with hemophilia should never take aspirin because it _____

    _____.

12. When a patient has an iron-deficiency anemia, treatment consists of _____

    _____

    _____.

13. When a patient is anemic, oxygen levels tend to drop because of the deficiency of _____

    present in the blood.

14. Side effects of oral iron therapy include _____

   _____.

15. Aplastic anemia may be caused by _____, a(n) _____, or a(n)

   _____.

16. A blood loss of _____ % is considered when postural hypotension occurs.

17. The classic signs and symptoms of hypovolemic shock are _____

   _____

   _____.

18. The patient experiencing hypovolemic shock is positioned _____

   _____.

19. Nutritional anemia is caused by inadequate _____, _____, or

   _____.

APPLICATION OF THE NURSING PROCESS

Directions: Write an expected outcome and list three nursing measures for each of the following nursing problems commonly found in patients with blood disorders.

1. Altered tissue perfusion due to decreased red blood cells and hemoglobin

   Expected outcome: _____

   _____

   a. _____

   b. _____

   c. _____

2. Potential for infection due to decreased or abnormal white blood cells

   Expected outcome: _____

   _____

   a. _____

   b. _____

   c. _____

3. Altered activity tolerance due to fatigue and weakness

   Expected outcome: _____

   _____

   a. _____

   b. _____

   c. _____

4. Potential for injury due to possible hemorrhage

   Expected outcome: _____

   _____

   a. _____

   b. _____

   c. _____

5. List interventions you would place on the teaching plan for a 35-year-old female patient who has iron-deficiency anemia.

   _____

   _____

   _____

   _____

   _____

   _____

TABLE ACTIVITY

Directions: Complete this table on the four types of anemia by filling in the blank columns. Include all answers that apply.

Anemia	Characteristic RBC	Etiology	Additional Effects
Iron-deficiency anemia			
Pernicious anemia			
Aplastic anemia			
Sickle cell anemia			

REVIEW QUESTIONS FOR THE NCLEX® EXAMINATION

Directions: Choose the best answer(s) for the following questions.

1. An important part of assessment of the patient with an iron-deficiency anemia is: *(Select all that apply.)*
   1. determining if there is a family history of this type of problem.
   2. determining if there is abnormally high blood loss with menstruation.
   3. asking if the patient takes any vitamins.
   4. determining if the patient is a strict vegetarian.
   5. checking to see if any drugs that cause hemolysis are being taken.
   6. obtaining a thorough dietary history of what the patient normally eats.

2. Nursing interventions for the patient admitted with severe anemia should include:
   1. implementation of strategies to conserve the patient's energy.
   2. obtaining blood specimens for diagnostic testing.
   3. administering ordered blood products.
   4. assessing the patient for signs of depression.

3. When the nurse administers a form of iron to the anemic patient, she keeps in mind that iron:
   1. comes in many different forms and strengths.
   2. should be given through a straw if in liquid oral form.
   3. usually leaves a bad aftertaste in the mouth.
   4. is more quickly effective in the intravenous form.

4. When a blood transfusion is given to a patient, it is important to: *(Select all that apply.)*
   1. verify the blood unit numbers and the patient's blood bracelet with another nurse.
   2. determine if anyone in the family has had a transfusion reaction.
   3. take baseline vital signs.
   4. prime the filter and IV tubing with normal saline.

5. A patient with chronic iron-deficiency anemia may have: *(Select all that apply.)*
   1. spoon-shaped nails.
   2. bloodshot eyes.
   3. fatigue.
   4. headache.

6. A treatment often used for polycythemia vera is:
   1. iron therapy.
   2. vitamin C.
   3. phlebotomy.
   4. aspirin.

7. Nursing interventions for the patient with idiopathic thrombocytopenic purpura must include measures to:
   1. prevent spontaneous bleeding.
   2. increase the number of red blood cells.
   3. prevent health care–associated infection.
   4. encourage better nutrition.

8. Teaching to prevent sickle cell crisis includes: *(Select all that apply.)*
   1. encouraging the patient to eat a diet with sufficient protein.
   2. teaching the patient to restrict fluids at night.
   3. teaching the patient to take folic acid regularly.
   4. encouraging avoidance of any recreational drug or alcohol.

9. A high-priority goal for the planning of care for the patient with aplastic anemia is:
   1. prevention of fatigue.
   2. assistance with activities of daily living (ADLs).
   3. prevention of infection.
   4. alleviation of pain.

10. When gathering data to support a diagnosis of leukemia, the nurse knows that the most common symptoms are:
    1. excessive bleeding, headaches, and chills.
    2. exposure to known toxic agents that cause the disorder.
    3. fatigue, malaise, and frequent infections.
    4. viral infection, nausea, and decreased hemoglobin.

11. One of the first signs of disseminated intravascular coagulation is:
    1. blood clotting that interferes with circulation in the extremities.
    2. chest pain from tiny blood clots throughout the lungs.
    3. continued bleeding from an injection site, ecchymoses, and petechiae.
    4. bleeding from the mouth, nose, and other body orifices.

12. When administering more than one unit of blood by transfusion, the nurse must:
    1. change the filter for each new unit to be transfused.
    2. wait at least 1 hour between administration of units.
    3. allow the second unit to warm to room temperature before hanging it.
    4. administer at least 250 mL of normal saline between units given.

13. Subtle signs of a transfusion reaction may be:
    1. somnolence and confusion.
    2. bradycardia and increased blood pressure.
    3. backache and a feeling of anxiety.
    4. irritability and headache.

14. The drug hydroxyurea (Hydrea):
    1. helps boost hemoglobin levels.
    2. separates neutrophils from the blood.
    3. treats all types of leukemia.
    4. reduces frequency of sickling episodes.

15. Which statement is true about bone marrow transplant?
    1. There is a 50% chance of HLA match between siblings.
    2. 200 mL of bone marrow is needed for the transplant.
    3. A potential complication for the donor is excessive blood clotting.
    4. Engraftment of the transplanted bone marrow takes 2–5 weeks.

16. In _____% of patients with chronic myelogenous leukemia, _____

    _____ is present.

17. The basis for having elderly adults take low-dose aspirin daily is:
    1. the blood of the elderly tends to coagulate more easily.
    2. aspirin stimulates the bone marrow to produce new cells.
    3. aspirin assists the uptake of iron from the intestinal tract.
    4. aspirin helps prevent the ecchymoses common in the elderly.

18. The order is to infuse 2 units of packed red cells. One unit contains 195 mL and the other contains 210 mL. The blood is to infuse over 4 hours. The blood IV tubing setup delivers 10 gtts/mL. At what rate should the infusion run? _____

CRITICAL THINKING ACTIVITIES

Scenario A: S.T. is a 37-year-old Hispanic man who has sickle cell disease. He has frequent episodes of pain. His anemia has been managed with transfusions on several occasions. He has signs of chronic renal failure. He has been prescribed pentoxifylline (Trental), oxycodone/acetaminophen (Roxicet, Percocet), and folic acid (Folvite). At the hematology clinic this morning, his Hgb was 6.9 g/dL. He was transfused with 2 units of packed red cells over 3 hours and then sent home. About an hour and a half later, he developed dyspnea. His wife called 911 and he arrived at the emergency department with oxygen by mask.

1.   How would you describe sickle cell disease? How is it related to race?

2.   What is the mechanism by which patients with sickle cell disease develop anemia?

3.   Why should the admitting nurse inquire about his pain and the need for medication?

Scenario B: P.W., age 12, has hemophilia B (Christmas disease). His mother brought him to the emergency department because of considerable pain and swelling in his left knee. He states that he bumped the knee on a desk at school. A CBC shows Hgb of 10.4 g/dL and a deficiency of clotting factor IX.

1.   Describe how this X-linked recessive trait for hemophilia is transmitted.

2.   Explain why this patient has a bleeding problem when injured.

3.   What is the expected treatment for P.W.?

STEPS TOWARD BETTER COMMUNICATION

VOCABULARY BUILDING GLOSSARY

Term	Definition
clump	(noun) a cluster, group of pieces; a small pile of things
	(verb) pieces gather or stick together in a group
dire (dīr)	very serious; having dangerous or threatening consequences
enhance'	increase, improve; give better opportunity
har'vest	to collect something for use
meti'culous	extremely careful
mit'igate	(verb) reduce, lessen, alleviate
modal'ity, -ies	a particular system or arrangement, a method
sic'kle	a crescent shape, like a new moon; a farm tool with a curved blade

COMPLETION

Directions: Fill in the blanks with the correct words from the Vocabulary Building Glossary to complete the statements.

1. When extensive bleeding occurs during surgery, extra fluids are given to _____ the effect of the blood loss.

2. When a patient develops leukopenia, the nurse must use _____ aseptic technique to prevent infection.

3. When an injury occurs to tissue, _____ clump to help stop bleeding.

4. An oxygen deficit will cause red blood cells to _____ in patients with sickle cell disease.

5. When leukemia is diagnosed, the patient and health care provider must choose an appropriate _____ of treatment.

6. The four types of leukemia are _____, _____, _____, and _____.

7. Using strict asepsis when caring for a patient with a blood dyscrasia will _____ the chances of preventing infection.

8. Before a bone marrow transplant, the health care provider must _____ marrow from a matching donor.

GRAMMAR POINTS

The word **"by"** + the **-ing** form of a verb is often used when talking about how something happens or the method of doing something. An object or phrase is usually required to complete the sentence.

Example: Nurses help patients by teaching about drug side effects.

Directions: Complete each sentence using "by" plus the -ing forms of the following verbs:

cautioning	undergoing
reporting	following
asking	suppressing
using	destroying
wearing	administering

1. After giving a narcotic, nurses help prevent patient falls _____ patients not to get up without assistance.

2. Patient information is relayed to the oncoming shift _____ on the condition, treatments, and complaints of patients by the nurses leaving.

3. A thorough history is obtained _____ the patient several specific questions.

4. A nurse complies with Standard Precautions _____ gloves whenever contact with body fluids is likely.

5. The nurse is protected from contamination _____ a waterproof gown, gloves, and goggles when irrigating a wound.

6. A patient fights leukemia _____ chemotherapy treatment.

7. The immunosuppressed patient prevents infection _____ strict guidelines to avoid contact with pathogens.

8. Many types of chemotherapy work _____ replication of the malignant cells.

9. Radiation therapy works _____ malignant cells.

10. Hypovolemic shock is treated _____ fluids and blood.

COMMUNICATION EXERCISE

Directions: With a partner, make a list of the most important points to use in teaching the patient with leukemia and the family about 1) prevention of infection, 2) prevention and treatment of bleeding episodes, and 3) appropriate nutrition. Then orally "teach" your partner about these issues.

_____

_____

_____

CULTURAL POINT

Be aware that some religions prohibit blood transfusions and other people are very cautious of the procedure. Approach a patient carefully to determine his or her feelings about transfusions.

The Cardiovascular System

chapter

17

Answer Key: Review the related chapter to answer these questions. A complete answer key was provided to your instructor.

REVIEW OF ANATOMY AND PHYSIOLOGY

Labeling

Structures of the Circulatory System

Directions: On the figure below, label the structures of the circulatory system. Then, using arrows, indicate the pathway that blood follows through the system. Explain the diagram and pathway to a partner.

superior vena cava   inferior vena cava   pulmonary artery to right lung
pulmonary veins from left lung   right atrium   right ventricle
left atrium   left ventricle   aorta
pulmonary veins from right lung   thoracic aorta   pulmonary artery to left lung

COMPLETION

Directions: Fill in the blanks to complete the statements.

1. Cardiac output depends on the heart _____, the amount of blood return-
   ing to the _____, the strength of _____, and the
   _____ to the ejection of the blood.

2. The right coronary artery supplies the _____, _____,
   _____, and the _____.

3. _____ equals the amount of blood pumped out of the heart each minute.

4. The aging heart becomes _____, resulting in decreased _____
   in the elderly.

5. _____ is the cramping pain in the leg muscles brought
   on by exercise.

6. A weight gain of 3 lbs or more in a(n) _____ period indicates fluid retention.

7. The health care provider prescribes furosemide (Lasix) oral liquid 20 mg PO every morning. The pharmacy delivers a 100-mL bottle of furosemide with a concentration of 40 mg/5 mL. How many mL
   should you give the patient? _____ mL

SHORT ANSWER

Risk Factors and Assessment for Cardiac Disorders

Directions: Read the clinical scenario and answer the questions that follow.

Scenario: Mr. Nielsen is a 58-year-old Caucasian banker. He reports that he was having difficulty doing his
usual 2-mile walk because of fatigue and shortness of breath. He has type 2 diabetes. He tells you, "At first,
I thought it was just stress and being sort of overweight, drinking too much beer, and eating too much rich
food. I decided to make an appointment because my wife reminded me that my father and grandfather died
of heart disease in their early 60s."

1. You are collecting information about cardiac risk factors from Mr. Nielsen. What are four nonmodifiable
   risk factors related to the development of heart disease?

   a. _____

   b. _____

   c. _____

   d. _____

2. List five modifiable risk factors that Mr. Nielsen has just indicated in the scenario. What information can you give him about modifying the factors that he has just mentioned?

   a. _____

   b. _____

   c. _____

   d. _____

   e. _____

3. What diagnostic tests would you expect Mr. Nielsen to undergo?

   a. Laboratory: _____

   b. Diagnostic: _____

   _____

   _____

4. List at least six things that should be included in the physical assessment of a patient like Mr. Nielsen, who may have a cardiac disorder.

   a. _____

   b. _____

   c. _____

   d. _____

   e. _____

   f. _____

COMPLETION

Diagnostic Testing for Cardiac Disorders

Directions: Fill in the blanks to complete the statements.

1. Ultrasound Doppler flow studies are conducted to detect a(n) _____ in the vessel or to determine the _____ of the vessel.

2. Coronary angiography requires injection of a(n) _____.

3. The purpose of a stress echocardiogram is to detect _____ _____.

4. Explain to the patient that during impedance plethysmography, he may feel some discomfort related to _____.

5. An elevated myoglobin level detects damage to _____, possibly from a(n) _____ infarction.

APPLICATION OF THE NURSING PROCESS

Changes with Aging

Directions: Read the scenario and provide the answers to the following questions.

Scenario: You are working in an extended-care facility and Ms. Wiabo is one of your elderly patients. Ms. Wiabo is in stable condition, but she has several chronic health problems, including hypertension and occasional problems with fluid retention.

1. List at least six changes in the cardiovascular system associated with aging.

   a. _____

   b. _____

   c. _____

   d. _____

   e. _____

   f. _____

2. List at least six interventions (including assessments) to use with patients like Ms. Wiabo who have fluid retention.

   a. _____

   b. _____

   c. _____

   d. _____

   e. _____

   f. _____

3. Which nursing diagnosis is top priority for Ms. Wiabo?
   a. Decreased self-esteem related to activity intolerance
   b. Insufficient knowledge related to disease process, medications, and self-care
   c. Potential for excess fluid volume related to heart failure
   d. Potential for social isolation related to being away from family

4. What is the best expected outcome for the nursing diagnosis chosen in question 3?
   a. Patient will verbalize signs and symptoms of medication side effects within 7 days.
   b. Patient will be able to perform ADLs within 2 months.
   c. Patient's urine output will be within normal range day to day.
   d. Patient will not gain more than 1 lb in any 24-hour period.

PRIORITY SETTING

Directions: Read the scenario and prioritize the steps to perform the procedure.

Scenario: You are preparing to take a routine blood pressure on an ambulatory patient at a clinic. You have never taken a blood pressure on this patient before and the patient does not remember his last blood pressure reading. You must use an ordinary manual blood pressure cuff (i.e., not a blood pressure machine). Put the following steps in the correct order to perform the procedure.

___3___ a. Palpate the brachial artery.

___2___ b. Select the correct cuff size.

___4___ c. Center the bladder cuff over the brachial artery.

___11___ d. Listen until the sounds stop.

___13___ e. Report abnormal findings to the RN or health care provider.

___7___ f. Release cuff and wait 30–60 seconds.

___10___ g. Deflate cuff slowly and smoothly to obtain a correct diastolic reading.

___12___ h. Record your findings as soon as you obtain the reading.

___5___ i. Support the patient's arm on which the cuff is placed at heart level.

___1___ j. Ensure the patient has not smoked or had caffeine for the past 30 minutes.

___8___ k. Place the bell of your stethoscope over the brachial artery.

___9___ l. Tighten the screw clamp; inflate cuff 30 mm Hg above the palpated pressure.

___6___ m. Obtain a palpated systolic blood pressure.

REVIEW QUESTIONS FOR THE NCLEX® EXAMINATION

Directions: Choose the best answer(s) for the following questions.

1. The patient with elevated cholesterol and obesity and who smokes would be at much less risk of a cardiac event if he or she:
   1. stopped smoking.
   2. lost weight.
   3. lowered cholesterol.
   4. exercised more.

2. The nurse knows that to correctly perform the procedure for taking an apical pulse, the pulse must be counted for:
   1. 15 seconds.
   2. 30 seconds.
   3. 1 minute.
   4. 2 minutes.

3. The nurse has observed that the patient's jugular veins are prominent when the patient is in an upright position. This finding is associated with which cardiovascular disorder?
   1. Congestive heart failure
   2. Cardiac dysrhythmia
   3. Angina pectoris
   4. Aortic aneurysm

4. When obtaining a patient's blood pressure, the nurse knows that if the blood pressure cuff is too narrow, the blood pressure will be:
   1. unaffected by the equipment.
   2. falsely elevated.
   3. lower than expected.
   4. the same in both arms.

5. When planning care for a patient with a cardiovascular problem, it is important to plan activities to:
   1. promote cardiac output.
   2. prevent venous occlusion.
   3. prevent edema and fluid retention.
   4. promote rest and relieve fatigue.

6. The nurse is evaluating the patient's peripheral pulses. Which intervention(s) should be included in a routine assessment?
   1. Note rate and rhythm and mark the location.
   2. Take radial pulse on the patient's dominant side.
   3. Compare pulses bilaterally; note volume and strength.
   4. Elevate the extremity and check the pulse.

7. What is considered the best indicator of fluid buildup?
   1. Pitting edema
   2. Decreased urinary output
   3. 3 lbs weight gain in 24 hours
   4. Low serum sodium

8. A patient has a nursing diagnosis of Altered skin integrity related to an ulcer from decreased circulation. An appropriate nursing intervention would be:
   1. increase fluid intake to 3000 mL per day.
   2. promote adequate protein in the diet.
   3. administer the prescribed diuretic to decrease edema.
   4. allow to ventilate feelings about the disease process.

9. When planning nursing care, the nurse knows that many heart medications need to be given as close to the prescribed time as possible. The best rationale for this practice is to:
   1. complete shift duties in a timely fashion.
   2. prevent adverse response to medications.
   3. avoid confusing your elderly patients.
   4. maintain a steady blood level of the drug.

10. Your patient was admitted for unstable angina and is complaining of chest pain. Put the following actions in priority order. __2 4 3 1__
    1. Administer the ordered nitroglycerin tablets.
    2. Assess the quality and character of the pain.
    3. Administer low-flow oxygen via nasal cannula.
    4. Assess vital signs.

11. The nurse is caring for a patient with Altered activity tolerance related to chronic heart failure. Which task(s) would be best to assign to the nursing assistant?
    1. Observe the patient for fatigue and shortness of breath when ambulating.
    2. Assist the patient with morning hygiene such as washing back and feet.
    3. Explain to the family why taking long walks on the hospital grounds is not feasible at this time.
    4. Obtaining assistive devices that would help the patient conserve energy and strength.

12. When working with patients with lower limb arterial disorders, you know that ___elastic___ ___stockings___ are contraindicated.

CRITICAL THINKING ACTIVITIES

Scenario: Ms. Eoyang is an elderly female patient who comes to the clinic after experiencing some mild chest pain. She is accompanied by her husband. You are attempting to perform the PQRST for pain assessment. Mr. Eoyang keeps answering for his wife, even though she is alert and oriented and seems capable of answering for herself. She sits quietly and smiles at you, but allows her husband to do the talking despite your best efforts.

1. What is the PQRST pain assessment? _____

   _____

   _____

   _____

2. What other assessment questions would you ask? _____

   _____

   _____

   _____

3. What are your personal feelings about this type of situation?_____

   _____

   _____

4. What factors (i.e., cultural, social, age, psychological) might help explain Mr. and Ms. Eoyang's behavior?

   _____

   _____

   _____

   _____

   _____

STEPS TOWARD BETTER COMMUNICATION

VOCABULARY BUILDING GLOSSARY

Term/Phrase	Pronunciation	Meaning
a whooshing or purring sound	whoosh' ing	a sound like quickly moving air
equipment used should be calibrated	cal' i bray ted	marked with correct units of measure
appear pale and mottled	mot' tled	marked with irregular patches of color
condition indicative of gangrene	in dic' a tive	showing signs of, suggesting
excoriations	ex co ri ay' shuns	scratches or abrasions on skin

Term/Phrase	Pronunciation	Meaning
it is a good gross assessment	gross ah ses' ment	general and broad, not specific
circulation is occluded by constriction	oc clud' ed	blocked
assessment and staging of edema	stay' jing	determining the extent or phase of a disease or condition
dependent edema	de pen' dent	hanging down, which can cause swelling
impede, impedance	im pede'	to block, to get in the way of
precipitate; precipitating event	pre cip' i tate	to cause to start
assess mentation	men tay' shun	mental activity
collaborate with patients/colleagues	col lab' o rate	to work together with in both planning and action

COMPLETION

Directions: Using the Vocabulary Building Glossary above, prepare five sentences. Leave the vocabulary word space blank, and ask a classmate to complete the sentence with the correct word.

1. _____

2. _____

3. _____

4. _____

5. _____

VOCABULARY EXERCISE

Descriptors, Descriptive Terms, Special Uses

Directions: The words listed below are used to describe the quality and character of a patient's pulse. If you are not sure of the meaning of some of the words, ask your instructor to explain or to let you hear an example.

Descriptors of pulse qualities:

full	fast	absent
strong	irregular	hammer-like
weak	regular	normal
thready	erratic	fleeting
bounding	diminished	moderate
rapid	distant	1+, 2+, 3+, 4+ (designates strength)
slow	barely palpable	

Directions: Evaluate the expected pulse of the following three people and write out your assessment findings using the descriptive terms.

Person 1: Radial pulse of someone who has just run a race: _____

Person 2: Pedal pulse of someone with arterial vascular disease: _____

Person 3: Apical pulse of a patient with heart disease who has a dysrhythmia: _____

_____

COMMUNICATION EXERCISE

History-Taking and Documenting Assessment

1. What are the things you would need to ask about in history-taking that would provide information about a cardiovascular patient? What objective observations could you make that would also provide information?

    _____

    _____

    _____

2. With a peer, practice cardiac assessment by asking questions about the risk factors in Table 17-1 in the textbook. Write out the questions you will use. Take turns asking and then answering the questions. Take notes and document your assessment findings. Ask your partner or the instructor to critique your documentation.

    _____

    _____

    _____

    _____

    _____

COMMUNICATION EXERCISE

Directions: With a partner, discuss some things you would say to a patient in each of these cases.

1. The patient is in pain and you want to interact therapeutically with active listening. _____

    _____

    _____

    _____

2. Mr. Johnson wants a hot water bottle on his feet because they are cold. _____

    _____

    _____

    _____

3. Ms. Bennett does not want anything to eat or drink, but her medications are to be taken with food.

_____

_____

_____

4. Explain to a family the risks to cardiac health that cannot be controlled or modified and those risks that can be modified.

_____

_____

_____

CULTURAL POINT

African Americans and females have different experiences with heart conditions and symptoms than those usually described for Caucasian males. Be sure that you learn what these differences are and pay attention to the symptoms of these patient groups.

Care of Patients with Hypertension and Peripheral Vascular Disease

chapter

18

Answer Key: Review the related chapter to answer these questions. A complete answer key was provided to your instructor.

COMPLETION

Hypertension

Directions: Fill in the blanks to complete the statements.

1. Long-term hypertension may lead to death from damage to the _____, _____, and _____.

2. Hypertension is a systolic pressure greater than _____ mm Hg or a diastolic pressure greater than _____ mm Hg.

3. Hypertension can be secondary to and symptomatic of other diseases, such as those affecting the blood supply to the _____ and _____.

4. Nicotine has a major impact on blood vessels and blood pressure by producing _____.

5. Hypertension is diagnosed when an elevated blood pressure is taken at least _____ and averaged on two different occasions, _____ weeks apart.

6. The health care provider examines blood vessels in the _____ to detect signs of persistent hypertension.

SHORT ANSWER

Hypertension

Directions: Read the scenario and answer the questions that follow.

Scenario: You are participating in a health fair that includes blood pressure screening for hypertension and dispensing information about healthy lifestyle habits. In addition, interested people are inquiring about how to recognize potential symptoms and various types of treatment, including medication for hypertension.

1. List four specific ways in which a person with mild hypertension might help reduce his blood pressure without taking any antihypertensive drugs.

   a. _____

   b. _____

   c. _____

   d. _____

2. List subjective symptoms and objective data that would be significant in the assessment of a patient with hypertension.

   a. Subjective symptoms: _____

   _____

   b. Objective data: _____

3. The target is to maintain a blood pressure at or below _____.

4. List specific patient information in each of the following areas for the patient with mild hypertension: self-care and keeping blood pressure under control.

   a. General lifestyle changes: _____

   _____

   _____

   _____

   _____

   _____

   b. Dietary advice: _____

   _____

   _____

5. List three drug classifications that may be used in the treatment of hypertension and give an example of each classification.

   _____

   _____

   _____

APPLICATION OF THE NURSING PROCESS

Caring for a Patient with Arterial Insufficiency

Directions: Read the scenario and provide the answers to the following questions.

Scenario: Ms. Thompson is a secretary and has worked for an engineering firm for 25 years. She has gained several pounds over the holidays and has started walking to try to lose some weight. She reports that she has noticed leg cramps after walking just a couple of blocks. The pain stops when she stops walking for several minutes. The health care provider tells her that she may have a mild arterial insufficiency that can be treated with exercise and possible medication if her symptoms worsen.

1. What questions would you ask her to determine risk factors for arterial insufficiency?

   a. _____

   b. _____

   c. _____

2. List five signs and symptoms that would indicate diminished *arterial* blood flow in the peripheral vessels.

   a. _____

   b. _____

   c. _____

   d. _____

   e. _____

3. You are assessing Ms. Thompson and checking the "5 Ps." What are the "5 Ps"?

   a. _____

   b. _____

   c. _____

   d. _____

   e. _____

4. The health care provider tells Ms. Thompson that she has intermittent claudication. You explain to her that intermittent claudication is characterized by:

   a. edema of the lower legs.
   b. cramping pain occurring with walking that eases with rest.
   c. warm, reddened areas on the lower legs.
   d. pale, cold feet.

5. What are three major nursing goals for patients like Ms. Thompson?

   a. _____

   b. _____

   c. _____

6. List five self-care measures that could be taught to Ms. Thompson to help her cope with impaired peripheral circulation.

   a. _____

   b. _____

   c. _____

   d. _____

   e. _____

7. Write evaluation criteria that would indicate that the interventions are successful and the expected outcome is being met for Ms. Thompson for the following expected outcome:

   Patient will verbalize three self-care measures to protect tissues from injury due to decreased arterial flow after a patient teaching session.

   a. _____

   b. _____

   c. _____

PRIORITY SETTING

Directions: Read the scenario and prioritize as appropriate.

Scenario: You are caring for Mr. Elisandro, who has been admitted for a diagnosis of deep vein thrombosis, and he is currently receiving IV heparin. He has a sequential compression device (SCD) in place with calf compression sleeves.

1. In the morning, you enter Mr. Elisandro's room and you find that the IV heparin has been turned off. Mr. Elisandro tells you that "somebody came in during the evening and took the IV pump away." What is your priority action?
   a. Quickly obtain a new pump and restart the heparin.
   b. Report the incident to the charge nurse.
   c. Obtain a health care provider's order for partial thromboplastin time (PTT) and activated partial thromboplastin time (aPTT).
   d. Check the provider's orders to see if heparin was discontinued.

2. Mr. Elisandro is lying in bed. His SCD calf compression sleeves are at the bottom of the bed. He tells you that the new nursing assistant removed them during morning hygiene 3 hours ago. What is your priority action?
   a. Replace the sleeves and activate the device; talk to the nursing assistant about the purpose of the SCDs.
   b. Instruct the nursing assistant on how to replace the compression sleeves.
   c. Teach the patient how to replace them and to call for assistance as needed.
   d. Report the incident to the nursing educator and the charge nurse.

3. While you are assessing Mr. Elisandro after lunch, you note several abnormal findings. Which assessment finding is the priority?
   a. Bleeding gums and petechiae
   b. Dyspnea and tachypnea
   c. Increasing pain in the calf
   d. Pitting edema of the affected limb

4. Based on your determination of the priority assessment finding (#3 above), which action will you take first?
   a. Check the PTT and aPTT results.
   b. Obtain equipment to give oxygen.
   c. Assess the quality/onset of calf pain.
   d. Measure the circumference of the limb.

REVIEW QUESTIONS FOR THE NCLEX® EXAMINATION

Directions: Choose the best answer(s) for the following questions.

1. When assessing a patient for possible peripheral vascular disease (PVD), which is a prime contributing factor?
   1. History of structural defects in the heart
   2. History of excessive alcohol intake
   3. History of inflammation of the veins
   4. History of cigarette smoking

2. A nursing assessment that is most important in the care of a patient with a deep vein thrombosis is to assess for:
   1. pale, cool extremity.
   2. decreasing level of consciousness.
   3. sudden shortness of breath.
   4. sudden acute pain.

3. A secondary cause of peripheral arterial disorders is:
   1. diabetes mellitus.
   2. a sedentary lifestyle.
   3. rheumatic fever.
   4. hypertension.

4. It is most important to teach the patient with chronic venous stasis to sit with the legs:
   1. crossed.
   2. straight.
   3. elevated.
   4. dependent.

5. The nurse is teaching the patient about dietary sources of potassium. Which food group is the best dietary source of potassium?
   1. Milk, cheese, and eggs
   2. Beef, turkey, and tomatoes
   3. Whole-grain bread and cereals
   4. Lettuce, cabbage, and onions

6. An acute sign of inadequate arterial blood supply to the feet is:
   1. excessive hair growth.
   2. reddened, warm skin.
   3. brittle, thick toenails.
   4. pale, cool, mottled skin.

7. The patient is taking digoxin and a thiazide diuretic. This combination of medications increases the risk for cardiac dysrhythmias related to:
   1. hypokalemia.
   2. hypotension.
   3. hyperkalemia.
   4. hypertension.

8. The patient with newly diagnosed Raynaud disease is being discharged. Which teaching is appropriate?
   1. Quit smoking and exercise regularly.
   2. Control blood pressure and lose weight.
   3. Avoid exposure to cold and quit smoking.
   4. Eat a heart-healthy diet and get enough rest.

9. The medication cilostazol (Pletal) is used for patients experiencing intermittent claudication to:
   1. relax vessel walls and increase blood flow to the legs.
   2. decrease the possibility of platelet aggregation.
   3. decrease foot and leg edema.
   4. dissolve any clots in the vessels of the legs.

10. Upon assessment, signs of abdominal aortic aneurysm include:
    1. higher blood pressure in the legs than in the arms.
    2. bounding popliteal pulses and warm, pink skin.
    3. an enlarged abdomen with decreased bowel sounds.
    4. back pain and possibly a visible pulsation of the abdomen.

11. Factors that contribute to the formation of varicose veins include: *(Select all that apply.)*
    1. gaining too much weight.
    2. family history of diabetes.
    3. family history of atherosclerosis or hypertension.
    4. standing regularly for long periods of time.
    5. congenital heart problems.
    6. pregnancy.

12. When providing postoperative care for a patient following a carotid endarterectomy, which assessment finding is the priority concern?
    1. Increasing hoarseness
    2. Loss of appetite
    3. Presence of a bruit
    4. Nausea

13. Teaching for a patient discharged on warfarin (Coumadin) includes keeping appointments for frequent laboratory tests to check the:
    1. serum heparin level.
    2. activated partial thromboplastin time or partial thromboplastin time.
    3. platelet aggregation test.
    4. International Normalized Ratio value and/or prothrombin time.

CRITICAL THINKING ACTIVITIES

Scenario: You are working with several patients who are to receive heparin. Perform the following math calculations to determine the correct dose or to verify the setting of the IV infusion.

1. The patient is on an IV heparin drip for treatment of a deep vein thrombosis. The IV heparin bag (25,000 units/250 mL) is in place with a pump. It is set to infuse at 8 mL/hour. The health care provider has ordered 800 units/hour. Is the pump setting correct or incorrect? _____

2. The health care provider orders 5000 units SQ heparin for postoperative prophylaxis. The pharmacy delivers a 10-mL vial of heparin sodium (5000 units/mL). How many mL should you give? _____

3. The pharmacy delivers a premixed bag of heparin 20,000 units/500 mL. How many units are in 1 mL? _____

4. The patient is on an IV heparin drip. The IV heparin bag (10,000 units/100 mL) is in place with a pump. It is set to infuse at 10 mL/hour. The health care provider has ordered 1000 units/hour. Is the pump setting correct or incorrect? _____

STEPS TOWARD BETTER COMMUNICATION

VOCABULARY BUILDING GLOSSARY

Term	Pronunciation	Definition
bar'orecep'tor	bar o re sep' tor	sensory receptor stimulated by changes in pressure
claudica'tion	klaw di kay' shun	pain in leg muscles
depen'dent	de pen'dent	hanging down
incom'petent	in com'pe tent	not able to perform the function or job

Term	Pronunciation	Definition
ischemia	is kee' me a	insufficient blood in a part
periph'eral	pa rif' ah ral	on the outer edges
poten'tiated	po ten' shee ay ted	made more powerful (two drugs may react together to be more powerful)
synco'pe	sing ko' pee	temporary loss of consciousness, fainting
tor'tuous	tor' chew us	twisted, winding
viscos'ity	vis cos' i tee	thickness of a liquid
noncompli'ant	non com ply'ant	does not follow instructions
"silent" symptoms		symptoms that the patient is unable to observe or feel
side effect		result of a treatment or medication that is in addition to the intended effect

COMPLETION

Directions: Fill in the blanks with the correct words from the Vocabulary Building Glossary to complete the statements.

1. When taking a blood pressure, the arm should be at the level of the heart rather than

   _____.

2. When the nurse assessed the patient's arm before trying to start an intravenous infusion, the veins were

   found to be _____.

3. The patient who is polycythemic has increased blood _____.

4. The patient with swollen, dusky feet probably has _____ vascular disease.

5. Many hypertensive patients are _____ with therapy because they do not notice any

   symptoms of high blood pressure.

6. The patient who has peripheral arterial vascular disease often experiences _____

   when walking.

7. A(n) _____ signals the brain about changes in blood pressure.

8. When a vein develops varicosities, it becomes _____.

9. The effect on blood pressure is _____ when an antihypertensive is combined with a

   diuretic medication.

10. Hypertension often causes only _____.

11. When a thrombosis occurs in a vessel, _____ develops distal to it.

12. Carotid occlusion may cause _____ in the patient.

13. Hypokalemia is a(n) _____ of many diuretics.

WORD ATTACK SKILLS

Combining Forms

These combining forms are used in words found in Chapter 18 in the textbook:

angi/o	vessel, channel
vaso	vessel, duct
sclero	hard, hardening
ven/o	vein
thromb/o	blood clot
sta/	make stand, stop
sten/	narrow, compressed

Directions: Write the meanings of the following words constructed from the combining forms above. Use your dictionary as necessary.

1. Vasospasm:_____

2. Vasodilator: _____

3. Vasoconstriction: _____

4. Vasopressor:_____

5. Vasomotor:_____

6. Sclerosis:_____

7. Venogram: _____

8. Venous: _____

9. Thrombectomy:_____

10. Thrombosis: _____

11. Thrombus: _____

12. Stasis: _____

13. Stent: _____

Student Name_____ Date_____

Care of Patients with Cardiac Disorders

Answer Key: Review the related chapter to answer these questions. A complete answer key was provided to your instructor.

COMPLETION

Cardiac Disorders

Directions: Fill in the blanks to complete the statements.

1. A(n) _____ is used for patients who have repeated episodes of life-threatening ventricular fibrillation or ventricular tachycardia.

2. The signs and symptoms of mitral stenosis include _____,
   _____, _____, and _____.

3. A myocardial infarction may lead to heart failure because damage to the muscle causes _____
   _____.

4. The primary problem for a patient with a heart valve disorder is _____
   _____.

5. A sign of pericarditis that can be heard during auscultation of the heart is _____
   _____.

6. _____ imbalances may cause serious cardiac dysrhythmias.

7. Untreated strep throat may lead to _____ and _____ disease.

8. An elderly patient may experience a failure of the SA node, which indicates the need for _____
   _____.

APPLICATION OF THE NURSING PROCESS

Care of the Patient with Heart Failure

Directions: Read the scenario and provide the answers to the following questions.

Scenario: Ms. Jackson, age 68, has heart failure. She has been admitted to the hospital for complaints of severe dyspnea, generalized edema, weakness, and fatigue. Her health care provider has ordered up to bathroom PRN, in chair for 30 minutes three times a day, and oxygen titrated to maintain oxygen saturation at 94% or above. Ms. Jackson is also receiving digoxin (Lanoxin) 0.25 mg daily, hydrochlorothiazide (a diuretic), and Isordil (a venous dilator). She is prescribed a heart-healthy diet.

1. List objective and subjective data that would help assess Ms. Jackson's status with regard to dyspnea, edema, and peripheral circulation.

    a. Dyspnea—Subjective data:_____

    _____

    Objective data: _____

    _____

    b. Edema—Subjective data: _____

    _____

    Objective data: _____

    _____

    c. Peripheral circulation—Subjective data: _____

    _____

    Objective data: _____

    _____

2. Upon admission, which nursing diagnosis is a priority for Ms. Jackson?
    a. Altered activity tolerance due to decreased perfusion
    b. Potential for injury due to complications of CHF
    c. Altered cardiac output due to ineffective cardiac pumping
    d. Altered gas exchange due to fluid in lung tissue

3. List three nursing actions you would expect to find on Ms. Jackson's nursing care plan for "Altered activity tolerance due to decreased perfusion" during her hospitalization.

    a. _____

    b. _____

    c. _____

4. An appropriate task to assign to the nursing assistant would be to:
    a. ask the patient if she needs extra pillows to prevent orthopnea.
    b. assist the patient to turn every 1–2 hours.
    c. determine if Ms. Jackson needs partial or full assistance with activities of daily living.
    d. check the sacral area for edema and skin breakdown.

5. Ms. Jackson lives with her husband, daughter, and four grandchildren. Before she is discharged, she will need instruction in self-care and her family will need instruction so they can give her support and encouragement. She has been told by her health care provider to work up to walking at least 1 mile per day, continue taking her digoxin and diuretic, stay on her heart-healthy diet, and lose 25 pounds. Identify at least five points that should be included in the teaching plan for Ms. Jackson and her family so that she can remain relatively symptom-free once she returns home.

a. _____

b. _____

c. _____

d. _____

e. _____

6. Which statement by Ms. Jackson indicates that she understands the implications of digoxin toxicity?
   a. "I will report nausea, vomiting, and anorexia."
   b. "I can eat bananas and citrus to counteract side effects."
   c. "I can skip a dose if I experience side effects."
   d. "I should carry digoxin immune fab (DigiFab) as an antidote."

7. Ms. Jackson is prescribed digoxin 0.25 mg daily. Available in the medication dispensing machine are Lanoxin tablets, 0.125 mg/tablet. Is this the correct medication? _____ If so, how many tablets should Ms. Jackson take? _____

PRIORITY SETTING

Directions: Read the scenario and prioritize as appropriate.

Scenario: You are caring for Mr. Hijazi, an elderly patient who was admitted for heart failure related to mitral valve disease. During the morning assessment, you find that his condition seems to have deteriorated compared to yesterday. You find several abnormalities.

1. Which assessment finding is the most important?
   a. Absent peripheral pulses
   b. Frothy sputum and orthopnea
   c. Diarrhea and nausea
   d. Fever and tachycardia

2. Based on your assessment findings, Mr. Hijazi appears to be having complications due to heart failure and he is exhibiting the signs and symptoms of acute pulmonary edema. Rank according to priority of action: _____
   a. Report your findings to the RN/health care provider.
   b. Administer oxygen and morphine per standing orders.
   c. Place the patient in high Fowler position.
   d. Provide reassurance and support.

REVIEW QUESTIONS FOR THE NCLEX® EXAMINATION

Directions: Choose the best answer(s) for the following questions.

1. Which would the patient most likely report when experiencing chronic atrial fibrillation?
   1. Low blood pressure
   2. Headaches and fatigue
   3. Feelings of palpitations
   4. An irregular pulse rate

2. Patients with a sore throat are screened for streptococcus infection because untreated strep can lead to:
   1. pericarditis.
   2. heart valve injury.
   3. dysrhythmias.
   4. heart failure.

3. A patient is receiving furosemide (Lasix). To evaluate the effectiveness of the medication, the nurse would check:
   1. urine output and breath sounds.
   2. pulse rate and potassium laboratory values.
   3. blood pressure and respirations.
   4. weight loss and appetite.

4. Early signs of heart failure include:
   1. weight gain and dyspnea on exertion.
   2. a wet cough and severely swollen ankles.
   3. cyanosis, fatigue, and dyspnea.
   4. an irregular pulse rate and elevated blood pressure.

5. When administering digoxin, the nurse should always first:
   1. assess the amount of weight gain or loss.
   2. question the patient about fatigue and dizziness.
   3. check apical pulse for 1 minute.
   4. be certain that the patient has a full stomach.

6. A patient with third-degree heart block will demonstrate:
   1. a very slow pulse.
   2. a spike in blood pressure.
   3. edema in the lower extremities.
   4. rapid breathing and diaphoresis.

7. Upon assessment of a patient with aortic stenosis, the nurse might find which sign that differs from other valve disorders?
   1. Cardiac murmur
   2. Pulsus paradoxus
   3. Dyspnea upon exertion
   4. Widened pulse pressure

8. The postoperative care of a patient who has received a permanent pacemaker includes: *(Select all that apply.)*
   1. monitor heart rate and rhythm and check vital signs.
   2. monitor for bleeding at the insertion site.
   3. check peripheral pulses proximal to the insertion site.
   4. check level of consciousness frequently in the immediate postoperative period.
   5. teach the patient to count his pulse for a full minute.
   6. teach the patient that full recovery takes about 12 weeks.

9. When planning care for a patient who needs dietary modifications to improve heart health, the nurse would include teaching to:
    1. include 12 g of fiber in diet each day.
    2. include only foods that contain no trans-fats.
    3. avoid drinking any coffee or iced beverages.
    4. decrease the sodium and fat intake.

10. You are helping a patient with atrial fibrillation ambulate and she wobbles and tells you, "I'm suddenly quite dizzy." Which action should you take first?
    1. Tell her to take a few slow deep breaths.
    2. Take her blood pressure.
    3. Assess her pulse rate and rhythm.
    4. Help her to sit down.

CRITICAL THINKING ACTIVITIES

Scenario: You are assigned to work on a telemetry unit. There is a telemetry technician who is monitoring the patients from a remote location; however, there is a monitor at the nurses' station that is displaying the ECG rhythm for each patient. Although the technician will call if they note a problem, the nurses are also responsible for recognizing dysrhythmias and responding accordingly.

Directions: Identify the ECG rhythms and answer the related questions.

1. Rhythm strip #1

   a. Identify this rhythm. _____

   b. What is the appropriate action to take? _____

   _____

2. Rhythm strip #2

   a. Identify this rhythm. _____

   b. Explain why patients who have this dysrhythmia may be on Coumadin.

   _____

   _____

3. Rhythm strip #3

   a. Identify this rhythm. _____

   b. What is the appropriate action to take? _____

   _____

4. Rhythm strip #4

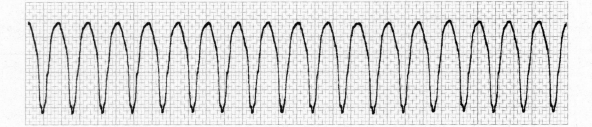

   a. Identify this rhythm. _____

   b. What are the medical treatments that could be ordered to treat this dysrhythmia?

   _____

   _____

5.   Rhythm strip #5

a.   Identify this rhythm. _____

b.   Explain in your own words why this rhythm may cause your patient to have a change in mental status.

_____

_____

STEPS TOWARD BETTER COMMUNICATION

VOCABULARY BUILDING GLOSSARY

Term	Pronunciation	Definition
inva′sive	in vay′sive	involving the puncture or cutting of the skin or putting an instrument into the body
telem′etry	te lem′ e tree	measuring data with radio waves and electronic equipment
engorg′ed	en gorj′ d	filled to the limit; swollen
bloated	blow′ tid	to be swollen; larger than normal
quiver	kwiv′ er	to vibrate with a small, rapid motion
hyper′trophy	hi per′ tro fee	extra growth; thickened
cardiomyop′athy	kar dee o mi op′ ah thee	disorder of heart muscle that prevents it from pumping effectively
a′trioventric′ular	a′ tree o ven trik′ you lar	relating to an atrium and ventricle of the heart
fib′rilla′tion	fib′ ri la′ shun	small, rapid, irregular muscle contractions; quivering
intersti′tial	in ter stish′ al	spaces in the tissue between the cells

COMPLETION

Directions: Fill in the blanks with the correct words from the Vocabulary Building Glossary to complete the statements.

1. During ventricular fibrillation, the heart _____.

2. The patient whose heart rate is being monitored is hooked up to a(n) _____ unit that transmits the ECG pattern to the monitor in the nurses' station.

3. _____ or increased growth of the left ventricle muscle may be hereditary.

4. When congestive heart failure occurs, the lung vessels become _____ with blood and fluid leaks into the interstitial spaces.

5. A cardiac catheterization is a(n) _____ type of test.

6. The major problems exhibited by patients with _____ are heart failure and dysrhythmias.

7. If the SA node fails to pace the heart, the _____ node may take over.

8. Patients can be treated for chronic atrial _____, but ventricular _____ is life-threatening.

9. The patient who experiences right-sided congestive heart failure develops a swollen liver and may feel _____.

10. Edema results if body fluids in the intravascular fluid compartment begin to leak into the _____ compartment.

WORD ATTACK SKILLS

Combining Forms

Here are some important combining forms found in this chapter:

cardi/o	heart
my/o	muscle
sin/o	a space or channel
vas/o	vessel
end/o	inside

COMMUNICATION EXERCISE

You are advising Ms. Perryman who has complained of pain in her legs due to varicose veins. She also has high blood pressure. (Practice the dialogue with a partner.)

Ms. Perryman:	My legs hurt—and look at these ugly varicose veins! My feet and legs hurt at the end of the day. They are swollen. And I get so tired!
Nurse:	Would you like me to work out a plan with you that might help?
Ms. Perryman:	Oh, yes! That would be wonderful.
Nurse:	I would like you to wear these support hose—but no tight underwear or pants or anything that would cut off the circulation. If you can put the hose on in the morning while you are still in bed it would help.
Ms. Perryman:	Why is that?
Nurse:	If you put them on before your legs swell, it helps keep the circulation flowing. When your legs hang off the edge of the bed they swell with the blood flowing to them.
Ms. Perryman:	That makes sense.
Nurse:	When you are sitting, I would like you to keep your feet elevated if you can. Do you get much exercise?
Ms. Perryman:	No, not very much.
Nurse:	Let's see if you can do more walking. You can begin with just 15 minutes at a time. If you could do swimming or water aerobics it would be a big help.
Ms. Perryman:	Where could I do that?
Nurse:	The YMCA and the parks department sometimes have programs. I can check into it and let you know. Are you a smoker?
Ms. Perryman:	No, not for years.
Nurse:	That's good, because smoking constricts the blood vessels even more. About your diet— if we can get you on a low-salt, low-fat, heart-healthy diet that will help a lot. I will show you how to read the food labels. That's it—diet, exercise, wearing support hose, and keeping your legs elevated.
Ms. Perryman:	That sounds like a lot to do.
Nurse:	Yes, it is, but you will feel so much better—and it could even save your life! Next week when I visit, we will see if we can tell the difference in your blood pressure, too.

Care of Patients with Coronary Artery Disease and Cardiac Surgery

chapter

20

Answer Key: Review the related chapter to answer these questions. A complete answer key was provided to your instructor.

TERMINOLOGY

Directions: Define the following terms relative to the heart.

1. Angina pectoris: _____

2. Coronary insufficiency: _____

3. Drug-eluting stent: _____

4. Myocardial infarction (MI): _____

5. Percutaneous coronary intervention (PCI):_____

6. Ischemia:_____

COMPLETION

Directions: Fill in the blanks to complete the statements.

1. As the coronary vessels narrow, the patient may experience symptoms of ischemia such as

   _____ and _____.

2. Women are more likely to experience heart attacks after reaching _____;

   however, poor _____ habits, _____ lifestyle, and

   _____ levels of stress contribute to development of cardiovascular disease ear-

   lier in life.

3. For women, the main symptoms of a heart attack may be diffuse chest pain, extreme fatigue, and tender-

   ness to touch or a burning or tingling sensation, which may be mistaken for _____

   _____.

4. Any activity that increases the heart's workload increases its need for _____.

5. The prognosis of the patient who suffers an acute MI depends on the _____ of

   the artery obstructed, the location, and the _____ of heart tissue that is dam-

   aged.

6. Coronary artery bypass graft is usually performed when _____ _____.

7. To lower cholesterol and maintain a healthy diet, it is recommended to eat fish at least _____ a week.

8. A thrombolytic agent must be administered within _____ hours of experiencing the symptoms of MI to prevent or decrease damage to the heart muscle.

9. After receiving a heart transplant, the patient must take _____ for life.

10. Two constant potential complications that the heart transplant patient must deal with are _____ and _____.

11. The health care provider prescribes IV fluid for a postoperative patient to infuse at 125 mL/hour. The drop factor is 10 gtts/mL. What is the drip rate? _____

12. Omega-3 fatty acids have been found to _____ in patients with hyperlipidemia.

13. If a person is suspected of having a heart attack at home, besides immediately calling 911 and having the person lie down, it is wise to give the person _____.

TABLE ACTIVITY

Cardiac Surgeries

Directions: Fill in the blocks below with the type of surgery or procedure that matches the description. The first block has been done for you.

Type of Surgery	Description
Coronary artery bypass graft (CABG)	Surgery bypasses the blocked artery, replacing it with sections of a vein or artery taken from another part of the patient's body.
	Surgery bypasses the blocked artery but does not require stopping the heart's activity, and therefore does not require using the heart-lung machine.
	A catheter is introduced through the femoral artery and a balloon catheter is used to open a coronary artery.
	Accomplished with a mechanical or biologic device.
	Performed for selected patients who have end-stage left ventricular failure resulting from cardiomyopathy.

APPLICATION OF THE NURSING PROCESS

Care of a Patient with Angina

Directions: Provide the answer to the following questions.

Scenario: Mr. Souza, age 62, is admitted to the hospital with chest pain. Over the past year, he has gradually become more fatigued and uncomfortable whenever he exerts himself. He now has pain in his chest even without exertion. His admitting diagnosis is unstable angina.

1. What specific questions would you ask when taking Mr. Souza's history that could be helpful in assessing his cardiovascular status?

    a. _____

    b. _____

    c. _____

    d. _____

2. Two nursing diagnoses on Mr. Souza's nursing care plan are Pain and Insufficient knowledge. List three specific nursing interventions appropriate for each nursing diagnosis.

    Pain due to decreased coronary artery circulation:

    a. _____

    b. _____

    c. _____

    Insufficient knowledge related to self-care:

    a. _____

    b. _____

    c. _____

3. Which objective finding indicates that Mr. Souza's level of physical activity is appropriate to his recovery?
    a. Patient asks for assistance when he becomes fatigued.
    b. Patient's heart rate and respiratory rate are stable after ambulation.
    c. Patient's activity is observed by the physical therapist.
    d. Family tells you that he is walking like he used to prior to hospitalization.

PRIORITY SETTING

Directions: Read the scenario and prioritize as appropriate.

Scenario: You are working in an extended-care facility. Mr. Ido is walking down the hall and reports to you that he is having angina. He has a PRN order for sublingual nitroglycerin and he asks you to assist him with the medication. Prioritize the steps in administering the nitroglycerin.

_____   a.   If the pain has not eased or if BP increases, administer a second tablet.

_____   b.   Give one tablet, placed under the tongue.

_____   c.   Notify the health care provider regarding pain.

_____   d.   Assist the patient to lie in bed.

_____   e.   Wait 5 minutes, reassess pain and blood pressure.

_____   f.   Obtain a baseline blood pressure.

_____   g.   After 5 minutes, reassess pain and recheck blood pressure.

_____   h.   Administer a third tablet if pain persists.

_____   i.   Recheck blood pressure; it should have decreased.

REVIEW QUESTIONS FOR THE NCLEX® EXAMINATION

Directions: Choose the best answer(s) for the following questions.

1. The risk factors that lead to a higher incidence of atherosclerosis include: *(Select all that apply.)*
    1. high levels of high-density lipoproteins.
    2. cigarette smoking.
    3. a history of hypertension and diabetes mellitus.
    4. age (> age 40), gender, and race.
    5. women on oral contraceptives or estrogen replacement therapy.

2. An elevated level of what is the most significant in diagnosing damage to the myocardium?
    1. Troponin
    2. Creatine phosphokinase (CPK)
    3. Creatine phosphokinase-MB (CK-MB)
    4. Lactate dehydrogenase (LDH)

3. A patient taking lovastatin (Mevacor) for treatment of hypercholesterolemia should have follow-up because of the potential for:
    1. nephrotoxicity.
    2. cardiotoxicity.
    3. hepatotoxicity.
    4. ototoxicity.

4. The patient presents in the emergency department (ED) with severe chest pain. Which drugs are likely to be administered during the initial emergency care?
    1. Morphine, oxygen, nitrates, aspirin
    2. Beta-blockers, clopidogrel (Plavix)
    3. Simvastatin (Lipitor), lorazepam (Ativan)
    4. Oxygen, dobutamine (Dobutrex)

5. Which statement by the patient indicates a need for additional teaching about taking his nitroglycerin?
   1. "I should try to sit or lie down before I take a tablet."
   2. "If I get a headache, I should not take any more."
   3. "I can take up to three tablets before I call my health care provider."
   4. "The tablets should be stored in a dark bottle."

6. When an elderly person sustains an MI, symptoms expressed are often:
   1. severe chest pain, nausea, and dizziness.
   2. dyspnea, nausea, confusion, and indigestion.
   3. pain in the arms and clammy skin.
   4. palpitations, chest pain, and fatigue.

7. The health care provider is considering using fibrinolytic therapy such as t-PA (Activase) for a patient who has come into the ED experiencing an MI. Which information is most important to relay to the provider?
   1. History of hypertension
   2. History of hemorrhagic stroke
   3. Symptom onset 3 hours ago
   4. Intraspinal surgery during childhood

8. Which criterion would indicate that the interventions after an MI are helping meet the expected outcome of "patient will suffer no further cardiac damage"?
   1. Lessened chest pain
   2. Conscious and interacting appropriately
   3. No ST elevation on the ECG rhythm strip
   4. No complaints of heartburn

9. For a patient who is taking a statin drug, an important teaching point to include would be to:
   1. report muscle tenderness or pain that persists for more than a few days.
   2. increase consumption of grapefruit juice to supply K^+.
   3. have follow-up appointments to monitor platelet count.
   4. discontinue medication when the target weight goal is met.

10. You are ready to begin your patient assessments after receiving report. Which patient will you assess first?
    1. A 36-year-old with mitral stenosis scheduled for a balloon valvuloplasty later in the morning
    2. An 82-year-old 2 days after coronary bypass surgery who has a temperature of 100.5° F
    3. A 52-year-old with cardiomyopathy who developed chest pain and shortness of breath during shift change
    4. A 63-year-old who had a coronary stent placed yesterday afternoon who has some bloody drainage on the procedure site dressing

11. There are several patients on a busy cardiac rehabilitation unit who need assistance. Which task would be appropriate to assign to the nursing assistant?
    1. Find out why a depressed patient is not doing his physical therapy.
    2. Answer a family member's question about how to contact a local support group.
    3. Escort a patient who has been discharged home to his wife's car.
    4. Listen to a patient who is complaining about the bad hospital food.

12. After an MI, the patient is monitored for cardiogenic shock. A sign that cardiogenic shock is impending might be:
    1. crackles in the lungs upon auscultation.
    2. slowing of the pulse rate.
    3. PVCs on the ECG.
    4. decreasing urine flow to 20 mL per hour.

CRITICAL THINKING ACTIVITIES

Scenario A: You are at the local park for a neighborhood picnic. You notice that Ms. Grandville, a middle-aged obese woman, is holding her hand over her chest. She tells you that she is "having a little indigestion from the potato salad;" however, you notice that she is breathing faster than normal and she appears anxious. On further questioning, she admits to chest pressure, but she says that she will just drive herself home and rest. She declines your offer to help or your advice about going to the hospital.

1. What coping mechanism is Ms. Grandville using to respond to the symptoms?

    _____

2. Explain in your own words how the use of this coping mechanism affects her decision-making.

    _____

    _____

    _____

3. Write a brief dialogue that you could use with Ms. Grandville so that she can make an informed decision.

    _____

    _____

    _____

    _____

    _____

    _____

Scenario B: You are making home visits to Mr. Ketauna, an elderly patient who has chronic cardiomyopathy. The family reports that Mr. Ketauna is mentally active, although he is somewhat depressed, because over the past several years his quality of life has steadily been decreasing. They are considering asking the health care provider if he would be a candidate for a heart transplant. You suggest that the family talk to the provider and you decide to do some research to help clarify their concerns.

1. List at least five of the criteria for heart transplant.

    a. _____

    b. _____

    c. _____

    d. _____

    e. _____

2. What are some of the ethical implications for the above criteria when trying to determine who will or will not receive an organ transplant?

_____

_____

_____

_____

_____

_____

_____

3. In your own words, discuss some adjustments that the family and the prospective recipient would have to make while waiting on the transplant list.

_____

_____

_____

_____

_____

_____

_____

_____

STEPS TOWARD BETTER COMMUNICATION

VOCABULARY BUILDING GLOSSARY

Term	Definition
col lat'er al	(adj.) parallel, secondary
com pen' sa tor y	(adj.) making up for, counterbalancing
com'pro mise	(noun) a settlement between two sides that both agree on; (verb) 1. to make such an agreement; 2. to expose to danger by unwise action
e'ti ol'o gy	(noun) the cause, origin
ex'tra cor por'e al	(adj.) outside the body
fi'brous	(adj.) made of fibers; long, thin strands of tissue
prog no'sis	(noun) an advance indication, a forecast or prospect of the probable outcome
wean, weaning (ween)	(verb) a gradual withdrawal

COMPLETION

Directions: Fill in the blanks with the correct words from the Vocabulary Building Glossary to complete the statements.

1. The pathology report will help determine the _____ of the disease.

2. _____ plaques build up in the arteries, occluding the blood flow.

3. The _____ for the patient depends on the size and location of the obstruction in the artery.

4. The oxygen demands from exertion may _____ the coronary circulation of an elderly person.

5. Patients whose bodies have a strong _____ mechanism may have a well-developed _____ circulation.

6. When the heart-lung machine is used to pump and oxygenate the blood, the procedure is called _____ circulation.

7. After surgery, _____ from the ventilator is begun if oxygenation is adequate.

MATCHING

Directions: Match the abbreviation on the left with the correct meaning on the right.

1. _____	CAD	a. Coronary care unit
2. _____	CHF	b. Percutaneous transluminal coronary angioplasty
3. _____	CK	c. Myocardial infarction
4. _____	CCU	d. Coronary artery bypass graft
5. _____	ECG	e. Congestive heart failure
6. _____	MI	f. Acute coronary syndrome
7. _____	CVP	g. Central venous pressure
8. _____	PAP	h. Metabolic equivalents
9. _____	PCWP	i. Creatine kinase
10. _____	PTCA	j. Coronary artery disease
11. _____	CABG	k. Pulmonary artery pressure
12. _____	IABP	l. Pulmonary capillary wedge pressure
13. _____	ACS	m. Intraaortic balloon pump
14. _____	MET	n. Electrocardiogram

COMMUNICATION EXERCISE

The following words are often used to describe the pain associated with these conditions:

angina pectoris: dull, tightness, ache

acute myocardial infarction: sudden, severe, crushing, burning, pressure, squeezing, knife-like (left arm more frequently indicated)

1. Can you give two reasons why people often have heart attacks while shoveling snow?

    a. _____

    b. _____

2. Unscramble this sentence:

    consumed Grapefruit when be not a juice should drug taking statin.

    _____

The Neurologic System

Answer Key: Review the related chapter to answer these questions. A complete answer key was provided to your instructor.

REVIEW OF ANATOMY AND PHYSIOLOGY

Terminology

Directions: Match the term on the left with the correct statement, function, or definition on the right.

1. _____ Pyramidal tracts
2. _____ Accommodation
3. _____ Subarachnoid space
4. _____ Nerve stimulus
5. _____ Neurotransmitter
6. _____ Dysphagia
7. _____ Myelin sheath
8. _____ Synapse
9. _____ Meninges
10. _____ Reflex arc

a. Space between two neurons
b. Covering of nerves that insulates them
c. Physical, chemical, or electrical event that changes cell membrane and conducts as an electrical impulse along nerve pathway
d. Path traveled by a stimulus from point of stimulus through the spinal cord and back to effector site
e. Protective membranes that cover the brain and help protect the spinal cord
f. Conduction pathways, beginning in the cerebral cortex and ending in the spinal cord, that control skeletal muscle movement
g. Space through which cerebrospinal fluid travels and where villi help regulate amount of circulating fluid
h. Secreted at the synapse
i. Eye lens adjustment for seeing at different distances
j. Difficulty swallowing

TABLE ACTIVITY

Directions: Fill in the column on the left with the function(s) of each division of the brain.

Division	Function
Cerebrum	
Cerebellum (Table 21-1)	
Diencephalon	
Thalamus	
Hypothalamus	

Brainstem (consists of three parts):
    Midbrain
    Pons
    Medulla oblongata	

SHORT ANSWER

Changes that Occur with Aging

1. The number of functioning dendrites decreases with aging. This causes _____
    _____ in the older person.

2. Cognitive function, gait, and balance in older adults can be affected by _____
    _____.

3. Continued intellectual function in the healthy elderly is promoted by _____
    _____.

4. With aging, there is often a decrease in _____ memory, but often
    _____ is unaffected.

SHORT ANSWER

Directions: Answer the following questions in the spaces provided.

1. List specific observations that should be made while conducting a routine "neuro check."

    a. Level of consciousness: _____

    _____

    _____

    b. Motor function: _____

    _____

    _____

    c. Pupillary reactions: _____

    _____

    _____

COMPLETION

Nursing Management

Directions: Fill in the blanks to complete the statements.

1. Pyramidal tracts control _____.

2. Reflexes cause _____ movements.

3. An abnormal response to scraping an object across the sole of the foot will result in _____ _____ of the toes (Babinski sign).

4. A diagnostic test for a possible herniated lumbar disc is called a(n) _____ _____.

5. Cranial nerves are found in _____ and they number _____.

6. A quick way to assess the facial nerve is to ask the patient to _____.

7. When the pupil of one eye is increasing in size, it indicates _____ _____.

SHORT ANSWER

Directions: Answer the following questions in the spaces provided.

1. List three specific things you might notice a patient doing that could indicate poor coordination and balance, and write them as if you were documenting them on the patient's medical record.

    a. _____

    b. _____

    c. _____

2. List four ways a patient can prevent neurologic disorders.

    a. _____

    b. _____

    c. _____

    d. _____

3. Describe what an electroencephalogram (EEG) is and what it is *not*.

    _____

    _____

    _____

    _____

4. List at least four pieces of information you think would be significant during an admission assessment of a patient's neurologic status. This information would be obtained while taking the patient's health history. One example would be recent infections affecting the sinuses or face.

    a. _____

    b. _____

    c. _____

    d. _____

REVIEW QUESTIONS FOR THE NCLEX® EXAMINATION

Directions: Choose the best answer(s) for the following questions.

1. Parasympathetic stimulation may cause a change in vital signs demonstrated by:
    1. increased pulse rate.
    2. slowed pulse rate.
    3. decreased blood pressure.
    4. decreased respiratory rate.

2. Promotion of blood pressure control can help prevent brain damage from:
    1. medications.
    2. stroke.
    3. myocardial infarction.
    4. atherosclerosis.

3. Tests for coordination and balance check areas controlled by:
    1. tendons and muscles.
    2. the pons and medulla.
    3. the left cerebral hemisphere.
    4. the cerebrum and cerebellum.

4. A test that measures electrical activity of skeletal muscle is _____.

5. You are caring for a patient who sustained a head injury in an accident. Assessment reveals that one pupil is larger than the other. What should you do?
    1. Since it is almost change of shift, wait and advise the oncoming nurse of the finding.
    2. Report it immediately because it could be a symptom of a life-threatening condition.
    3. Report it immediately because it is a sign that the patient has indulged in recreational drug abuse.
    4. Give the patient some water because it is a sign of dehydration.

6. When assessing the accident patient for possible increased intracranial pressure, the nurse should assess the blood pressure for:
    1. a steady falling of systolic and diastolic pressure.
    2. signs of a paradoxical pulse.
    3. a drop in diastolic pressure with a rise in systolic pressure.
    4. steady rise in both systolic and diastolic pressure.

7. When a patient with a neurologic problem is confined to a wheelchair and has a nursing problem of potential for altered skin integrity, it is important to teach the patient to:
    1. shift weight in the chair every 15 minutes.
    2. flex and extend the arms at least every 2 hours.
    3. deep-breathe and cough periodically.
    4. watch calorie intake so that weight doesn't increase.

8. A bedside neuro check includes:
    1. take vital signs, perform a speech check, assess the cranial nerves, and perform a motor function test.
    2. check grip strength, take the vital signs, perform a speech check, and assess the cranial nerves.
    3. check vital signs, assess LOC, assess pupil reaction, and perform a motor function test.
    4. check vital signs, assess LOC, perform a speech check, and perform a motor function test.

9. Measures that help a patient with dysphagia include: *(Select all that apply.)*
    1. check swallowing ability before feeding.
    2. purée foods to ease swallowing.
    3. maintain an upright position for 30 minutes after eating.
    4. keep a nonstressful atmosphere at mealtime.
    5. feed at a steady pace.
    6. refrain from talking while the patient is eating.

10. A high priority of nursing care for the patient who is confused is:
    1. enhancing mobility.
    2. providing safety.
    3. adequate nutrition.
    4. promoting sleep and rest.

CRITICAL THINKING ACTIVITIES

1. Why is positioning so important for the patient who is unconscious?

2. What would you teach a patient who is about to have an electromyelogram (EMG)?

STEPS TOWARD BETTER COMMUNICATION

VOCABULARY BUILDING GLOSSARY

Term	Pronunciation	Definition
myriad	mir'i ad	many, a vast number
mechanism	mek'an ism	a method, a process by which something happens
nystagmus	nis tag'mus	rapid, involuntary movement of the eyeball
widened pulse pressure		greater difference between systolic and diastolic pressures
mnemonic	ne mon'ik	a device to aid the memory and recall facts

COMPLETION

Directions: Fill in the blanks with the correct words from the Vocabulary Building Glossary to complete the statements.

1. When checking the eyes, if _____ is found, it indicates an abnormality.

2. A(n) _____ of causes can affect the neurologic system and cause problems.

3. A(n) _____ occurs when the systolic pressure goes up and the diastolic goes down.

4. A verse or an abbreviation (e.g., PERRLA) is a good _____ to help recall facts or lists of things.

5. Excess carbon dioxide in the blood is one of the _____ that can cause intracranial pressure to rise after a head injury.

WORD ATTACK SKILLS

Prefixes

A. *Directions: Form a word combining the correct prefix below with the word stem listed. Write the meaning of the word. Use a dictionary as necessary.*

Prefix	**Meaning**
a-, in-, an-, im-	no, not, without, lack of
dys-, dis-, mal-	bad, difficult, wrongly

Word Stem	**Combined Word**	**Meaning**
1. -orders	_____	_____
2. -paired	_____	_____
3. -voluntary	_____	_____
4. -noxia	_____	_____
5. -oriented	_____	_____
6. -effective	_____	_____
7. -orientation	_____	_____

B. *Directions: Several words in this chapter have the same prefix. Write the meanings for the following words by attaching the prefix cereb- (brain), dys- (bad, difficult), or hemi- (half, partly) to the suffix listed. Use your dictionary as needed, especially to check correct spelling.*

Suffix	**Word**	**Meaning**
1. -brum	_____	_____
2. -bellum	_____	_____
3. -bral	_____	_____
4. -paresis	_____	_____
5. -plegia	_____	_____
6. -phasia	_____	_____

COMMUNICATION EXERCISES

Dialogue Practice

Directions: Discuss with a partner.

A. With a partner, use the guidelines in the Focused Assessment box in the textbook to perform an assessment. Practice asking each question. Practice charting your assessment.

B. As a second-language learner, do you think the steps to help an aphasic person (self-talk, parallel talk, expansion, and modeling) would help someone learning a new language? Why or why not? What happens in each of the steps?

Explanations

What would you say to a patient who asked why the health care provider does a knee jerk (patellar reflex) test?

Orientation and Function Questions

Directions: Make a short list of questions you could ask an alert patient to assess his mental function.

_____

_____

_____

_____

_____

Care of Patients with Head and Spinal Cord Injuries

chapter **22**

Answer Key: Review the related chapter to answer these questions. A complete answer key was provided to your instructor.

COMPLETION

Head and Spinal Cord Injuries

Directions: Fill in the blanks to complete the statements.

1. When a concussion occurs, the signs and symptoms include _____, balance problems, _____ , _____ and _____ .

2. In open head injury, there is _____ of the scalp, and _____ of the skull.

3. Elderly people are more susceptible to subdural hematoma after a bump on the head because the brain tends to _____ within the cranial vault and _____ may be torn.

4. A(n) _____ hematoma results after a head injury from rapid leakage of blood from the _____, which quickly elevates _____ _____.

5. Ecchymosis behind the ear is termed _____ and indicates _____ _____.

6. Initial measures after a head injury include securing a(n) _____ and elevating _____.

7. To determine if there is a cerebrospinal fluid leak after a head injury, _____ and _____ should be tested.

8. An early sign of increased intracranial pressure (ICP) is _____ and _____ consciousness.

9. Traumatic spinal cord injuries occur from compression, _____, or tearing of the cord.

10. Following the immediate flaccid paralysis that may occur with spinal cord injury, _____ often occurs.

11. When positioning the spinal cord–injured patient, to prevent muscle spasms, avoid _____.

12. Autonomic dysreflexia is dangerous because it can cause sudden _____

    _____.

13. A common problem in spinal cord–injured patients is _____ reflux that predisposes to

    _____.

14. Quadriplegia occurs when spinal cord injury occurs at the level _____.

15. If a patient has a cervical spine injury and is in a halo traction device, you should never _____

    _____ device.

SHORT ANSWER

Intracranial Pressure

Directions: Answer the following questions in the spaces provided.

1. The classic signs of increasing ICP are _____, _____,

    _____, and _____.

2. The earliest sign of increasing ICP is usually a change in _____

    _____.

3. When nursing interventions that may increase ICP are necessary, it is wise to

    _____.

4. A priority concern for the nurse caring for a patient after intracranial surgery is _____

    _____.

5. Pathophysiologically, a head injury causes swelling and pressure against cerebral veins and

    arteries that interfere with the flow of blood, causing _____ and

    _____ of the tissues.

6. Herniation of brain tissue through the tentorial notch causes changes in the

    _____ and _____ characteristic of increased ICP.

7. Pupil changes occur with increasing ICP because _____

    _____.

8. Positioning of the patient with increased ICP is extremely important to help

    _____ and reduce _____

    _____.

9. Cushing's Triad is a sign of increased ICP and includes:

    a. _____

    b. _____

    c. _____

Other indications of rising ICP are:

d. _____

e. _____

f. _____

g. _____

COMPLETION

Spinal injury

1. The four main objectives in nursing care of the patient with a spinal cord injury are_____
_____
_____.

2. To prevent further injury in a patient with a spinal cord injury, you should _____
_____.

3. Because drug metabolism is altered in patients with spinal cord injury, check for _____
_____.

Back Pain and Herniated Disk

Directions: Fill in the blanks to complete the statements.

1. Health care workers are prone to back pain just from _____.

2. Back pain and disorders can be prevented by proper _____ and the use of
_____ and _____.

3. In the elderly, one reason for degeneration of the spinal vertebrae is _____.

4. *Chronic back pain* is defined as pain that lasts for more than _____ or occurs on a(n)
_____.

5. Signs of a herniated lumbar disk may include pain radiating down _____ into the
_____, _____, or _____.

6. Signs of a herniated cervical disk may include pain in the _____ and
_____, radiating down the arm with _____ and _____.

7. Patients who are experiencing back pain should not _____ or _____ for
long periods of time.

8. Surgical removal of a damaged disk may be performed by a percutaneous laser _____.

9. If a spinal fusion is necessary, a(n) _____ must be performed.

10. After spinal surgery, the patient is taught to carry items _____.

APPLICATION OF THE NURSING PROCESS

Directions: Write a brief answer to each question.

Scenario: Your patient has sustained a closed head injury in an automobile accident and was admitted to the ICU. The priority nursing problem on the care plan is potential for injury due to possible increased intracranial pressure.

1. Write two appropriate expected outcomes for this diagnosis for this patient.

    a. _____

    b. _____

2. Nursing interventions that would be carried out to help the patient achieve the expected outcomes would be:

    _____

    _____

    _____

3. Criteria by which you would evaluate whether the expected outcomes have been met are:

    _____

    _____

PRIORITY SETTING

You are assigned the following patients:

   a. Mr. Hopper, age 23, who has a C-5 injury sustained in a diving accident and is in cervical tongs and on a specialty bed.
   b. Ms. Hernandez, age 48, who has a ruptured disk at L-5. She has just had a diskectomy this morning.
   c. Ms. Chinn, age 72, who suffered a back injury and a pelvic fracture in an automobile accident. She is on bedrest and has paresthesia in her right leg and foot.

Mr. Hopper is complaining of muscle spasms and pain. Ms. Hernandez calls complaining of nausea. Ms. Chinn calls and asks for help, explaining that she has experienced some incontinence and the bed is wet.

In which order would you attend to these patients' needs? _____

REVIEW QUESTIONS FOR THE NCLEX® EXAMINATION

Directions: Choose the best answer(s) for the following questions.

1. Discharge teaching for the patient who has sustained a concussion should include instructions to:
    1. take the prescribed analgesic for headache every 4 hours.
    2. lie down flat at home and move around as little as possible.
    3. force fluids to prevent dehydration and infection.
    4. report immediately any severe headache or persistent vomiting.

2. Planning for the patient who has sustained a spinal injury would include listing which nursing problem as the highest priority in the care plan?
   1. Altered sensory perception due to spinal contusion
   2. Potential for infection due to trauma to spinal column
   3. Incontinence due to paraplegia
   4. Potential for injury due to inability to move

3. The first priority in assessing the patient with head trauma at an accident scene is determining:
   1. whether spinal injury is present.
   2. the level of consciousness using the Glasgow coma scale.
   3. whether the airway is patent.
   4. whether hypotension is present.

4. Mary took a fall while skiing and bumped her head on a small tree. She got right up and stated that she was fine. However, shortly afterwards Mary began suffering from a headache. What should her family do?
   1. Give Mary two Tylenol and see if it resolves the headache.
   2. Give Mary two ibuprofen because it would help reduce any inflammation Mary is experiencing.
   3. Call 911 as Mary experienced a head injury earlier and may be developing complications such as a subdural hematoma.
   4. Wait to see if any other symptoms such as nausea and vomiting develop, and if they do, take her to an urgent care center.

5. Mannitol is an osmotic diuretic that helps decrease ICP. Nursing interventions for the patient receiving this drug include: *(Select all that apply.)*
   1. monitor intake and output.
   2. observe for chest pain.
   3. monitor for increasing salivation.
   4. watch for electrolyte imbalances.
   5. check skin turgor.

6. A patient with a daughter who is engaged to be married suffered an accident that left him paraplegic. What comment indicates the patient is in the stage of bargaining?
   1. "I am saddened that I will miss being able to dance with my daughter at her wedding."
   2. "I do not deserve to be paralyzed for my daughter's wedding!"
   3. "If God will let me just walk my daughter down the aisle for her wedding, I'll never complain about being in this chair again!"
   4. "Maybe I will be able to have special braces so that I will be able to operate a Segway as a way of 'walking' my daughter down the aisle."

7. Mr. Pineda suffered a closed head injury and has increased ICP. The health care provider has prescribed mannitol 1 g/kg IV every 6 hours. Mr. Pineda weighs 194 lbs. How many grams of mannitol would be the correct dose to be given every 6 hours? _____ g

8. What is a priority nursing intervention for the patient with a spinal cord injury who is quadriplegic?
   1. Preventing overdistention of the bladder
   2. Assessing skin integrity every shift
   3. Using an abdominal binder to raise blood pressure
   4. Providing frequent massage of the legs

9. Autonomic dysreflexia can lead to:
   1. heat stroke from loss of thermoregulation.
   2. paralytic ileus.
   3. severe muscle cramps.
   4. severe hypertension.

CRITICAL THINKING ACTIVITIES

Scenario A: Mr. Schultz sustained a head injury in a bicycle accident. He was admitted to the ICU from the emergency department as his level of consciousness was decreasing. He is arousable, but very drowsy. His vital signs are BP 132/84, P 78, R 16, T 98.8° F (37.1° C). Vital and neuro signs are ordered every hour. A pulse oximeter is attached and he is placed on a cardiac monitor.

1. He had a head CT without contrast in the ED. What information is obtained from this test?

His pulse pressure shows widening after 3 hours and he is more difficult to arouse.

2. What medications would you expect he might receive?

His condition worsens and one pupil begins to dilate. He is placed on mechanical ventilation.

3. When suctioning his endotracheal tube, why is it especially important to oxygenate him thoroughly beforehand?

Scenario B: Mr. Schultz was found to have a subdural hematoma. A craniotomy was performed and the hematoma evacuated. You are caring for him postoperatively.

1. What would you pay particular attention to when positioning him?

2. Why is it important to maintain a quiet, nonstimulating atmosphere for this patient?

3. Besides increasing ICP, what is the next complication against which you would direct your nursing care?

STEPS TOWARD BETTER COMMUNICATION

VOCABULARY BUILDING GLOSSARY

Term	Pronunciation	Definition
contrecoup	con'tra coo'	a counter or opposite blow—the contents of the cranium hit the inside of the skull, then bounce back and hit the other side, causing a second injury or contrecoup
noxious	nok'shus	unpleasant and harmful; foul-smelling
precipitating	pre sip'i tay' ting	causing
"goose bumps"		roughness of the skin as the hairs stand erect, caused by cold or fear
"log rolling"		the method of moving or turning a patient by rolling him to one side by using a blanket beneath him to wrap and roll him so that the body moves as one unit; also describes the exchange of assistance to take such action

COMPLETION

Directions: Fill in the blanks with the correct words from the Vocabulary Building Glossary to complete the statements.

1. Bleeding into the brain is a(n) _____ factor for an increase in ICP.

2. The patient who has a spinal cord injury is repositioned on the side by _____ him as a single unit.

3. Mr. Eagle hit his head hard on the windshield, his head bounced backwards, and he ended up with an injury on the front of the brain and a(n) _____ injury on the back of the brain.

4. _____ odors in the room of a patient after brain surgery may cause the ICP to rise.

5. A reaction seen with autonomic dysreflexia is _____ on the skin.

WORD ATTACK SKILLS

Directions: In the combined word form find and then write the word stem that joins with the prefix to make the combined word. Write the meaning. Use a dictionary as needed. Two examples are provided.

Prefix	Word Stem	Combined Word	Meaning
dys-	-reflexia	dysreflexia	disordered response to stimuli
under-	-lying	underlying	at the base or bottom of, a cause
oto-	_____	otorrhea	_____
rhino-	_____	rhinorrhea	_____
contra(e)-	_____	contralateral	_____
	_____	contrecoup	_____
ipsi-	_____	ipsilateral	_____
hema-	_____	hematoma	_____
hemo-	_____	hemodynamic	_____
hypo-	_____	hypothermia	_____
	_____	hypoxia	_____
hyper-	_____	hyperextension	_____
	_____	hyperreflexia	_____
un-	_____	uninterrupted	_____
poly-	_____	polyuria	_____
vaso-	_____	vasoconstriction	_____
	_____	vasodilation	_____
im-	_____	immobility	_____
in-	_____	innervation	_____
	_____	inability	_____
over-	_____	overdistended	_____
re-	_____	rehabilitation	_____

COMMUNICATION EXERCISE

Dialogue Practice

Write out what you might say to the mother of a 16-year-old boy who suffered a head injury to reassure her and involve her in the plan to help her son. Cover why she shouldn't try to keep him awake (sleep is helpful for healing, but he will be aroused periodically to check the level of consciousness). Explain to her how she can help with passive range-of-motion exercises and with keeping his hands in good anatomic position.

Documentation

Document what you told her below.

_____

_____

_____

_____

CULTURAL POINTS

Many cultures have taboos about discussing sexual matters with outsiders or with someone of the opposite sex who is not a spouse. Even in cultures where sex is discussed openly, people may hesitate to talk about their personal situations and concerns. As a nurse, you will need to be able to interact with patients about sexual problems.

The patient with a spinal cord injury who is paraplegic will surely have sexual concerns. After reading the section in your text about paraplegia, jot notes about the likely concerns your paraplegic male or female patient might have. Think about how you would communicate with each patient about sexual concerns.

To overcome your own shyness or inhibitions in discussing sexual matters, ask a classmate to interact with you so that you can practice what you would say to your patient.

Care of Patients with Brain Disorders

chapter

23

Answer Key: Review the related chapter to answer these questions. A complete answer key was provided to your instructor.

COMPLETION

Seizure Disorders and Epilepsy

Directions: Fill in the blanks to complete each statement.

1. Seizures may occur anytime the _____ is deprived of

   _____.

2. During a tonic-clonic seizure, the person usually loses _____ and may be

   _____.

3. Seizures are classified based on _____.

4. The goal of anticonvulsant therapy is to control the seizures by using the _____

   amount of the drug with the _____ side effects.

5. Focal seizures affect _____, leading to _____.

6. IV phenytoin must be mixed with _____ only.

SHORT ANSWER

Directions: Complete the following statements.

1. Other than epilepsy, seizures can be caused by: _____

   _____

   _____

2. Generalized seizures are characterized by:_____ .

3. Automatisms are: _____ .

4. The manifestations of epilepsy depend on: _____

   _____

5. Status epilepticus is dangerous because:_____

   _____

6. When a seizure occurs, note: (*List five observations.*) _____

_____

_____

_____

_____

MATCHING

Cerebrovascular Accident

Directions: Match the term in the first column with the brief definition in the second column.

1. _____ Aphasia
2. _____ Dysphasia
3. _____ Apraxia
4. _____ Hemiplegia
5. _____ Atrophy
6. _____ Ataxia
7. _____ Hemiparesthesia
8. _____ Diplopia
9. _____ Dysarthria
10. _____ Agnosia

a. Loss or impairment of acquired motor skills
b. Unsteadiness or lack of coordination
c. Inability to recognize an object by sight, touch, or hearing
d. Reduced sensation on one side
e. Difficulty speaking
f. Impairment of or difficult speech
g. Paralysis of arm and leg on one side
h. Double vision
i. Muscle wasting
j. Loss of ability to communicate by either spoken or written word

COMPLETION

Directions: Fill in the blanks to complete the sentence.

1. Transient ischemic attacks (TIAs) are warnings that _____ and the patient should be evaluated by medical personnel.

2. Individuals most at risk for stroke include those with _____, a history of _____, and _____.

3. When a stroke is suspected, ask the person _____, _____ _____, _____, and answer a simple question.

4. The symptoms of a stroke caused by thrombosis occur _____, whereas those caused by embolus occur _____.

5. An individual who experiences a cerebrovascular accident (CVA) in the right hemisphere of the brain often has paresis or paralysis on the _____ side.

6. A patient who has had a subarachnoid hemorrhage is at risk for developing _____.

7. The patient with a leaking cerebral aneurysm often presents with _____ _____.

8. An embolus causing a stroke often arises from the _____ in a patient who has _____.

9. Structures that can cause an intercerebral hemorrhage are a(n) _____ and a(n) _____.

10. A subarachnoid hemorrhage often causes _____ of neurologic _____ and loss of _____.

COMPLETION

Brain Tumor

Directions: Fill in the blanks with the correct words to complete the statement.

1. A sign of a brain tumor in up to 50% of adults is _____.

2. An infratentorial brain tumor often causes a loss of _____ and _____.

3. First signs of a brain tumor may include loss of muscular strength and coordination, _____ loss, _____, _____, or difficulty speaking clearly.

4. Diagnostic tests to verify presence of a brain tumor are _____, _____, and _____.

5. Two complications of a brain tumor are _____ and _____ _____.

Infections and Inflammatory Disorders of the Nervous System

Directions: Fill in the blank(s) with the correct words to complete the sentence.

1. Meningitis is a(n) _____ of the _____ covering the _____ and _____.

2. Bacterial meningitis frequently follows a(n) _____ infection.

3. Classic signs of meningitis are _____ _____.

4. A(n) _____ rash on the chest and extremities accompanies _____ meningitis.

5. Meningitis is confirmed by a(n) _____, where CSF pressure is _____ and glucose is _____.

6. For the patient with meningitis, it is important to watch for _____, as well as neurologic deficits and seizures.

7. The signs and symptoms of viral meningitis are _____, _____, _____, and _____.

8. A nonvector-transmitted form of encephalitis is _____.

9. Encephalitis is spread by vectors such as _____ and _____.

10. Postviral encephalitis is a(n) _____ disorder.

TABLE ACTIVITY

Directions: Fill in the nursing implications for the following medications commonly used for a patient after a CVA.

Drug	Action	Nursing Implications
t-PA (alteplase; tissue plasminogen activator)	Converts fibrin to plasminogen, causing lysis of thrombus or embolus of CVA	
Aspirin (Ecotrin)	Decreases platelet aggregation	
Phenytoin (Dilantin)	Alters ion transport, inhibiting spread of seizure activity to motor cortex	
Nimodipine (Nimotop)	Inhibits calcium ion flux across cellular membrane; decreases or prevents cerebral vasospasm	

PRIORITY SETTING

Scenario: A patient who has been diagnosed with a thrombotic CVA was admitted yesterday and is assigned to you. The patient has left-sided hemiplegia, particularly of the arm. It is now 7:30 AM. Breakfast is served at 8:00 AM. According to the orders and care plan, you are to carry out the following. Indicate in what order you would perform each task.

_____ a. Neurologic check q2h

_____ b. Vital signs q4h

_____ c. IV of 0.9% NS at 50 mL/hr

_____ d. Blood glucose via glucometer AC and HS

_____ e. Urine sample to lab for urinalysis

_____ f. Monitor for seizure activity

_____ g. Up in chair three times a day with assistance

_____ h. Assist with bath

REVIEW QUESTIONS FOR THE NCLEX® EXAMINATION

Directions: Choose the best answer(s) to each of the following or supply the missing words to complete the statement.

1. During a seizure, it is important for the nurse to observe:
    1. the type of aura the patient experiences.
    2. where movement occurs and how it progresses.
    3. the quality and rate of respirations during the seizure.
    4. the position of the patient's arms and legs during the seizure.

2. During a generalized seizure, you could expect the patient to experience: *(Select all that apply.)*
    1. loss of muscle tone.
    2. tonic-clonic movements.
    3. automatisms.
    4. absence for a few seconds.
    5. possible urinary incontinence.
    6. unilateral movements of limbs.

3. The teaching plan for the patient with epilepsy should include: *(Select all that apply.)*
    1. refrain from drinking alcohol.
    2. wear a Medic-Alert bracelet or necklace.
    3. do not go anywhere by yourself.
    4. don't become overly tired.
    5. eat bananas to replace potassium loss.
    6. swim only with a partner.

4. Besides small emboli or small blood vessel rupture, a TIA may be caused by _____

    _____.

5. Hydrocephalus is a complication after an intercerebral bleed because:
    1. blood in the cerebral ventricular system interferes with the resorption of CSF.
    2. excessive amounts of CSF are produced after an intercerebral bleed.
    3. excessive hormone production increases the production of CSF.
    4. the ventricles become blocked by blood clots.

6. A post-CVA patient is experiencing motor difficulties on the right side of the body. You know that:
    1. the accident occurred on the left side of the brain.
    2. the accident occurred on the right side of the brain as the patient experiences the deficit of the same side as the insult.
    3. it was caused by a subarachnoid hemorrhage.
    4. because the motor symptoms are on the right side, there will be no bowel or bladder dysfunction.

7. One of the best things for building the self-esteem of the neurologically impaired person is:
    1. to establish small, accomplishable goals.
    2. time to adapt to body changes.
    3. a way to be a productive member of society.
    4. contact with friends and family.

8. Your patient describes that she experiences visual disturbances as shimmering arc-shaped lights in her field of vision and blocks in her vision similar to a blind spot. This is followed by a one-sided headache. She is experiencing: *(Select all that apply.)*
    1. an aura-type disturbance prior to onset of a migraine headache.
    2. optic neuritis.
    3. retinal detachment.
    4. visual disturbances called a *scotoma*.

9. An effective treatment to stop a migraine headache for many people is to:
    1. place an ice bag on the throbbing area of the head.
    2. lie down in an odor-free, darkened room with the eyes closed.
    3. sit very still in an upright position with the eyes closed.
    4. apply heat packs to the forehead and neck.

10. A patient experiencing status epilepticus is receiving phenytoin IV. He is to receive 18 mg/kg in 24 hours. He weighs 162 lbs. The total amount he should receive is _____. If he is to receive this medication mixed with 500 mL of 0.9% NaCl every 8 hours, each 500 mL IV bag should contain _____ mg of phenytoin.

CRITICAL THINKING ACTIVITIES

Scenario A: Ms. Rosario has been found to have an aneurysm in the brain. She has had headaches for many years, but they have become much worse lately. She also has type II diabetes and hypertension for which she takes several medications. She has been admitted to your unit.

1. How might this aneurysm be treated?

2. If the aneurysm begins to leak, what symptoms might Ms. Rosario have?

3. What would you expect the treatment of this patient to be?

4. What is your priority nursing responsibility?

Scenario B: Mr. Tompkins, age 76, suffered a CVA with right hemiplegia. He is in the recovery stage and has been admitted to the rehabilitation institute. He is achieving some feeling in his right arm and leg, but is still unable to walk or use his arm effectively.

1. What particular deficits might this type of CVA have caused that will affect his everyday living?

2. What therapies would you expect him to undergo at the rehabilitation institute?

3. What would you do when he has crying spells?

4. What medications would you expect to be administering related to the CVA?

Scenario C: Mr. Hiroshi, age 66, is experiencing sharp, intense paroxysms of facial pain that last for a couple of minutes. The pain occurs on the right side of the face.

1. What questions would you ask Mr. Hiroshi to assess his problem?

2. What do you expect the diagnosis might be?

3. If this is a facial nerve problem, what treatment might you expect the health care provider to prescribe?

STEPS TOWARD BETTER COMMUNICATION

VOCABULARY BUILDING GLOSSARY

Term	Pronunciation	Definition
seizure	see' zur	sudden attack or occurrence of a disease; convulsion; caused by abnormal electrical activity in the brain
spasm	spa' zim	strong involuntary contractions
untoward [effects]	un tord'	inconvenient, awkward, unexpected
groggy	grog' ee	weak and unsteady, possibly confused (may come from "grog," an alcoholic drink)
intractable [seizures]	in trak' ta bel	unmanageable, hard to control
susceptible	su sep' ti bel	likely to be affected by
debilitating	de bil' ih ta ting	making weak, or feeble; losing energy and ability
ischemia	is ke' mia	deficiency of blood, or obstruction
aura	or' a	atmosphere surrounding something; a radiation of light

COMPLETION

Directions: Fill in the blanks with the correct words from the Vocabulary Building Glossary to complete the statements.

1. When the patient woke up, he seemed a little _____ and wasn't ready to eat his breakfast.

2. The child's legs seemed to be in _____ and she couldn't straighten them.

3. A person who is poorly nourished is more _____ to disease.

4. The man was found on the floor having an apparent _____.

5. The severe seizures are _____ and need to be better controlled.

6. The man was discouraged because his stroke was so _____.

7. The woman usually was warned that a migraine was coming on by the _____ she saw beforehand.

8. The family was surprised by the _____ effects of their father's illness.

COMMUNICATION EXERCISE

Explanations

A. *Directions: Can you put these symptoms in lay terms so that the patient's family can understand them?*

"Homonymous hemianopsia, hemiplegia or hemiparesis, agnosia, apraxia, aphasia, and dysphagia are some of the problems caused by a CVA."

_____

_____

_____

_____

_____

_____

B. *Directions: Explain the difference between a shunt and a stent.*

_____

_____

PRONUNCIATION SKILLS

Directions: Practice pronouncing these words aloud.

Symptomatology	Sym tow ma tol'o gee
Electroencephalogram	E lec trow' en sef'a low gram
Homonymous hemianopsia	Ho mon'i mus hem'ee ah nop'see a
Cytomegalovirus encephalitis	Cy tow meg'ah low vir'us en sef'a ly'tis

MATCHING

Directions: Choose from the list of definitions at right, and write in the blank space the correct meaning for each word on the left.

1. Idiopathic   _____   No known cause

2. Neoplasm   _____   Narrowing of the blood vessels

3. Flaccid   _____   Tumor

4. Vasoconstriction   _____   Both sides

5. Bilateral   _____   Limp, hanging loose, weak, soft

COMMUNICATION EXERCISE

Directions: Write a short dialogue or monologue of what you would say to the patient or family in each of these cases. Practice your dialogue with another student.

Provide encouragement for a stroke patient with left-sided hemiparesis who is learning how to walk again. Show patience and encouragement. What would you say if the patient becomes frustrated and angry? Write out some ideas of how you would provide encouragement and how you would handle the anger.

_____

_____

_____

_____

Care of Patients with Peripheral Nerve and Degenerative Neurologic Disorders

chapter

24

Answer Key: Review the related chapter to answer these questions. A complete answer key was provided to your instructor.

COMPLETION

Degenerative Neurologic Disorders

Directions: Fill in the blanks to complete the statements.

1. Substances that seem to play a role in the occurrence of Parkinson disease are

   _____.

2. In patients with Parkinson disease, there is a deficiency of _____ in the brain

   causing problems with _____ and _____.

3. Four drugs that help control tremor, rigidity, and drooling in patients with Parkinson disease are

   _____, _____, _____, and

   _____.

4. Signs and symptoms of multiple sclerosis depend on the extent to which inflammation and destruction

   of the _____ have occurred.

5. Multiple sclerosis is a disease of the central nervous system and its symptoms are caused by

   _____ of the nerve fibers.

6. The four types of clinical progression of multiple sclerosis are _____,

   _____, _____, and _____.

7. Alzheimer disease progresses at _____ and eventually results in

   _____.

8. Amyotrophic lateral sclerosis is a(n) _____ neuromuscular disease char-

   acterized by degeneration of the _____ in the anterior horns of the

   _____ and the lower cranial nerves.

9. Guillain-Barré syndrome usually follows a(n) _____, but can occur after

   _____ immunization.

10. Pathologic changes that occur with Guillain-Barré syndrome are _____,

    _____, _____, and _____.

11. When the lower brainstem becomes involved in Guillain-Barré syndrome, the

    _____ are affected.

12. Guillain-Barré syndrome is characterized by the appearance of a(n) _____

    _____.

13. The patient with Guillain-Barré syndrome suffers paresthesias, muscular aches and cramps, and

    _____.

14. Postpolio syndrome may occur _____ years later and problems may be

    _____ or _____.

15. Huntington disease is genetically transmitted and is characterized by _____.

16. Huntington disease causes deterioration in _____ capacity and

    _____ disturbances.

17. Myasthenia gravis is a(n) _____ disease manifested by fatigue

    and muscle exhaustion aggravated by _____ and relieved by

    _____.

18. The purpose of plasma exchange as a treatment for myasthenia gravis is to mechanically remove

    _____.

TABLE ACTIVITY

Directions: Complete the following table comparing three neurologic diseases: Parkinson disease, multiple sclerosis, and myasthenia gravis.

	Parkinson Disease	Multiple Sclerosis	Myasthenia Gravis
Definition			
Clinical manifestations			
Cause			
Diagnostic measures			
Medical management			
Special nursing concerns and patient problems			

PRIORITY SETTING

Scenario: You are assigned to a variety of patients who have several medications to be administered at 8:00 AM. Breakfast is served at 8:00 AM. You plan to start dispensing the medications ordered for 8:00 AM at about 7:45 AM in order to get them all administered on time. Consider the nursing implications of the diagnoses and the drugs to be administered. Decide on the order of priority in which you will give each patient's medications and indicate the numerical order in the blanks provided.

The patients and medications are:

_____ a. Ms. Hubers, diagnosis of type 2 diabetes and pneumonia. She is to receive Diabinese and Biaxin.

_____ b. Mr. Hunter, diagnosis hypertension and heart failure. He is to receive digoxin, furosemide, and losartan.

_____ c. Ms. Johnson, diagnosis myasthenia gravis. She is to receive Mestinon.

_____ d. Mr. Takura, diagnosis Parkinson disease. He is to receive Sinemet, Cogentin, and Metamucil.*

*What special nursing implication regarding the administration of Metamucil should be considered?

_____

_____

REVIEW QUESTIONS FOR THE NCLEX® EXAMINATION

Directions: Choose the best answer(s) for the following questions or fill in the blank with the correct answer.

1. Interventions for the patient with moderate Parkinson disease might include: *(Select all that apply.)*
   1. allowing extra time to perform tasks.
   2. medicating 15 minutes before meals.
   3. allowing rest periods during meals.
   4. propping up with pillows when resting.
   5. ambulating at least twice a day.
   6. providing an alternative to oral communication.

2. An expected outcome for the patient with Parkinson disease who has a nursing problem of potential for injury would be:
   1. patient will not experience a fall while ambulating before discharge.
   2. patient will not develop a respiratory infection this month.
   3. patient's rigidity will decrease with medication within 2 weeks.
   4. patient will not sustain skin impairment from bedrest before discharge.

3. Patients taking levodopa to control Parkinson disease should be assessed for the side effect of:
   1. headache.
   2. gastrointestinal bleeding.
   3. muscle aches.
   4. orthostatic hypotension.

4. While assessing patients for Parkinson disease, which risks should be taken into consideration? *(Select all that apply.)*
   1. History of prior head injury
   2. Gender
   3. Age
   4. Family history

5. Assessment findings of weakness of a leg, blurred vision, spasticity of muscles, and a positive Lhermitte sign for a patient will most likely lead to a diagnosis of:
   1. Parkinson disease.
   2. multiple sclerosis.
   3. myasthenia gravis.
   4. amyotrophic lateral sclerosis.

6. When planning nursing care for a patient with multiple sclerosis, remember that the patient:
   1. fatigues very easily and has the most strength in the afternoon.
   2. may exhibit periods of elated behavior.
   3. will experience more fatigue in a hot environment.
   4. needs increased calories in the diet.

7. Treatment for myasthenia gravis may consist of: *(Select all that apply.)*
   1. high-dose steroids.
   2. anticholinesterase therapy.
   3. IVIG therapy.
   4. plasmapheresis.

8. A nursing intervention for safety of the patient with Guillain-Barré syndrome is to:
   1. keep intubation equipment and an Ambu bag at the bedside.
   2. keep the head of the patient's bed elevated 15–30 degrees at all times.
   3. have the patient perform range-of-motion exercises at least three times a day.
   4. keep the room darkened and the environment quiet to prevent agitation of the patient.

9. When assessing a patient with amyotrophic lateral sclerosis, the nurse would find:
   1. difficulty breathing.
   2. bilateral tremors.
   3. ascending paralysis.
   4. weakness of voluntary muscles.

10. Huntington disease is genetically transmitted and usually causes death within _____ years after signs appear.

CRITICAL THINKING ACTIVITIES

Scenario A: Ms. Johnson, age 33, has just been diagnosed with multiple sclerosis. Her health care provider thinks she has the relapsing-remitting type. She is a graduate student at the university. She has been having trouble with her vision.

1. What can she expect with this type of multiple sclerosis?

2. How would you help her decide what to do about her vision problems, as they are interfering with her studying?

3. Her health care provider has talked with her about using beta-interferon to help control her disease. What could you tell her about this medication?

Scenario B: Mr. Katsigris, age 46, has recently been diagnosed with myasthenia gravis. He is not familiar with the disease and has many questions.

1.   What could you tell him about the disease?

2.   What are the biggest dangers with this disease?

3.   What would you tell him about the usual treatment for the disease?

STEPS TOWARD BETTER COMMUNICATION

VOCABULARY BUILDING GLOSSARY

Term	Pronunciation	Definition
collaborate	co lab'o rate	to work together
ascending	a send' ing	going upward
dyspepsia	dis pep'si a	indigestion
plateau	plat oh'	a level time after an increase; a fairly level area of high ground
drooling		water or saliva coming out of the mouth, usually due to lack of muscle control

COMPLETION

Directions: Fill in the blanks with the correct words from the Vocabulary Building Glossary to complete the statements.

1.   _____ the stairway takes much more energy than descending the stairs.

2.   The nursing staff and the physical therapists agreed to _____ on solving the problem.

3.   Because of his stroke, Mr. Branson's facial muscles were paralyzed and he had difficulty preventing himself from _____.

4.   The patient's rehabilitation efforts seemed to reach a(n) _____ that was difficult to get beyond.

5.   Ms. Johnson's _____ made her irritable after meals.

GRAMMAR POINTS

Collaborate is the base verb meaning to work together; **collaborator** is a noun (one of the people who does the working together); **collaboration** is a noun referring to the action of working together; and **collaborative** is an adjective describing the kind of action.

Similarly, **drool** is the base verb; **drooler,** a noun, would be a person (not commonly used); **drooling** would be the noun describing the action (from the participle).

COMMUNICATION EXERCISES

A. Dialogue Practice

Think Critically

A patient comes into the clinic complaining about hand tremors and "stiffness" of the joints that started recently, excessive sweating, and some urinary incontinence. You notice that her gait is abnormal. What would be a priority question you would ask her as you start taking her history?

Use the above as the basis for a dialogue. With a partner, practice asking the questions in the Focused Assessment box in the textbook.

B. Explanations

With a partner, practice explaining to a patient with myasthenia gravis why wearing a Medic-Alert emblem/bracelet is a good idea.

CULTURAL POINTS

Directions: For discussion in a group:

People with the disorders described in this chapter have a number of physical manifestations relating to their illness (tremors, lack of muscle control, strange gaits, tics, etc.). How do you think these physical manifestations affect their feelings about going out in public? How are people with such disorders received by the people they meet or who observe them? What nursing problems could this cause?

If there are people in your class from other cultures, ask how people with physical disorders would be treated in their culture. Are there differences among the cultures?

What might you—as a medical person—be able to do to help the situation?

The Sensory System: Eye

chapter

25

Answer Key: Review the related chapter to answer these questions. A complete answer key was provided to your instructor.

REVIEW OF ANATOMY AND PHYSIOLOGY

Terminology

Directions: Match the term on the left with the correct definition, function, or statement on the right. (Answers may be used more than once.)

1. _____ Pupil
2. _____ Ciliary body
3. _____ Iris
4. _____ Anterior chamber
5. _____ Posterior chamber
6. _____ Eyelashes
7. _____ Lacrimal gland
8. _____ Tears
9. _____ Suspensory ligaments
10. _____ Ectropion

a. Secretes tears that moisten, lubricate, and cleanse the eye
b. Sits between lens and retina and contains vitreous humor
c. Connect the iris to the choroid
d. Contain an enzyme that kills bacteria
e. Between the lens and the cornea
f. Eversion of the lower lid that may occur with aging
g. Secrete aqueous humor
h. Central opening allowing light into interior
i. Connect the ciliary body and lens
j. Help trap foreign particles, keeping them out of the eye
k. Colored portion of the eye

LABELING

Directions: Label the following structures on the diagram of the eye.

sclera
pupil
Schlemm's canal
ciliary process
cornea
conjunctiva
anterior chamber
choroid
lens
optic disk
posterior chamber
iris
optic nerve
retina
vitreous body

TABLE ACTIVITY

Directions: Complete the following table, providing the signs and symptoms and treatments for selected eye diseases.

Disease	Signs and Symptoms	Medical Treatment and Nursing Interventions
Blepharitis: Infection of glands and lash follicles along lid margin		
Chalazion: Internal stye; infection of meibomian gland		
Hordeolum: External stye; infected swelling near the lid margin on inside		
Conjunctivitis: Inflammation of the conjunctiva; "pink eye" is a specific type caused by chemical irritants, bacteria, or virus		
Keratitis: Inflammation of the cornea		
Corneal abrasion or ulceration		

APPLICATION OF THE NURSING PROCESS

Directions: Write a brief answer to each question.

1. List the five danger signals of eye disease that should be looked for upon assessment of each patient.

    a. _____

    b. _____

    c. _____

    d. _____

    e. _____

2. List five guidelines for assisting a blind person.

    a. _____

    b. _____

    c. _____

    d. _____

    e. _____

3. What are four important steps in administering eyedrops?

    a. _____

    b. _____

    c. _____

    d. _____

COMPLETION

Directions: Fill in the blanks with the correct words to complete the statements.

1. The term for inability to see objects close at hand is _____.

2. Keratitis may be caused by _____ or _____.

3. If a chemical splashes into the eye, the eye should be treated with _____ for at least _____ with _____ or _____.

4. If a foreign body is stuck into the eye, the best thing to do is to _____, _____ the eye, and to _____.

5. A cataract causes a blurring of vision because the _____ becomes _____.

6. Cataract surgery is performed when the loss of vision _____ the person's life.

7. Glaucoma is often _____ until damage to vision has occurred from _____ and pressure on the _____.

8. The characteristic sign of narrow-angle glaucoma is _____ _____.

9. Drugs used in the treatment of glaucoma act to _____ of _____ or decrease _____.

10. Uncontrolled glaucoma causes _____.

11. The sudden occurrence of flashes of colored light is a sign of _____.

12. Retinopathy is often a disorder that occurs in patients with diabetes mellitus and is either from

_____ of blood vessels or _____ of blood vessels with

_____.

13. Early symptoms of macular degeneration are inability to see _____ of

_____ and _____.

14. The patient who has just had eye surgery should be positioned with the head

_____ and should not lie on the _____ side.

15. When administering preoperative mydriatic eyedrops, you should wait _____ minutes between the instillation of one drop and the other.

APPLICATION OF THE NURSING PROCESS

Directions: Write a brief answer to each question.

1. List nursing problems frequently encountered for patients with disorders of the eye.

    a. _____

    b. _____

    c. _____

    d. _____

    e. _____

2. Give four assessment findings that may indicate the presence of a cataract.

    a. _____

    b. _____

    c. _____

    d. _____

3. Your clinical patient is scheduled for same-day surgery in the ambulatory surgery unit. Eyedrops are ordered to be instilled three times at 15-minute intervals. The patient has just been admitted to the unit. An IV is to be started, a gown put on by the patient, the preoperative checklist is to be completed, and the patient is to be ready for surgery in 60 minutes. In what order of priority should these actions take place?

    _____

    _____

    _____

    _____

    _____

    _____

SHORT ANSWER

Retinal Detachment and Eye Surgery

Directions: Read the clinical situation and write brief answers to the questions that follow.

Scenario: Mr. Cox, age 82, is scheduled for a scleral buckle for a retinal detachment. He will be hospitalized at least overnight.

1. Considering the procedure Mr. Cox is undergoing, what should be included in his teaching plan to prepare him for the early postoperative period?

    a. _____

    b. _____

    c. _____

    d. _____

    e. _____

2. What safety precautions should be taken during Mr. Cox's hospital stay?

    a. _____
        _____

    b. _____
        _____

    c. _____
        _____

    d. _____
        _____

3. Name three instructions that should be included in Mr. Cox's discharge teaching specific to the type of surgery he had.

    a. _____
        _____

    b. _____
        _____

    c. _____
        _____

4. List five goals or expected outcomes for nursing interventions in the postoperative care of all patients who have had surgery of the eye.

a. _____

b. _____

c. _____

d. _____

e. _____

TABLE ACTIVITY

Directions: List at least three of each type of medication and complete its action.

Classification	Examples	Action
Drugs Used for Glaucoma		
Miotics		
Carbonic anhydrase inhibitors		
Sympathomimetics		
Alpha$_2$ adrenergic agonist		
Antiinflammatories		
Drugs to Facilitate Diagnosis and Surgery		
Antiinfective Optic Medications		

REVIEW QUESTIONS FOR THE NCLEX® EXAMINATION

Directions: Choose the best answer(s) for each of the following questions.

1. Fluorescein angiography is used as an assessment tool by the health care provider. Teaching for the patient about the procedure includes stating:
    1. "the optic nerve will be visualized to determine any problems."
    2. "eye muscle testing will occur during the test."
    3. "the test helps measure visual acuity."
    4. "dye will be injected intravenously and the blood vessels in the fundus examined."

2. When assessing a patient for vision problems, subtle signs of decreasing vision are:
    1. becoming less interested in a hobby such as sewing.
    2. developing a bruise on the shin from the open door to the dishwasher.
    3. seeing better when using prescribed glasses.
    4. wanting a light on in the room when watching television.

3. Beginning usually around age 40, patients often develop an eye condition known as *presbyopia*. This condition is when:
    1. there is increased pressure within the eyeball.
    2. the ciliary muscle has less ability to allow the eye to accommodate, resulting in close vision impairment.
    3. protrusion of the eyeball prevents close focus.
    4. close vision improves while distant vision becomes more difficult.

4. An intervention for setting up a dinner tray for a blind person would be to:
    1. place the person's hands on each side of the plate.
    2. describe where each type of food is located using the "clock" method.
    3. allow the person to cut up the meat.
    4. make certain there are no shadows in the room.

5. Community teaching for the prevention of eye problems should include: *(Select all that apply.)*
    1. wearing a hat when outdoors.
    2. wearing sunglasses that block UVA and UVB rays when outdoors.
    3. using eyedrops when returning inside from being in the sun.
    4. eating a diet rich in fruits and vegetables that contain antioxidants.
    5. obtaining regular glaucoma screening after age 40.
    6. cleansing the eyes with eyedrops regularly.

6. Ms. Messina is scheduled for a cataract extraction with intraocular lens implant of the right eye. Assessment of Ms. Messina during preoperative care would include: *(Select all that apply.)*
    1. food likes and dislikes for dietary selections.
    2. degree of retained vision and history of previous hospitalizations.
    3. ability to instill eyedrops and perform self-care.
    4. ability to understand and follow directions postoperatively.

7. Planning for safety needs for a patient with a right cataract extraction and intraocular lens implant in the immediate postoperative period would include: *(Select all that apply.)*
    1. placing the call light cord and console on her left side.
    2. unplugging the television so that she is not tempted to watch it.
    3. keeping her in bed for 12 hours.
    4. medicating quickly if she becomes nauseous from anesthesia.

8. The priority measures a diabetic patient must take following surgery for diabetic retinopathy are: *(Select all that apply.)*
    1. lay flat for 12 hours.
    2. maintain strict control of blood glucose levels.
    3. maintain blood pressure within a normal range.
    4. avoid watching television for more than 1 hour per day.

9. The *most* important nursing intervention in the recovery period before discharge from the day surgery unit to ensure success of eye surgery is:
    1. medicating for pain before it becomes severe.
    2. answering the call light promptly.
    3. assisting the patient to walk to the bathroom.
    4. positioning the patient per orders.

10. The nurse's *most* important evaluation criterion for interventions to prevent complications of glaucoma surgery is:
    1. checking the degree of eye pain.
    2. checking security of the eye dressing.
    3. assessing the amount of nausea.
    4. checking the amount of redness of the operative eye.

11. The therapeutic response expected of dorzolamide (Trusopt) is:
    1. dilation of the pupil.
    2. constriction of the pupil.
    3. decreased intraocular pressure.
    4. decreased production of aqueous humor.

12. Mr. Schultz has come to the emergency department with severe eye pain. He is diagnosed with closed-angle glaucoma. The health care provider orders IV Diamox 150 mg in 200 mL of D_5W to be given over 15 minutes. The vial of the drug contains 500 mg in 2 mL. How many mL would be added to the D_5W for this infusion? _____

CRITICAL THINKING ACTIVITIES

1. Develop a teaching plan on protecting vision for a community or school group.

2. Explain the Amsler Grid test to your elderly relatives and/or neighbors and perform an assessment for macular degeneration using the grid.

STEPS TOWARD BETTER COMMUNICATION

VOCABULARY BUILDING GLOSSARY

Term	Pronunciation	Definition
acuity	ah kyou' i tee	clearness, sharpness
ap'titude	ap' tĭ tūd	good ability to do or learn something
bear in mind		remember; think about; consider
opaque	o pāk'	light cannot go through it
phenom'enon	fah nom' ah non	an unusual or interesting fact or occurrence
take it for granted		to not think about something, especially a gift or normal behavior, such as sight, food, or family; to assume a condition will always exist

COMPLETION

Directions: Fill in the blanks with the correct words from the Vocabulary Building Glossary to complete the statements.

1. Joan has a special _____ for nursing.

2. Seeing flashing lights after a retinal detachment is an odd _____.

3. The nurse should always _____ that asepsis is always important in caring for patients with an eye surgery.

4. A cataract makes the lens of the eye _____.

5. After age 60, Joe noticed that the _____ of his eyesight had decreased.

6. People with good eyesight may _____ and neglect proper vision screenings.

VOCABULARY EXERCISE

Review of Terms and Combining Forms

kerat/o	cornea
phot/o	light
optic, opt/o	vision
opia	vision
humor	any fluid or semifluid in the body
ophthalm/o	eye
superior	above
inferior	below
lateral	toward the side
medial	central, in the middle

PRONUNCIATION SKILLS

conjunctiva	kun junk′ ti vuh
amblyopia	am blē ō′ pē uh
trabec′ uloplasty	trah bek′ you low plas tee

ABBREVIATIONS

ARMD	age-related macular degeneration
LVES	low-vision enhancement system
OD	right eye
OS	left eye
OU	both eyes

One way to remember this is to think that right eye (OD) comes first in the alphabet; left eye (OS) comes second in the alphabet, and both eyes (OU) comes last.

Directions: Practice pronouncing the above words and abbreviations with a peer. Have your partner write down the words or abbreviations as you say them. Check the list for accurate enunciation.

COMMUNICATION EXERCISE

With a peer, practice assessment by using the information in the Focused Assessment boxes in the textbook to take a history. Ask your partner questions to help clarify points that require more explanation.

The Sensory System: Ear

Answer Key: Review the related chapter to answer these questions. A complete answer key was provided to your instructor.

REVIEW OF ANATOMY AND PHYSIOLOGY

Labeling

Directions: Label the diagram of the ear with the following parts. (Not all parts may be used.)

pinna
semicircular canals
auditory meatus
cochlea
eustachian tube

malleus
vestibular nerve CN VIII branch
incus
cochlear nerve CN VII
stapes

tympanic membrane
vestibule
facial nerve

SHORT ANSWER

Prevention of Hearing Loss

Directions: Write a brief answer for each question.

1. How can people protect themselves from hearing damage?

   a. _____

   b. _____

   c. _____

2. What are four signs of hearing loss?

   a. _____

   b. _____

   c. _____

   d. _____

3. What are five common medications that are potentially ototoxic and may cause hearing loss?

   a. _____

   b. _____

   c. _____

   d. _____

   e. _____

TABLE ACTIVITY

Conductive Versus Sensorineural Hearing Loss

Directions: Complete the following table comparing conductive and sensorineural hearing loss.

Characteristic	Conductive	Sensorineural
Location of dysfunction		
Common causes		
Treatment		

COMPLETION

The Ear and Hearing Loss

Directions: Fill in the blanks with the correct words to complete the statements.

1. Tuning fork tests measure hearing by _____ or _____ conduction.

2. A simple hearing test is the _____ test.

3. The Romberg test is performed by having the person stand _____ _____.

4. When eardrops are administered, they should first be _____ or they may cause discomfort or dizziness.

5. When eardrops are instilled, the patient should remain in the lateral position for _____ minutes.

6. When communicating with a hearing-impaired person, it is best to position yourself _____ of the person.

7. When working with a patient who has a hearing aid, the nurse should make certain that the aid _____.

8. Many people do not know that hearing aids from a reputable dealer usually have a(n) _____ _____.

9. People who are deaf may _____ themselves because of embarrassment and frustration over difficulty communicating.

10. Exposure to environmental loud noise causes a(n) _____ hearing loss that is often not correctable.

CRITICAL THINKING ACTIVITIES

1. Formulate a teaching plan for college students on how to protect hearing.

2. Plan how you would handle the situation if you go to a concert, dance, or other place that has music that is playing too loudly.

COMPLETION

Directions: Fill in the blanks with the correct words to complete the statements.

1. Causes of labyrinthitis include bacterial meningitis, chronic otitis media, or _____.

2. Symptoms of labyrinthitis are loss of hearing in the affected ear, severe dizziness with nausea and vomiting, and _____.

3. A tympanoplasty involves surgical reconstruction of the _____ and _____ to restore middle ear function.

4. Besides difficulty hearing, ear problems and deafness are often accompanied by _____, which can cause considerable fatigue in the person.

5. Otosclerosis is generally a(n) _____ degeneration of the _____.

6. Hereditary deafness is usually due to changes in the _____ of the ear and causes a(n) _____ hearing loss.

7. Conductive hearing loss can often be helped by a(n) _____ or corrected with _____.

REVIEW QUESTIONS FOR THE NCLEX® EXAMINATION

Directions: Choose the best answer(s) for each of the following questions.

1. When assessing a patient who complains of a mild hearing loss, the nurse should first:
   1. schedule an audiogram.
   2. inspect the ear canal for cerumen.
   3. inquire about past episodes of upper respiratory infection.
   4. irrigate the ear canal for clearer vision of the eardrum.

2. For the patient undergoing assessment for a hearing loss, the nurse would explain that electronystagmography is performed in conjunction with:
   1. caloric testing.
   2. the tuning fork test.
   3. the Rinne test.
   4. an audiogram.

3. The order of sound transmission from the outer ear to the brain is:

   a. pinna
   b. tympanic membrane
   c. middle ear
   d. organ of Corti
   e. vestibulocochlear nerve
   f. medulla oblongata

   1. a, b, c, d, e, f
   2. f, b, c, d, e, a
   3. d, e, f, b, a, c
   4. e, a, f, b, c, d

4. Decreases in hearing often occur with aging because of: *(Select all that apply.)*
   1. vascular changes from diabetes.
   2. loss of elasticity of the tympanic membrane.
   3. nerve cell atrophy in the ear and brain.
   4. arteriosclerosis and decreased blood flow.

5. When irrigating the ear canal to remove cerumen, aim the stream of water above or below the impaction to allow _____ to push out the cerumen.

6. When assessing a patient who is complaining of ear pain, the most important question would be:
   1. "Have you been listening to loud music?"
   2. "Have you had a recent upper respiratory infection?"
   3. "Are you prone to form a lot of wax in your ears?"
   4. "What have you taken for your pain?"

7. The nurse would expect to implement which order for the patient with Ménière disease?
   1. Cefazolin (Kefzol) 1 g q6h IV
   2. Furosemide (Lasix) 20 mg three times a day
   3. Morphine 4 mg IV q4h PRN pain
   4. Ondansetron (Zofran) 4 mg IV q6h PRN nausea and vomiting

8. The teaching plan for the discharged patient who has Ménière disease and is prescribed meclizine would probably include which information about the drug?
   1. It is a cholinergic medication.
   2. It is a vitamin-drug combination.
   3. There are antihistamine side effects.
   4. It can be taken when you have glaucoma.

9. Otosclerosis is a hereditary condition which causes degeneration of bone in the inner ear. This may result in profound hearing loss. Treatment for this condition includes: *(Select all that apply.)*
   1. correction through use of a hearing aid.
   2. a change in diet.
   3. surgical correction involving replacing the stapes with a prosthetic device (stapedectomy).
   4. sodium.

10. The patient who has had a stapedectomy should be instructed to:
    1. keep the head elevated when in bed.
    2. sneeze and cough with the mouth closed.
    3. apply the ear protector for sleep.
    4. sleep with the affected ear up.

11. When teaching the elderly patient about care of his hearing aid, you would include which action(s)? *(Select all that apply.)*
    1. Keep the battery in the hearing aid.
    2. Clean the ear mold regularly with alcohol.
    3. Never put the hearing aid in water.
    4. Open the battery cover when the hearing aid is not in the ear.

12. Meclizine (Antivert) is a drug that is used for patients with Ménière disease. This drug is used to reduce dizziness and is a(n):
    1. antihistamine.
    2. corticosteroid.
    3. antihypertensive.
    4. beta blocker.

13. Ms. Jaiswal just had a stapedectomy. She has an IV of $D_5\frac{1}{2}NS$ hanging and there are 660 mL left in the bag. It is prescribed to run at 100 mL/hour. The IV tubing delivers 10 drops per mL. You should set the drip rate at _____ gtts/min.

SHORT ANSWER

Tinnitus and Hearing Loss

Directions: Write a brief answer to each question.

1. What are four medical or nursing interventions that might be helpful to the patient with vertigo?

   a. _____

   b. _____

   c. _____

   d. _____

2. What are four possible causes of tinnitus?

   a. _____

   b. _____

   c. _____

   d. _____

3. Can you list four suggestions you might make to help a person deal with chronic tinnitus?

   a. _____

   b. _____

   c. _____

   d. _____

4. Name two types of therapy that might be useful in the rehabilitation of a person with a hearing loss.

   a. _____

   b. _____

CRITICAL THINKING ACTIVITIES

Case Study: Otosclerosis

A 62-year-old female patient is at the ear, nose, and throat clinic regarding her hearing loss, which is getting worse. She has had a progressive loss of hearing since her late 40s. She wears bilateral hearing aids. She can hear better in her left ear than her right ear. Her mother had hearing loss starting in her 40s as well. Her evaluation has determined that she has otosclerosis. Treatment options are discussed and she has made a decision to have a stapedectomy of the right ear.

1. Why is it significant that her mother had early hearing loss?

2. What diagnostic tests would you expect she underwent during the evaluation?

3. Why is the stapedectomy to be done on the right ear rather than the left ear?

4. What preoperative teaching would you do? What would you cover?

Postoperatively, she is nauseous and states that she is quite dizzy when she tries to sit upright. She has meclizine, Percocet, and Zofran prescribed.

5. Which medication would you administer for the nausea? Which for the dizziness?

6. What safety interventions should you implement?

When the external ear dressing is removed, the patient states she can't hear a thing out of the left ear and becomes upset and tearful.

7. What is the probable cause of her inability to hear in that ear now? What could you say to her at this time that might calm her down?

STEPS TOWARD BETTER COMMUNICATION

VOCABULARY BUILDING GLOSSARY

Term	Pronunciation	Definition
am'plified	am' plah fīd	increased, made louder or bigger
catch-all	kach' awl	containing a wide variety of different things
enun'ciate	ee nun' cee āt	to speak clearly
pitch	pich	degree of highness or lowness of a sound
prompt	prom' t	quickly; on time; exactly when needed

COMPLETION

Directions: Fill in the blanks with the correct words from the Vocabulary Building Glossary to complete the statements.

1. The patient could hear low sounds but had difficulty hearing sounds with a high

   _____.

2. When a patient has a hearing loss, it is important that the nurse _____ words.

3. _____ music at concerts may be damaging to the ear and cause a loss of hearing.

4. The term *hearing loss* is a(n) _____ for several different types of physiologic problems.

5. An ear infection should receive _____ medical attention.

GRAMMAR POINTS

Review of Terms and Combining Forms

acoust/o	hearing
aural	relating to the ear
myring/o	eardrum
os, oste/o	bone
ot/o	ear
tax/o	order, coordination
toxic, tox/o	poison
tympan/o	eardrum

PRONUNCIATION SKILLS

vestib'ulococh'lear	ves tib' you lo kok' lee ar
eusta'chian	you sta' che an
sup' purative	sup' u rah tiv
labyrinthi' tis	lab ĭ rin thy' tis
tonometry	tō nom' uh trē

ABBREVIATIONS

AD	right ear
AS	left ear
AU	both ears
ENT	ear, nose, and throat
OM	otitis media

Practice pronouncing the above words and abbreviations with a peer. Have your partner write down the words or abbreviations as you say them. Check the list for accurate enunciation.

The Gastrointestinal System

chapter

27

Answer Key: Review the related chapter to answer these questions. A complete answer key was provided to your instructor.

REVIEW OF ANATOMY

Directions: Label the structures on the diagram of the digestive system.

Anus
Esophagus
Gallbladder
Large intestine
Liver
Mouth (oral cavity)
Pancreas
Parotid gland
Rectum
Small intestine
Stomach
Sublingual gland
Submandibular gland
Tongue

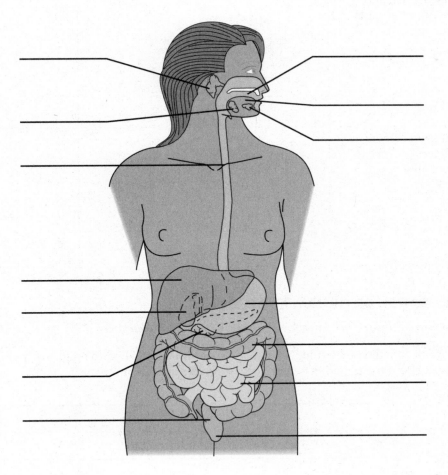

TABLE ACTIVITY

Causes and Prevention of Digestive Disorders

Directions: Complete the following table by giving the pathology and preventive measures for various causative factors in the development of digestive disorders.

Causative Factors	Pathology (What Occurs)	Preventive Measures
Psychological and emotional stress and tension		
Mechanical and chemical irritants		
Infectious agents: bacteria, viruses, parasites		

APPLICATION OF THE NURSING PROCESS

Directions: Provide a brief answer to each of the following questions.

1. Your patient is scheduled for a diagnostic workup related to epigastric pain. What questions should you ask about the patient's health history and family health history?

   a. _____

   b. _____

   c. _____

   d. _____

   e. _____

   f. _____

2. Why is checking the color of the urine a part of the gastrointestinal assessment? _____
    _____

3. What assessment data might indicate that bile is not reaching the intestine?_____
    _____

4. When a patient is experiencing nausea and vomiting, what would be an appropriate nursing diagnosis?
    _____

5. When the nursing diagnosis is Constipation due to unknown cause, what would be an appropriate ex-
    pected outcome?

    _____

    _____

6. List three specific nursing interventions for the patient who suffers from constipation.

    a. _____

    b. _____

    c. _____

7. How would you evaluate whether the above interventions were effective?

    _____

    _____

    _____

8. The patient is scheduled for an esophagogastroduodenoscopy (EGD). How would you explain this pro-
    cedure to the patient? What special care would he or she need before and after the procedure?

    a. Procedure: _____

        _____

        _____

    b. Care before EGD: _____

        _____

        _____

    c. Care after EGD: _____

        _____

        _____

PRIORITY SETTING

Directions: You are assigned to a newly admitted elderly patient who is suffering from abdominal pain and vomiting.

1. When examining the abdomen, you would perform the steps in a particular order. What order should the examination be performed?

   _____

   _____

2. As you are performing the abdominal assessment, the patient begins to vomit. What is the priority action?
   a. Assess the emesis for blood, bile, or undigested food particles.
   b. Offer the patient tissues, an emesis basin, and mouth care.
   c. Elevate the head of the bed or assist to a side-lying position.
   d. Administer a PRN antiemetic medication.

3. The patient tells you that the pain is "really bad" and seems to be getting worse. What is the first action that you should perform?
   a. Check the time and dose of last administered pain medication.
   b. Reassure the patient that everything that can be done has been done.
   c. Ask the patient to further describe and locate the pain.
   d. Report the worsening of pain to the health care provider or RN.

REVIEW QUESTIONS FOR THE NCLEX® EXAMINATION

Directions: Choose the best answer(s) for the following questions.

1. The health care provider schedules a patient for a colonoscopy. In preparing him for this procedure, you explain that:
   1. he will be sedated to minimize discomfort.
   2. the procedure takes only about 6 minutes.
   3. he may have a liquid breakfast before the procedure.
   4. he can go back to work as soon as the procedure is over.

2. The nurse is caring for several patients with gastrointestinal problems. Which patient is most likely to need a guaiac (Hemoccult) test?
   1. Patient reports dark amber-colored urine.
   2. Patient reports black discoloration of stool.
   3. Patient vomits small amounts of yellow emesis.
   4. Patient complains of right upper quadrant pain.

3. Which healthy lifestyle choice can decrease the risk of pancreatic cancer?
   1. Eat a well-balanced diet.
   2. Obtain 30 minutes of exercise at least 3 times a week.
   3. Refrain from drinking any alcohol.
   4. Refrain from smoking cigarettes.

4. When patients undergo diagnostic tests of the gastrointestinal system, elderly patients in particular must be closely watched for:
   1. dehydration and electrolyte imbalance.
   2. nausea and vomiting.
   3. diarrhea.
   4. constipation from contrast media.

5. Hyperactive bowel sounds in one quadrant and absent bowel sounds in other quadrants plus nausea and vomiting may indicate:
    1. pancreatitis.
    2. cholecystitis.
    3. gastrointestinal bleeding.
    4. intestinal obstruction.

6. Your patient is receiving an IV of $D_5\frac{1}{2}NS$ 1000 mL ordered to run at 150 mL/hr. The IV tubing delivers 15 drops per mL. You would set the IV to run at _____ gtts/min.

7. Your patient is to have a liver biopsy. What teaching point(s) should be included in the instructions? *(Select all that apply.)*
    1. Nothing is allowed by mouth for 4–8 hours prior to the procedure.
    2. Local or general anesthesia will be used.
    3. Patient will be positioned on the right side for the procedure.
    4. The procedure takes about an hour.
    5. It will be necessary to lie on the right side for 1–2 hours postprocedure.
    6. Heavy lifting or strenuous activities are to be avoided for 1–2 weeks.

8. The nurse hears in report that a patient is suspected of having ascites. Which action is the nurse most likely to initiate for this specific condition?
    1. Elevate the head of the bed 30–45 degrees.
    2. Assess for pain every 30–60 minutes.
    3. Perform serial measurements of abdominal girth.
    4. Slightly elevate legs and buttocks to help expel flatus.

9. The patient is supposed to be NPO for 12 hours prior to diagnostic testing. The nursing assistant reports that the patient just drank a soda and ate a sandwich. What should the nurse do first?
    1. Explain the purpose of NPO to the patient.
    2. Make an incident report that includes all the relevant facts.
    3. Cancel the test and reschedule it for the next day.
    4. Notify the charge nurse and the diagnostic technician.

CRITICAL THINKING ACTIVITIES

Scenario: A 78-year-old patient is admitted with nausea, vomiting, diarrhea, and dehydration. An IV of D_5RL is started at 125 mL per hour. The patient also has hypertension and osteoarthritis of the knees. The vomiting has stopped, but the patient is still somewhat nauseous.

1. Considering the nausea and vomiting, what measures would you take to help rehydrate the patient?

2. Considering the diagnosis of hypertension, what fluids would you need to use with caution in this patient?

3.   What nursing measures would you institute because of the diarrhea?

STEPS TOWARD BETTER COMMUNICATION

VOCABULARY BUILDING GLOSSARY

Term	Pronunciation	Definition
absorption (noun)	ab sorp' shun	the uptake of a substance into or across tissues
alleviate; alleviating (verb)	a lee'vee ate	to lessen, to make less severe
assimilation (noun)	as sim i lay' shun	the transformation of food into tissue
atrophy (verb)	a' tro fee	to dry up, become withered, waste away

COMPLETION

Directions: Fill in the blanks with the correct words from the Vocabulary Building Glossary to complete the statements.

1.   Taste buds may _____ as a person ages.

2.   Every attempt is made to _____ pain.

3.   Formed stool is the result of _____ of water from fecal material as it passes through the large intestine.

MATCHING

Directions: Match the abbreviation or word on the left with the correct term on the right.

1. _____   ERCP
2. _____   BE
3. _____   HIDA
4. _____   UGI
5. _____   NPO
6. _____   GI
7. _____   Mastication
8. _____   Peristalsis
9. _____   Metabolism

a.   Upper gastrointestinal
b.   Gastrointestinal
c.   Nothing by mouth
d.   Barium enema
e.   Endoscopic retrograde cholangiopancreatography
f.   Hepatobiliary iminodiacetic acid scan
g.   Converting nutrients to energy
h.   Chewing
i.   Rhythmic squeezing action

COMMUNICATION EXERCISE

Scrambled Sentences

Directions: Arrange the words in the correct order to make a sentence.

1. avoided Heavy weeks. are or to be 1–2 activities for lifting for strenuous

   _____

2. be anesthetic or will general used. local A

   _____

3. history have digestive Do a family of problems? you

   _____

CULTURAL POINT

Certain diseases have a genetic predisposition. This means people may tend to inherit that disease from their parents. Because of this, people of certain races or ethnic groups may be more likely to get a particular disease. Genetic predisposition is one reason why taking a family medical history is so important. If you are working in an area with a particular ethnic population (Jewish, Native American, Asian, etc.) be sure to inform yourself and be on the lookout for the related symptoms of diseases that are genetically predisposed in that group. Working with the groups toward education and prevention is also recommended.

Care of Patients with Disorders of the Upper Gastrointestinal System

chapter

28

Answer Key: Review the related chapter to answer these questions. A complete answer key was provided to your instructor.

REVIEW OF ANATOMY AND PHYSIOLOGY

Completion

Upper Gastrointestinal Disorders

Directions: Fill in the blanks to complete the statements.

1. A common surgical procedure for obesity that can be done laparoscopically is _____ _____.

2. In North America, an emphasis on a slim body has been an influence that has contributed to the development of _____ in young women.

3. A risk factor for cancer of the esophagus is gastric _____ and the development of _____.

4. A hiatal hernia is a defect in the wall of the _____.

5. About 90% of patients who have GERD have a(n) _____.

6. The main cause of gastritis is _____.

7. Decreased blood pressure and increased pulse do not occur in the patient with a GI bleed until he has lost more than _____ of his blood.

8. When GI bleeding first occurs, the hemoglobin and hematocrit readings may not show a drop for _____ hours.

9. Dumping syndrome sometimes occurs after the patient has had a(n) _____ _____.

10. Gastritis associated with _____ is common in the patient with kidney failure.

11. The surgical procedure of hemiglossectomy is performed for the treatment of _____ _____.

SHORT ANSWER

Ulcer Disease

Directions: Read the clinical situation and answer the questions that follow.

Scenario: Ms. Galt, age 41, works two jobs to support herself and her children. Recently, she has been skipping meals to save time and money. In the past few months, she has had frequent bouts of heartburn, has lost 15 pounds, and occasionally vomits up blood-streaked, partially digested food. She was seen by a health care provider at her neighborhood clinic who told her she may be developing a peptic ulcer and that she should eat more regularly and take an antacid when she has heartburn.

1. Although she is suffering from anxiety about her home situation, Ms. Galt's ulcer is not diagnosed as a stress ulcer. How does a stress ulcer differ from a peptic ulcer?

    _____

    _____

Ms. Galt continues to have epigastric pain and becomes too sick to work. She is scheduled for a diagnostic workup.

2. What daily pattern of pain would you expect Ms. Galt to describe when asked about her pain?

    _____

    _____

3. What type of diagnostic test would most likely be performed first? _____

    _____

4. What are the three major complications of peptic ulcer?

    a. _____

    b. _____

    c. _____

5. Her health care provider prescribes esomeprazole (Nexium) for Ms. Galt. List the three results that are expected from this drug.

    a. _____

    b. _____

    c. _____

6. Ms. Galt is also told to take an antacid four times a day, to avoid foods that disagree with her, and to return to the outpatient clinic in 3 months for follow-up. What information do you think Ms. Galt will need to take care of herself properly, recover from her illness, and return to work?

    a. _____

    b. _____

    c. _____

    d. _____

    e. _____

7. Some patients are not able to respond to medical management and must have surgery. List four surgical procedures that might be performed to treat gastric and duodenal ulcers.

a. _____

b. _____

c. _____

d. _____

APPLICATION OF THE NURSING PROCESS

Directions: Provide answers to the following questions.

Scenario: Mr. Timmons has cancer of the stomach. He has been vomiting and unable to eat and was admitted to the hospital yesterday. He has lost 7 lbs in the last week. He was started on total parenteral nutrition (TPN) yesterday afternoon.

1. Which nursing diagnosis would be appropriate for this problem?
   a. Altered nutrition due to vomiting and inability to keep food in the stomach
   b. Potential for altered electrolyte balance related to nausea and vomiting
   c. Fluid loss related to vomiting
   d. Potential for deficient fluid volume due to vomiting

2. Write an expected outcome for the correct nursing diagnosis for Mr. Timmons' problem.

   _____

3. List three interventions appropriate for Mr. Timmons related to the administration of TPN.

a. _____

b. _____

c. _____

4. What are comfort interventions often used for the patient who is vomiting?

   _____

   _____

   _____

5. What evaluation criteria would be needed to determine whether the interventions are effective and the expected outcome is being met?

   _____

   _____

PRIORITY SETTING

Scenario: You are caring for the following patients: Ms. Schultz, a confused elderly patient with gastroenteritis and dehydration; Mr. Hooper, a 45-year-old working man with a bleeding peptic ulcer; and Ms. Peterson, a 48-year-old woman who is second-day postoperative after an abdominal surgical procedure for weight control. Which patients have needs that can be delegated to the nursing assistant? Indicate the order you would attend to the following needs of these patients. It is presently 7:45 AM.

_____   a.   Ms. Schultz urgently needs to go to the bathroom.

_____   b.   Mr. Hooper has just vomited again and has called for his nurse.

_____   c.   Ms. Peterson is calling for more pain medication.

_____   d.   Ms. Peterson needs assistance with her bath.

_____   e.   Mr. Hooper is scheduled for a gastroscopy at 9:30 AM and needs to be prepared.

_____   f.   Ms. Schultz has not yet been assessed for this shift.

REVIEW QUESTIONS FOR THE NCLEX® EXAMINATION

Directions: Choose the best answer(s) for the following questions.

1. A nurse hears in report that a patient has stomatitis. Which intervention is the nurse most likely to initiate for this patient?
    1. Check for tube gastric residual before feeding.
    2. Assess for a typical 24-hour eating pattern.
    3. Offer frequent mouth care and artificial saliva.
    4. Perform a physical assessment with a skinfold measurement.

2. The nurse is caring for a patient with a gastrostomy tube. Which nursing intervention is appropriate?
    1. Flush the tube after each feeding.
    2. Instruct the patient to take some practice swallows.
    3. Give only thickened liquids.
    4. Handle the tube using sterile technique.

3. Prior to administering an enteral feeding through a feeding tube, the nurse checks for residual. What is the best rationale for performing this nursing action?
    1. Checking for residual is likely to be in the procedural manual.
    2. The appearance of residual should be documented.
    3. Excessive volume can cause regurgitation and aspiration.
    4. The nutritionist bases formula recommendations on residual content.

4. Following a stroke, a patient has dysphagia and a nursing diagnosis of Altered swallowing ability. What would be the best outcome statement?
    1. Patient will receive puréed foods and thickened liquids.
    2. Patient will increase swallowing muscle strength.
    3. Patient will control breathing while swallowing.
    4. Patient will not aspirate when swallowing.

5. A patient is second-day postoperative for gastrointestinal surgery and has a nasogastric (NG) tube attached to suction. There is little drainage in the suction container after 4 hours. What should the nurse do first?
    1. Check to see that the NG tube is still in the correct place by checking the mark near the nose.
    2. Try to aspirate some stomach contents.
    3. Irrigate the tube with the ordered amount of solution.
    4. Instill 2 mL of air into the pigtail of the NG tube with a dry syringe.

6. A patient is suspected of having esophageal cancer. Which diagnostic test is the health care provider most likely to order to make the definitive diagnosis?
   1. Esophageal manometry with 24-hour pH monitoring
   2. Gastric analysis and serum tests for *H. pylori*
   3. Upper GI series and check body mass index
   4. Esophagogastroduodenoscopy with biopsy

7. Your patient who has had gastric surgery has an NG tube attached to suction. You have irrigated the tube twice with 30 mL of sterile water. At the end of the shift, there is 420 mL of drainage in the container. The NG output for the shift is _____ mL.

8. Proton pump inhibitors such as rabeprazole (AcipHex) work by:
   1. increasing HCl secretion in the stomach.
   2. neutralizing stomach acid.
   3. both neutralizing and suppressing stomach acid.
   4. suppressing the secretion of stomach acid.

9. A nursing implication for esomeprazole (Nexium) is to:
   1. administer the drug only with food.
   2. not to administer the drug with digoxin (Lanoxin).
   3. administer the drug along with an antacid.
   4. do not administer the drug along with orange or grapefruit juice.

10. When caring for a patient with nasogastric suction, you would test the drainage for blood if you found:
    1. copious greenish drainage in the container.
    2. material resembling coffee grounds in the tubing.
    3. complaints of continued nausea by the patient.
    4. a rising blood pressure and pulse rate.

CRITICAL THINKING ACTIVITIES

Scenario A: Mr. Sims comes to the ambulatory clinic because he is having severe heartburn (GERD). He was diagnosed with a hiatal hernia a year ago. You are assigned to take his history and will do the teaching reinforcement that he needs.

1. What questions would you ask him?

2. Describe the specific teaching you would do for this patient.

Scenario B: The nurse is working in clinic that specializes in treating obesity. The nurse is responsible for assessing patients and teaching about weight management, risk factors, and treatment options.

1. Some factors of obesity are controllable, some are not. What factors contribute to obesity? *(Select all that apply.)*
   1. A high-protein, moderate-fat diet
   2. Vitamin and supplement intake
   3. A diet high in calories and fat
   4. Family genetic make-up
   5. Large dinner plates and growing portion sizes
   6. Prepackaged foods and "fast food"

2. What are the complications of obesity? *(Select all that apply.)*
   1. Hypertension
   2. Diabetes mellitus
   3. Multiple sclerosis
   4. Asthma
   5. Cholelithiasis
   6. Coronary artery disease
   7. Arthritis of the knees

3. A person is considered obese if he or she weighs more than _____ percent above ideal weight for height and body type. *(Fill in the blank.)*
   1. 10%
   2. 30%
   3. 5%
   4. 20%

4. What data would the nurse gather specific to the assessment of a patient with obesity?

5. Discuss five nonsurgical treatment approaches that may be recommend for weight loss.

STEPS TOWARD BETTER COMMUNICATION

VOCABULARY BUILDING GLOSSARY

Term	Pronunciation	Definition
regurgitation	ree gurj ah ta' shun	bringing food from the stomach back to the mouth; repeating something without thinking about it
dumping	dump'ing	dropping a mass suddenly
intrinsic factor	intrin'sik fak'tor	glycoprotein necessary for the absorption of vitamin B_{12} from the gastrointestinal system
manifested	man'ifested	showing symptoms of something
adverse	ad'verse	negative, unfavorable
adhere	ad heer'	to follow, to stick to
abound	ah bownd'	exist in great numbers; to be multiple
despite	des pyt'	in spite of; not prevented by

COMPLETION

Directions: Fill in the blanks with the correct words from the Vocabulary Building Glossary to complete the statements.

1. Sometimes after a subtotal gastrectomy and vagotomy, _____ syndrome occurs.

2. Recurrent stomach pain, nausea, and _____ may be signs of peptic ulcer.

3. Patients who lack _____ tend to develop pernicious anemia.

4. People trying to lose weight often have problems trying to _____ to their diet.

5. People who regularly take antacids _____ in our society.

MATCHING

Directions: Match the abbreviation on the left with the correct term on the right.

1. _____ GI   a. Milliliter
2. _____ NG   b. Hemoglobin
3. _____ NSAIDs   c. Gastrointestinal
4. _____ mL   d. Nasogastric
5. _____ Hb or Hgb   e. Nonsteroidal antiinflammatory drugs

PRONUNCIATION SKILLS

Directions: With a peer, take turns pronouncing these words to increase your ability to speak English clearly.

gas'troesophage'al (gas' tro ee sof ah jee' al)   pertaining to the stomach and esophagus

hy'poglyce'mic (hi' po gli see' mik)   having low serum glucose

mal'occlu'sion (mal' ah cloo' zhun)   top and bottom teeth do not come together properly

meta'bolism (mah tab' ah lizm)   process of building up and breaking down tissue

The pronunciation of the letters **"ai"** in the two words constraint and contraindicated are different. In the first word, they make the long **"a"** sound because they are in the same syllable and are pronounced together (as in p<u>ai</u>n and compl<u>ai</u>n). In the second word, they are pronounced separately because they are in different syllables:

con str<u>ai</u>nts (kon strants')

con tr<u>a i</u>n di ca ted (kon' trah in' di ka' ted)

Care of Patients with Disorders of the Lower Gastrointestinal System

Answer Key: Review the related chapter to answer these questions. A complete answer key was provided to your instructor.

SHORT ANSWER

Assessment and Pathophysiology

Directions: Provide brief answers for the following questions.

1. The cause of irritable bowel syndrome is unknown, but several things seem to trigger episodes, including:

   _____

   _____

2. The pathophysiologic explanation for diverticulitis is:_____

   _____

   _____

3. If an elderly person develops appendicitis, the presenting signs and symptoms may differ from those in a younger adult. The older adult may present with only _____

   _____.

4. Peritonitis may occur when the appendix ruptures. The pathophysiologic explanation is:

   _____

   _____

   _____

5. Hemorrhoids may be internal or external and usually present with:_____

   _____

COMPLETION

Lower Gastrointestinal Disorders

Directions: Fill in the blank to complete the statement.

1. Severe malabsorption problems of the small intestine often necessitate _____

   _____.

2. An abdominoperineal resection requires a(n) _____ colostomy.

3. If a hernia becomes incarcerated, it can cause _____ of the protruding part.

4. Instead of surgery, hemorrhoids can sometimes be removed by _____ or _____.

5. A diet high in _____ is thought to contribute to the formation of cancer of the colon.

LABELING

Ostomies

Directions: Write the correct names of the procedures depicted in the three drawings below.

1. _____   2. _____   3. _____
   _____

COMPLETION

Directions: Fill in the blanks to complete the statements.

1. The discharge from an ascending colostomy is normally _____.

2. A potential problem for the patient with a sigmoid colostomy is _____.

3. An ascending colostomy is usually _____.

4. The discharge from an ileostomy is _____.

5. An ileostomy is often performed on the patient who has _____.

6. A continent ileostomy is drained by _____.

7. It is easier to establish a pattern of evacuation to control the flow of fecal material through a(n) _____ colostomy.

8. In a double-barreled colostomy, the distal stoma leads to the rectum and should discharge only small

amounts of _____.

9. The colonoscopy shows a small, apparently localized tumor in the upper sigmoid colon. The treatment

of choice for this tumor would be _____.

SHORT ANSWER

Directions: Write a short answer for each of the following questions.

1. What are two major principles that should be followed to protect the skin around the stoma from irritation and breakdown?

a. _____

b. _____

2. What is the major reason for irrigating a colostomy? _____

_____

3. What three nursing interventions may help prevent cramping, nausea, and dizziness during a colostomy irrigation?

a. _____

b. _____

c. _____

4. What three nursing interventions may help a patient prevent or overcome repeated expulsion of gas
from the colostomy?

a. _____

b. _____

c. _____

5. What three nursing interventions may help a patient prevent or overcome obstruction of the ileostomy?

a. _____

b. _____

c. _____

6. List four nursing interventions that might be helpful in assisting the patient to adjust psychologically
to an ostomy.

a. _____

b. _____

c. _____

d. _____

COMPLETION

Medications

Directions: Fill in the answers to the following questions.

1. List two important points the nurse should teach the patient who has diphenoxylate hydrochloride (Lomotil) prescribed.

    a. _____

    b. _____

2. What is a contraindication to using a stool softener? _____

    _____

3. Name a major problem with the use of contact laxatives. _____

    _____

4. Give an important nursing implication for administering a histamine receptor antagonist to a patient who is also taking an antacid.

    _____

5. How should a patient who has an antispasmodic prescribed be taught to take it? _____

    _____

6. What should the diabetic patient taking an oral hypoglycemic drug and sulfasalazine be specifically told to prevent a problem?

    _____

    _____

PRIORITY SETTING

Scenario: You are assigned the following patients: Ms. K., a newly admitted female, 68 years old, with probable intestinal obstruction; Mr. P., a 46-year-old male 1 day postoperative for a ruptured appendix and peritonitis; Ms. T., a 72-year-old female with diverticulitis and dehydration; and Ms. S., a 56-year-old female patient with Crohn disease on total parenteral nutrition (TPN). You have just received shift report for the previous shift. Place the following tasks and needs in the order in which you would attend to them.

_____   a. Ms. T. is calling for pain medication.

_____   b. Assessment (data collection) for Ms. T.

_____   c. Wound irrigation and dressing change for Mr. P.

_____   d. Assessment (data collection) for Mr. P.

_____   e. Ms. K. is vomiting, coughing, and calling for help.

_____   f. Assessment (data collection) for Ms. K.

_____   g. Assessment (data collection) of Ms. S. including blood sugar determination.

REVIEW QUESTIONS FOR THE NCLEX® EXAMINATION

Directions: Choose or supply the best answer(s) for the following questions.

1. The patient has a diagnosis of irritable bowel syndrome. What symptoms is the patient mostly likely to display?
   1. Constipation and/or diarrhea, abdominal pain, bloating
   2. Abnormal pouching out from the abdominal wall or in the groin area
   3. Frequent high-pitched bowel sounds in the area of peristaltic contractions
   4. Rapid dehydration and only slight abdominal distention

2. A female patient, age 26, has been diagnosed with ulcerative colitis. She is hospitalized for intestinal surgery. When gathering data on this patient, the nurse would expect to obtain a history of:
   1. alternating bowel pattern of diarrhea and constipation.
   2. intolerance to milk and milk products.
   3. episodes of bloody, mucoid diarrhea.
   4. excessive smoking and/or alcohol use.

3. In planning care for a patient with ulcerative colitis, there is a nursing diagnosis of Altered nutrition. Which intervention is most appropriate?
   1. Offer small, frequent amounts of high-protein, high-calorie food.
   2. Help the patient list effective coping mechanisms to deal with weight loss.
   3. Encourage large amounts of favorite and culturally acceptable foods.
   4. Advise the patient to exercise less and adopt a sedentary lifestyle.

4. The nurse is assessing a patient's abdomen and observes an outpouching of tissue on the abdomen. What should the nurse do *first*?
   1. Immediately report the finding to the RN or the health care provider.
   2. Ask the patient if this outpouching has recently occurred after lifting.
   3. Push on the outpouching to determine if there is a reducible hernia.
   4. Suggest that the patient make an appointment with a surgeon.

5. What evaluation finding indicates that therapy for intestinal inflammation is effective?
   1. Decrease in the number of diarrheal stools
   2. Decrease in appetite and food consumption
   3. Decrease in hemoglobin and hematocrit
   4. Decrease in weight and energy

6. Treatment of ulcerative colitis sometimes involves resting the bowel. In this event, the patient is placed on:
   1. long-term intravenous fluids.
   2. a bland diet for several weeks.
   3. a low-residue diet for 3 weeks.
   4. TPN.

7. When a patient is receiving TPN, the nurse incorporates which safety factor into the plan of care?
   1. Never speeding up the TPN solution if it falls behind schedule
   2. Carefully monitoring and assessing intake and output
   3. Changing the peripheral IV site every 48 hours
   4. Monitoring for signs of hypoglycemia during each nursing shift

8. The nurse is caring for a postsurgical patient who had abdominal perineal resection with a permanent colostomy. Why is a permanent colostomy necessary?
   1. The recovery time is lengthy and prohibits the reconnection of the colon.
   2. The anus is surgically removed in this procedure.
   3. The lower colon and anus are nonfunctional due to the disease process.
   4. Bowel rest enhances chemotherapy and radiation treatments.

9. A sign of colon cancer that a patient might experience is:
   1. nausea.
   2. excessive gas.
   3. pain after eating.
   4. black stool.

10. Which ostomy patient is most at risk for alteration in skin integrity related to contact with digestive enzymes at the ostomy site?
    1. Patient with an ileostomy
    2. Patient with sigmoid colostomy
    3. Patient with a double-barreled colostomy
    4. Patient with a continent ileostomy

11. The patient has an order to "force fluids." The intake and output records indicate the following for this shift:

	Intake	Output
0730		650 mL
0800	250 mL	
0900	220 mL	
1000	175 mL	420 mL
1100	225 mL	
1200	110 mL	
1300	455 mL	
1400	180 mL	675 mL
1500	220 mL	

    The intake and output for the shift are: I = _____ O = _____

12. A patient with diverticulitis and dehydration is receiving intravenous fluid. The order reads D_5NS 1000 mL at 150 mL/hr. The available IV tubing delivers 10 gtts/mL. The IV should run at _____ gtts/min.

13. The nurse is caring for a patient who had intestinal surgery. In the immediate postoperative period, what is the priority nursing diagnosis?
    1. Potential for fluid volume deficit
    2. Potential for nausea
    3. Potential for infection
    4. Altered body image

14. The nurse is observing the new stoma of a patient who recently had a colostomy. Which finding is the nurse most concerned about?
    1. There is slight bleeding around the stoma and the stem.
    2. The stoma has a cherry-red color and appears moist.
    3. The stoma has a deepening purplish color.
    4. There is no fecal output on the second postoperative day.

15. The patient with diverticular disease states, "Why can't I eat raspberries? I love them." What is the best nursing response to the patient's question?
    1. The berries can cause a bowel obstruction.
    2. The red color will come out in your stool and look like blood.
    3. The seeds will scratch the mucosa and cause bleeding.
    4. The seeds can get caught in the pouchings and cause inflammation.

16. The nursing student is caring for a patient with a possible appendicitis. The nurse would intervene if the student performed which action?
    1. Suggests that the patient rest with the right thigh drawn up
    2. Checks the patient's vital signs, including temperature
    3. Applies a warm pack to the right lower quadrant for comfort
    4. Explains that food and fluids are not allowed at this time

17. The patient reports that after a bowel movement, the stool is floating in the water. What is the significance of this finding?
    1. A stool specimen should be collected for culture and sensitivity.
    2. The patient may not be eating enough fiber in the diet.
    3. There may be a problem with the digestion of fat.
    4. Potentially there is insufficient bile to aid digestion.

CRITICAL THINKING ACTIVITIES

Scenario: Ms. Rubens has had inflammatory bowel disease for the past 5 years. Her specific diagnosis is Crohn disease. She is tired of feeling ill all the time, the diarrhea episodes, and inability to work full-time. The infliximab (Remicade) infusions don't seem to help much anymore. She is presently anemic, has lost 10 lbs in the past few months, and is seeking treatment that will help her have an improved lifestyle. She enters the hospital for hyperalimentation with TPN.

1. When you come onto your shift and are assigned this patient, which laboratory values would you check in the medical record?

2. How do the signs and symptoms of Crohn disease differ from those of ulcerative colitis?

3. Why is surgery not a first choice for patients with Crohn disease?

4. What type of drug is infliximab? What are its major side effects?

STEPS TOWARD BETTER COMMUNICATION

VOCABULARY BUILDING GLOSSARY

Term	Pronunciation	Definition
adhere	ad heer'	to follow, to stick to
adverse	ad'verse	negative, unfavorable
manifested	man'ifested	showing symptoms of something
mush		a soft, wet mass; consistency of cooked cereal
constraints	kon strayn'ts	limitations
"worry wort"		person who worries about everything
offend'ing	ah fend' ing	causing a problem
gur'gle	ger' gul	sound of water or liquid bubbling (as in boiling or moving over stones)
bout	bowt	a short, difficult period
empathy	em' pa thee	understanding another person's feelings
effluent	ef' floo ent	material discharged or flowing out
blanching	blanch' ing	turning white or light-colored

COMPLETION

Directions: Fill in the blanks with the correct words from the Vocabulary Building Glossary to complete the statements.

1. The patient's stool was the consistency of _____.

2. Because the patient worried about every little thing, she was called a(n) _____.

3. The _____ from a new ileostomy must be carefully measured.

4. The patient was having trouble with his ileostomy because he did not _____ to the dietary guidelines.

5. Ostomy patients worry about _____ those around them with bad odors.

6. The patient's intestinal disease was _____ by frequent bouts of bloody diarrhea.

7. While auscultating bowel sounds, the nurse heard a(n) _____ in the left upper quadrant.

8. The nurse checked the reddened area on the patient's buttocks for _____ when she turned him to determine if a pressure ulcer was developing.

9. The patient who ignores signs of colon cancer may have a(n) _____ outcome.

10. The patient with diverticulitis was experiencing another _____ of severe abdominal pain.

11. The nurse must try to develop _____ for patients who are experiencing a tremendous body image change due to an ostomy.

MATCHING

Directions: Match the abbreviation on the left with the correct term on the right.

1. _____ BM
2. _____ IBS
3. _____ IBD
4. _____ TPN

a. Inflammatory bowel disease
b. Bowel movement
c. Total parenteral nutrition
d. Irritable bowel syndrome

PRONUNCIATION SKILLS

Directions: Practice pronouncing these words with a peer to increase your ability to speak English.

def'ecate (def' ah kayt)   eliminate stool

incon'tinence (in kon' tah nens)   no control over passage of urine or stool

piloni'dal (py lo nydal)   having a core of hair

sa'crococcyg'eal (sa' kro kok sij' ee al)   pertaining to the sacrum and coccyx

CULTURAL POINT

There are a variety of common terms that patients may use for digestive functions. Proper medical terms are listed below in dark print; the other terms are not medical terms and are impolite, but you should understand the meaning when you hear them.

bowel movement (BM), **defecate**, **stool**, **feces**, shit, crap, excreta, poop, dump

gas, **flatus**, **flatulence**, pass gas, pass wind, fart, poop

diarrhea, the runs, the trots

Care of Patients with Disorders of the Gallbladder, Liver, and Pancreas

Answer Key: Review the related chapter to answer these questions. A complete answer key was provided to your instructor.

COMPLETION

Gallbladder Disease

Directions: Fill in the blanks to complete the statements.

1. The most frequent cause of cholecystitis is _____.

2. _____ is the presence of gallstones within the gallbladder or in the biliary tract.

3. Treatment of cholelithiasis using medications has the goal of _____ _____.

4. Four types of people most at risk for developing cholelithiasis are those who:

    a. _____

    b. _____

    c. _____

    d. _____

5. List four diagnostic tests that may be ordered to diagnose cholelithiasis or gallbladder disease.

    a. _____

    b. _____

    c. _____

    d. _____

Diseases of the Liver and Pancreas

Directions: Fill in the blanks to complete the statements.

1. Ascites is the result of a condition in which there is _____ of the portal circulation.

2. Medical treatment of ascites includes restriction of _____ and _____ and administration of _____.

3. The insertion of a large needle into the peritoneal cavity to remove ascitic fluid is called a(n)

   _____.

4. A transjugular intrahepatic portosystemic shunt (TIPS) procedure involves placing stents to bypass

   some of the portal circulation for the purpose of _____

   _____.

5. Neurologic changes that occur as a result of liver failure constitute a condition called _____

   _____.

6. Jaundice occurs when _____ flow out of the liver is blocked and

   _____ is entering the bloodstream.

7. In liver failure, mental status changes that can progress to coma are thought to be due to excess

   _____ in the blood, which alters brain cell function.

8. The patient with cirrhosis needs to be protected from exposure to _____.

9. The most deadly of all complications of cirrhosis of the liver is _____

   _____.

10. Both hepatitis B and cirrhosis increase the risk of _____.

11. If the tumor is confined to the liver, _____ is an option.

12. Three causes of pancreatitis are _____, _____,

    and _____.

13. When powdered pancreatic enzymes are given with food, the powder should be mixed in

    _____; it should not be allowed to remain on the

    _____ because it will cause irritation.

14. Cancer of the pancreas is twice as frequent among _____.

REVIEW QUESTIONS FOR THE NCLEX® EXAMINATION

Directions: Choose the best answer(s) for the following questions.

1. The nurse is caring for a patient who is known to be infected with hepatitis A. Which infection control
   precautions should the nurse implement? *(Select all that apply.)*
   1. Wear a mask when entering the patient's room.
   2. Wear a gown when delivering the patient's meal tray.
   3. Wear a gown and gloves when bathing the patient.
   4. Wear latex gloves when emptying the bedpan after a bowel movement.
   5. Wear a face shield during dressing changes.
   6. Wear protective shoe covers when assisting patient with ambulation.

2. The nurse is caring for a patient with acute pancreatitis. What is the priority nursing diagnosis?
   1. Potential for infection
   2. Acute pain
   3. Alteration in gas exchange
   4. Nutrition deficit

3. The nurse is caring for several patients. The post-cholecystectomy patient is requesting assistance with ambulation. The patient with pancreatitis wants medication for nausea. The cirrhosis patient has just noticed considerable blood in his stool. The patient with possible cancer of the liver is complaining of pain. Which patient should the nurse attend to *first*?
   1. The post-cholecystectomy patient
   2. The patient with cirrhosis of the liver
   3. The patient with pancreatitis
   4. The patient with possible cancer of the liver

4. Which medication is used to decrease ammonia levels in the patient with liver failure?
   1. Vasopressin (Pitressin)
   2. Esomeprazole (Nexium)
   3. Furosemide (Lasix)
   4. Lactulose (Cephulac)

5. Hepatitis virus is transmitted by various routes. Which virus is transmitted by the gastrointestinal route?
   1. Hepatitis A
   2. Hepatitis B
   3. Hepatitis C
   4. Hepatitis D

6. Which condition is most likely to be associated with complaints of pain radiating to the back at the level of the shoulder blade?
   1. Cholelithiasis
   2. Cirrhosis of the liver
   3. Pancreatitis
   4. Cancer of the pancreas

7. When are the symptoms of cholecystitis usually the most noticeable?
   1. After eating a fatty meal
   2. During exercising or exertion
   3. After drinking excessive alcohol
   4. Upon waking in the morning

8. The patient is diagnosed with liver failure and the ammonia level is elevated. Which potential problem would be most relevant?
   1. Acute confusion
   2. Decreased cardiac perfusion
   3. Infection
   4. Shock

9. The *highest* priority of nursing care for the patient with pancreatitis would be:
   1. providing supplemental enzymes for digestion of food.
   2. providing skin care to relieve pruritus.
   3. medicating for nausea whenever needed.
   4. providing adequate pain control.

10. Important nursing actions for the patient with symptoms of hepatitis are: (*Select all that apply.*)
    1. encourage as much rest as possible.
    2. encourage a high-protein diet.
    3. offer six small meals a day to counteract anorexia.
    4. reinforce teaching of hand hygiene.
    5. suggest diversional activities such as computer games.

11. Which of these signs and symptoms could signal liver transplant rejection?
    1. Change in color of stool or urine
    2. Depression and anxiety
    3. Right upper quadrant pain that is worse after eating
    4. Preference for fetal position to relieve pain

12. Which description of pain would the nurse expect to find when assessing a patient who is diagnosed with acute pancreatitis?
    1. Acute, steady abdominal pain localized to the epigastrium
    2. Acute pain with abdominal rigidity below the umbilicus
    3. Generalized dull abdominal pain with marked ascites
    4. Right quadrant or flank pain with low-grade fever

13. What assessment findings are likely for a patient who has acute pancreatitis? *(Select all that apply.)*
    1. Abdominal tenderness and guarding
    2. Fever
    3. Weight loss
    4. Dark, foamy urine
    5. Mild jaundice
    6. Nausea, vomiting, and weakness

14. What are the main symptoms of pancreatic cancer?
    1. Epigastric pain and weight loss
    2. Rectal bleeding and frequent diarrhea
    3. Increase in appetite and excessive thirst
    4. Intolerance to fatty foods with vomiting

15. The nurse is supervising a postcholecystectomy patient who is selecting foods from a hospital menu. The nurse would intervene if the patient made which selection?
    1. Oatmeal with skim milk
    2. Biscuits with gravy
    3. Toast with strawberry jam
    4. Coffee and orange juice

CRITICAL THINKING ACTIVITIES

Directions: Read the clinical scenario below and answer the questions that follow.

Scenario: Mr. Poe, age 29, is admitted to the hospital with possible viral hepatitis. He was in an automobile accident 6 weeks ago and had received two units of blood. One week ago, he returned from a vacation at the seashore where he had eaten a significant amount of shellfish. Within the past few days, he has felt very weak and tired and finally went to his health care provider, who hospitalized him.

1. What would you look for in Mr. Poe's health history that would be helpful to the health care provider in diagnosing his illness?

    a. _____

    b. _____

    c. _____

    d. _____

2. List subjective and objective data that would indicate inflammation or damage to Mr. Poe's liver.

   Subjective data: _____

   _____

   Objective data: _____

   _____

   _____

Within a few days of admission, Mr. Poe began to exhibit signs of severe jaundice. His diagnosis was type B viral hepatitis with liver damage.

3. List specific nursing actions that can be taken to help Mr. Poe with each of the following problems.

   a. Fatigue: _____

   _____

   _____

   b. Bleeding tendency: _____

   _____

   _____

   c. Nausea, vomiting, and anorexia: _____

   _____

   _____

4. What special precautions to prevent the spread of infection would you expect to be necessary in the care of Mr. Poe?

   _____

   _____

   _____

   _____

5. An IV infusion is ordered for Mr. Poe. The order reads D_5W 1000 mL at 100 mL/hr. The tubing set delivers 15 drops per mL. How many drops per minute should the IV run to infuse within the allotted time?

   _____

6. What might be given to individuals who were in close contact with Mr. Poe to provide them with passive immunity against type B hepatitis?

   _____

   _____

7. If Mr. Poe were to become a carrier of type B hepatitis, he would be at high risk for developing what conditions?

   a. _____

   b. _____

   c. _____

8. What should Mr. Poe know to avoid future liver damage from hepatotoxins? _____

   _____

   _____

   _____

STEPS TOWARD BETTER COMMUNICATION

VOCABULARY BUILDING GLOSSARY

Term	Pronunciation	Definition
accessory	ek ses' ah ree	additional, supplemental
geared (to/for/toward)	geer' d	aimed, intended for, adapted for a particular situation
prevalent	prev'alent	common, often occurs, widespread
plugged up		stopped by a blockage

COMPLETION

Directions: Fill in the blanks with the correct words from the Vocabulary Building Glossary to complete the statements.

1. Hepatitis is quite _____ among travelers.

2. The gallstone _____ the common duct, causing a backup of bile in the gallbladder and liver.

3. Much of the care of the patient with hepatitis A is _____ toward preventing the spread of infection.

4. The pancreas is a(n) _____ organ of the digestive system.

PRONUNCIATION SKILLS

These words are somewhat difficult to pronounce:

cholelith'iasis (ko le li thy' ah sis)
cholan'giopan'creatog'raphy (ko lan' jee o pan' cree ah tog' rah fee)
phagocyte (fah' go syt)
phagocytic (fah' go sit' ic)

Directions: Practice pronouncing the above words with a peer partner.

Short "i" Sound

Short i (ĭ) is the sound of the letter **"i"** in the words *it, is, infect, minute,* and *liver.* It is usually written with the letter "i," but sometimes with the letter "y."

*Directions: Draw a line under the letters in the following words that have the sound of short **"i."** Then practice pronouncing the words aloud.*

liver, filter, topic, digestive, insulin, lipid, sluggish, lipase, nutrition, cirrhosis, irritation, toxins, cholelithiasis, fluid deficit, bilirubin, Pitressin infusion, carcinogenic, phagocytic

WORD ATTACK SKILLS

Combining Forms

These combining forms are used frequently in Chapter 30:

chol/e	bile
lith/o	stone
-iasis	condition
-angi/o	vessel
pancreat/o	pancreas
-graphy	recording

Directions: Using vertical lines, break each word into its word elements (parts) and give the meaning of the word.

1. cholelithiasis: _____

2. cholangiopancreatography: _____

GRAMMAR POINTS

When asking questions during assessment about things that happened *in the past over a period of time,* it is often necessary to use the verb construction *have* plus the past participle form of the verb (the present perfect tense). *Examples:*

Have you had any pain?

Have you had any injuries?

Have you had any problems with…?

Have you used cleaning agents containing carbon tetrachloride?

How long have you taken this medication?

Have you taken any other drugs?

Have you been exposed to pesticides or toxins?

Have you been exposed to hepatitis?

Have you been tired lately?

How long have you been drinking?

This is different from talking about something *that happened in the past and was completed*. These statements use the simple past form of the verb. *Examples:*

Did you see the doctor recently?

I saw him last week.

When did you have the accident?

I had it last year in February.

The Musculoskeletal System

Answer Key: Review the related chapter to answer these questions. A complete answer key was provided to your instructor.

REVIEW OF ANATOMY AND PHYSIOLOGY

Completion

Changes Occurring with Aging

Directions: Complete the following statements.

1. As we age, bone density decreases because of _____.

2. Kyphosis in the elderly is because of thinning of the _____ and collapse of

   the _____.

3. The bones of the elderly break more easily because they are _____ and

   _____.

4. Stiffness and crepitation in the joints are a result of joint _____ and erosion

   from _____.

5. Nighttime muscle cramping in the elderly is increased because of _____

   and accumulation of _____.

SHORT ANSWER

Causes and Prevention of Musculoskeletal Disorders

Directions: Provide short answers to complete the following statements.

1. Poor nutrition can contribute to musculoskeletal problems because there may be _____

   _____.

2. Malignant tumors can contribute to musculoskeletal disorders in which two ways?

   a. _____

   b. _____

3. Five measures that can help prevent musculoskeletal disorders are:

    a. _____

    b. _____

    c. _____

    d. _____

    e. _____

MATCHING

Diagnostic Tests

Directions: Match the procedure on the left with the most appropriate phrase on the right.

1. _____ Bone scan
2. _____ Arthroscopy
3. _____ Arthrocentesis
4. _____ Synovial analysis
5. _____ Culture
6. _____ Goniometry
7. _____ Muscle strength

a. Measurement of range of motion of a joint
b. Apply ice or cold packs, support joint with pillows
c. Grading ranges from 0 (paralysis) to 5 (normal)
d. After procedure, watch for signs of infection, hemarthrosis, swelling, and injury to joint or loss of feeling
e. Normal findings are clear, viscous fluid containing no or very few blood cells
f. After procedure, monitor site of venipuncture for signs of inflammation and hematoma
g. Examination of bone tissue to identify infecting organism

APPLICATION OF THE NURSING PROCESS

Directions: Answer the questions that follow.

1. List three significant findings the nurse might record when taking a history during assessment of a patient with a complaint of back pain.

    a. _____

    b. _____

    c. _____

2. List three observations that the nurse can make about a patient's ability to move and walk.

    a. _____

    b. _____

    c. _____

3. Three nursing problem statements concerning physical aspects that would probably be found on the care plan for the patient who has severe rheumatoid arthritis affecting the hands, knees, and hips are:

    a. _____

    b. _____

    c. _____

4. Expected outcomes for the above nursing problem statements might be:

a. _____

b. _____

c. _____

COMPLETION

Directions: Fill in the blanks to complete the statements.

1. Joint mobility is maintained by regularly performing _____ exercises.

2. A patient who is immobilized for a long period of time loses _____ from his bones.

3. Lengthy immobilization tends to cause muscle to _____.

4. If ankylosis of a joint is unavoidable, the joint is _____ so that the extremity will have maximum function.

5. _____ exercise is helpful in preventing osteoporosis.

6. Proper exercise and positioning of joints for an immobile patient is extremely important because a contracture can begin to occur within as little as _____.

PRIORITY SETTING

Directions: You are assigned to ambulate an 82-year-old female patient who is recovering after a pelvic fracture. She had been on very limited activity and is still somewhat weak. Place the actions into the order in which you would carry them out. She uses a cane to ambulate.

_____ a. Plan how far you will go with her as she will have to come back as well.

_____ b. Have her stand still to dispel any dizziness.

_____ c. Check the orders.

_____ d. Assist to sit in the chair.

_____ e. Assess her ability to move, stand, and ambulate.

_____ f. Attach the gait belt to her.

_____ g. Assist to sit up in bed.

_____ h. Identify the patient.

_____ i. Ambulate back to the room.

_____ j. Perform hand hygiene.

_____ k. Hand her the cane.

_____ l. Assist to stand.

_____ m. Ambulate the correct distance.

_____ n. Assist to sit on the side of the bed.

REVIEW QUESTIONS FOR THE NCLEX® EXAMINATION

Directions: Choose the best answer(s) to the following questions.

1. Magnetic resonance imaging (MRI) is used to help diagnose a variety of musculoskeletal problems. What instructions would you give the patient who is to undergo an MRI? *(Select all that apply.)*
   1. A consent must be signed for this procedure.
   2. You must remove all metal from your body.
   3. You will be given a contrast medium to drink.
   4. You will need to remain perfectly still for 15–60 minutes.
   5. If you are claustrophobic, you may ask for a sedative beforehand.

2. When assessing whether crutches have been fitted to the patient properly, you know that when walking with them, the: *(Select all that apply.)*
   1. axillary bar should be two finger-breadths below the axilla.
   2. elbow should be flexed at a 45-degree angle.
   3. elbow should be flexed at a 30-degree angle.
   4. crutches should be about 16 inches shorter than the patient's height.
   5. axillary pad should fit snugly into the axilla.

3. The patient is selecting foods from a menu to demonstrate knowledge of dietary calcium sources. Which selection indicates that the patient needs additional information about the absorption of calcium from food sources?
   1. Green leafy vegetables
   2. Canned sardines
   3. Cheese and yogurt
   4. Milk

4. A way to try to prevent musculoskeletal disorders including rheumatoid arthritis is:
   1. exercise regularly throughout life.
   2. refrain from smoking or stop smoking.
   3. decrease the amount of fat consumed in the diet.
   4. maintain good posture at all times.

5. When checking the joints during a focused assessment, you should: *(Select all that apply.)*
   1. palpate them for tenderness.
   2. position them to full extension and flexion.
   3. inspect them for swelling or deformity.
   4. assess for warmth over the joint.
   5. determine range of motion without pain.

6. The nurse is assigned to care for several orthopedic patients. In planning care, it is appropriate to assign which task to unlicensed assistive personnel?
   1. Assess for pain in the patient who had an arthrocentesis.
   2. Take vital signs on each patient who has returned from a procedure.
   3. Determine whether the patient who had an arthroscopy is having any drainage.
   4. Assist the patient with a hip replacement to get out of bed for the first time.

7. When a walker is used for ambulation, it is important that it be appropriate height for the patient. Most walkers have adjustable legs. When walking with it, the walker height is correct when the patient's elbow is:
   1. locked to sustain the weight of the upper body.
   2. bent at 15–30 degrees.
   3. at a 45-degree angle to swing the walker forward.
   4. just slightly bent.

8. Because the patient is immobilized, the health care provider has ordered Lovenox, low–molecular-weight heparin injections. The prescription reads: enoxaparin sodium 60 mg subcut per day in 2 divided doses. On hand is enoxaparin sodium 30 mg/mL. How much medication would you draw up for each injection? _____ mL
    1. 1 mL
    2. 2 mL
    3. 0.5 mL
    4. 0.1 mL

9. An elderly patient with arthritis has a nursing diagnosis of Functional incontinence. Which intervention should the nurse use?
    1. Instruct the nursing assistant to report number of linen changes.
    2. Instruct the patient to call for assistance in getting to the toilet.
    3. Closely monitor the intake and output to observe for fluid balance.
    4. Suggest incontinence briefs until bladder control is achieved.

10. The nurse observes that an elderly patient has decreased strength, unsteady balance, slow reflexes, and a gait disturbance. What is the priority problem?
    1. Potential for falls
    2. Altered mobility
    3. Altered activity tolerance
    4. Altered self-care ability

CRITICAL THINKING ACTIVITIES

Scenario A: You are to teach a patient about proper and safe use of crutches. The patient cannot bear weight on the left leg.

1. Describe how you would teach the patient to go up and down stairs.

2. What safety measures would you teach?

Scenario B: You are assigned a patient who has rheumatoid arthritis who is recovering from an appendectomy. You need to have the patient exercise his joints.

1. How would you prepare the patient to do the exercises?

2. What would you do to prevent excessive pain during the exercise sessions?

STEPS TOWARD BETTER COMMUNICATION

VOCABULARY BUILDING GLOSSARY

Term	Pronunciation	Definition
deficit	def' ah sit	not enough, insufficient, less than required
distal		farthest away from, remote
dowager	dow' ah jer	an older widow, one who usually has money and owns property
initiate	in i' shee ayt	to start, begin, commence
flaccid	flas' id	limp, soft, hanging loose, drooping
trigger	trig' ger	initiate, cause to begin

COMPLETION

Directions: Fill in the blanks with the correct words from the Vocabulary Building Glossary to complete the statements.

1. When an injury has occurred to an extremity, the nurse checks the pulse _____ to the area of trauma.

2. An abnormal finding in a musculoskeletal assessment would be _____ muscles in the right lower extremity.

3. Accidentally brushing against the weights of a traction device may _____ pain for the patient.

4. Osteoarthritis often causes a(n) _____ in joint motion.

5. Sometimes the nurse must _____ action to obtain heat or cold treatments for a patient who needs them.

6. The bent-forward position of the elderly lady showed that she had a(n) _____ hump.

COMMUNICATION EXERCISE

Directions: Here are some examples of what to say if a patient were to ask you the following questions.

1. What is the difference between a tendon and a ligament?

   Ligaments hold the joint together. Tendons anchor muscle to bone.

2. What is the purpose of cartilage?

   Cartilage provides a cushion between the bones of the joint.

3. What is the difference between a sprain and a strain?

   A sprain involves stretching or tearing of ligaments around a joint. A strain involves pulling and tearing of a muscle or a tendon or both.

WORD ATTACK SKILLS

Directions: Study the word parts and answer the related questions.

1. ankyl/o   crooked or bent

   Can you think of a joint whose name came from this word element? _____

2. ab-   from

   ad-   to, toward

   re-   gain, do again

   -sorb   to attract or retain substances

Directions: Write the meanings of the following words:

   a. Absorb: _____

   b. Adsorb: _____

   c. Resorb: _____

3. -esthesi/o   sensation

   If *anesthesia* means without pain and *paresthesia* means having numbness or tingling, what does *para-* mean? _____

Pronunciation

Directions: Practice pronouncing the following words with a peer.

throm'bophlebit'is (throm' bo flee by' tus)

ankylo'sis (ang' kee lo' sis)

kypho'sis (ki fo' sis)

crepi'ta'tion (krep' i tay' shun)

Also practice pronouncing the terms given in the Focused Assessment box in the textbook.

Descriptive Terms

Directions: Here are some terms commonly used to describe findings of physical assessment:

Posture: erect, slumped, rounded-shouldered, straight

Gait: normal, rolling, heel-toe, toe-heel, ataxic, ambling, slow, rapid, bouncy

Range of motion: full, limited, diminished, little, restricted

Spine: normal curve, S-shaped, abnormally curved, tender, rounded

Joints: normal, reddened, swollen, painful, deformed, immovable, contracted, freely movable

Skeletal muscles: good tone, well-developed, underdeveloped, tense, hard, soft, poor tone, atrophic, painful

COMMUNICATION EXERCISE

Assessment Questions: History-Taking

Using the Focused Assessment box, practice asking and answering the questions with a peer. Answer either from your own experience or with imaginary answers. When you are the "patient," do not look in the book. Your responsibility is to listen and ask for repetition and clarification when you do not understand your partner, who is practicing the role of nurse.

Care of Patients with Musculoskeletal and Connective Tissue Disorders

chapter

32

Answer Key: Review the related chapter to answer these questions. A complete answer key was provided to your instructor.

COMPLETION

Musculoskeletal and Connective Tissue Disorders

Directions: Fill in the blanks to complete the statements.

1. Subluxation is a partial dislocation that usually occurs from _____.

2. With the pain of chronic osteoarthritis, the patient should not take more than _____ mg of acetaminophen a day.

3. The most common cause of below-the-knee amputation is _____.

4. In addition to increasing calcium and vitamin D, one of the best ways for women to prevent osteoporosis is to perform _____.

5. The most common cause of osteomyelitis is _____.

6. The muscles most commonly afflicted with muscle strain are the _____, _____, and _____ muscles.

SHORT ANSWER

Arthritis

Directions: Answer the following questions about arthritis in the spaces provided.

1. List four questions the nurse might ask when assessing the status of a patient with arthritis.

    a. _____

    b. _____

    c. _____

    d. _____

2. What are some objective data the nurse might collect when assessing a patient with arthritis?

    a. _____

    b. _____

    c. _____

3. List some interventions for patient with arthritis and a nursing problem of altered activity tolerance.

   a. _____

   b. _____

   c. _____

   d. _____

   e. _____

4. Summarize important teaching points for applications of cold and heat for your patient with arthritis.

   _____

   _____

   _____

   _____

LABELING

Fractures and Immobilization

Directions: Review the drawings below and identify each of the following types of fractures: comminuted, compound, greenstick, longitudinal, oblique, simple, spiral, and transverse.

1. _____

2. _____

3. _____

4. _____

5. _____

6. _____

7. _____

8. _____

APPLICATION OF THE NURSING PROCESS

Matching

Directions: Match the problem on the left with the appropriate nursing assessment or intervention on the right.

1. _____ Swelling and increased pressure within a fascial compartment

2. _____ Inadequate immobilization

3. _____ Numbness and tingling with increased pain with motion of fingers

4. _____ Infection of a pin site or fracture site

5. _____ Tachypnea, disorientation, crackles and wheezing, and rash with lesions that do not blanch with pressure

a. Patient complains of grating sensation and unrelenting pain, especially with motion.
b. Notify the health care provider promptly; this is symptomatic of fat embolism. This is a rare but potentially fatal condition.
c. Presents as dull pain that becomes progressively worse, fever, purulent drainage, foul odor. Initiate wound and skin precautions.
d. Notify provider that arm cast is too tight.
e. Test for sensation and do a capillary refill time test.

Short Answer

Directions: Provide a short answer to the following questions or provide the information requested.

1. The following problem statements might be on the nursing care plan for the patient who has had a joint replacement. For each nursing problem, write an expected outcome.

   a. Altered mobility due to surgical procedure on knee

   _____

   b. Potential for decreased perfusion due to possible thrombus formation

   _____

   c. Pain due to surgical procedure and rehabilitation exercises

   _____

2. Interventions to assist in improving mobility would include:_____

   _____

   _____

3. Interventions to help prevent thrombus formation for this patient would include:

   a. _____

   b. _____

   c. _____

   d. _____

4. Other interventions besides analgesic administration to assist the patient with pain could include:

_____

_____

_____

5. What observations would indicate that expected outcomes are being met?

_____

_____

PRIORITY SETTING

Scenario: You are assigned the following patients:

   a. Mr. Hubbard who has just had a right knee replacement and is using a continuous passive motion machine.
   b. Ms. Tashiro who has been admitted for a left hip replacement.
   c. Mr. Rodriguez who was in a motorcycle accident and has multiple injuries including a broken leg that is immobilized with a full leg cast.
   d. Ms. Ahmed who is 2 days postoperative for an amputation of her left foot. She is diabetic.

1. Indicate the priority order in which you would do your initial shift rounds. _____

2. Which patient requires the most thorough assessment at first visit? _____

3. All the call lights are on later in the morning. Mr. Hubbard is asking for pain medication. Ms. Tashiro needs assistance to the bathroom. Mr. Rodriguez says he doesn't feel well and sounds anxious. Ms. Ahmed says her left foot is itching and would someone please help her. Which patient would you attend to first? _____

   Why?_____

_____

_____

_____

REVIEW QUESTIONS FOR THE NCLEX® EXAMINATION

Directions: Choose the best answer(s) for the following:

1. A patient is in her first postoperative day after a total hip replacement as treatment for degenerative arthritis. The patient's operated limb must be kept in what position?
   1. Adduction
   2. Externally rotated
   3. Internally rotated
   4. Abduction

2. You must watch the patient with a fracture of the femur for a fat embolism. Signs and symptoms include:
   1. increased blood pressure, rapid pulse, and fever.
   2. altered mental status, petechiae on chest, and dyspnea.
   3. increased pain in the leg, foot swelling, and rapid pulse.
   4. increased WBCs, hypotension, and difficulty breathing.

3. When a patient with a new hip is being prepared for discharge, you should give which instructions to avoid dislocation of the prosthesis? *(Select all that apply.)*
   1. Sit only on low chairs.
   2. Use a raised toilet seat.
   3. Do not lie on your back in bed.
   4. Use a pillow between your knees when lying down.
   5. Do not cross your legs at the knee or ankle.
   6. Be careful not to bend at the hip more than 90 degrees.

4. A patient is discharged with a synthetic cast applied. What will he need to know to take care of himself and the cast? *(Select all that apply.)*
   1. How to assess the neurovascular status of the part encased in the cast
   2. How to dry the cast if it becomes wet
   3. Signs of infection under the cast
   4. Importance of reporting a broken or loose cast
   5. How to cut a window in the cast if there is pain or swelling
   6. Ways to safely scratch at the itching that will develop

5. The nurse is caring for several patients with hip or femur fractures on an orthopedic unit. Which patient should the nurse attend to *first*?
   1. Patient complains of difficulty breathing, feeling very hot, and a fine red rash on the chest.
   2. Patient states that pain at the surgical site is unrelieved by medication or repositioning.
   3. Patient reports that there is an odor coming from the cast and the foot is red and swollen.
   4. Patient says that if no one comes to help her to the bathroom, she is going to call the supervisor.

6. The nurse is at a park and observes a workman who sustains an accidental amputation of a finger. The nurse would intervene if a bystander performs which action?
   1. Rinses visible debris from the detached digit
   2. Wraps the digit in a clean, damp cloth
   3. Immerses the digit in a cup of cold water
   4. Places the digit in a plastic bag and attaches a name tag

7. The patient has suffered a fracture of the humerus in an accident and has a new cast. Compartment syndrome is a potential complication. A typical sign or symptom would be:
   1. rash on the distal extremity.
   2. swelling of the fingers.
   3. pain unrelieved by analgesia.
   4. fever and restlessness.

8. The patient who returns to the floor after a reduction and internal fixation of the right hip has an IV running. The order for the next IV reads: D_5NS 1000 mL at 125 mL/hr. The IV tubing has a drop factor of 15 gtts/mL. The IV should be set to run at ___36___ gtts/min.

9. Patients with rheumatoid arthritis who are receiving Enbrel or other biologic response modifiers must be watched for complications such as: *(Select all that apply.)*
    1. hearing loss.
    2. serious infection.
    3. severe edema.
    4. blood dyscrasias.
    5. signs of demyelination.
    6. skin eruptions.

10. Disease-modifying antirheumatic drugs prevent joint and cartilage destruction by:
    1. suppressing the immune system.
    2. stimulating cortisol production.
    3. providing collagen to the joints.
    4. blocking pain transmission.

11. The nurse is caring for a patient with a newly applied cast to the lower extremity. The patient continues to complain of pain despite medication and repositioning. What should the nurse do *first*?
    1. Call the health care provider to obtain an order for additional medication.
    2. Use distraction techniques such as computer games or puzzle books.
    3. Assess the temperature of the toes, sensation to touch, and capillary refill.
    4. Tell the patient that the medication has not had enough time to work.

12. An elderly orthopedic patient refuses to perform the coughing and deep-breathing exercises. He says, "I have a broken hip. There is nothing wrong with my breathing." What should the nurse do *first*?
    1. Document that the patient was instructed in the techniques but refused to do them.
    2. Obtain an incentive spirometer and ask the patient to try using it instead of the exercises.
    3. Use active listening and be supportive of the patient's right to refuse a therapy.
    4. Explain how immobility contributes to developing pneumonia or atelectasis.

CRITICAL THINKING ACTIVITIES

1. Your neighbor says she has an odd spot on her calf and asks you to look at it. She has a red spot that seems to have a reddish ring around it. What questions would you ask her? What advice will you give her after you collect the data?

2. Your older brother calls complaining of excruciating pain in his left big toe and asking for advice. What would you say to him?

3. What would you teach a patient about measures to prevent gout attacks?

4. Your neighbor sprains her ankle. What type of self-care remedies can you recommend while she is waiting to get an appointment with her health care provider?

5. Explain what happens when a bone heals and why it is important to establish and maintain a sturdy union of broken bone fragments.

STEPS TOWARD BETTER COMMUNICATION

VOCABULARY BUILDING GLOSSARY

Term	Pronunciation	Definition
knit	nit	to grow together in small bits; to make clothing (sweaters) by connecting loops of yarn with long needles
impede'	im peed'	to slow, or get in the way of
imped'iment	im ped' ah ment	something that blocks or gets in the way of action
debris'	dah bree'	pieces left of something broken

COMPLETION

Directions: Fill in the blanks with the correct words from the Vocabulary Building Glossary to complete the statements.

1. Swelling under a cast may _____ blood flow.

2. Before a compound fracture is set, the surgeon cleans out any _____ in the wound.

3. A splint often causes less _____ to moving about than a cast.

4. If properly immobilized, the bone disrupted by a fracture will _____.

GRAMMAR POINTS

Giving Instructions

The words you use when talking to patients are critical to their understanding of what things are important and necessary for them to do. Here are some terms with the meanings they will have for the patient:

You can/you may indicate that the action is *optional*, the patient is responsible for choosing to do what he or she is capable of doing.

You should/you will indicate that the action is *recommended*, or is important to do.

Notice that using *should not* or *will not* (the negative) is usually stronger than the positive:

You can't/you shouldn't/you may not indicate the action is *required* or *necessary*.

You have to/you must/you mustn't/never indicate the action is *absolutely necessary*.

Here are some examples of each category.

Optional:

You can exercise your knee joint as many times a day as you want as long as it doesn't cause swelling.

You may apply ice packs to your back for the pain for 20 minutes of each hour.

If you like, **you can** use a heating pad for the discomfort.

Recommended:

Range-of-motion exercises **should** be done three or four times a day.

You should keep a pillow wedged between your legs when you lie on your side after hip surgery.

You shouldn't cross your legs after hip surgery.

Required:

Don't poke anything down into the cast.

Be sure to keep your leg cast dry.

You may not smoke or have caffeine for 8 hours before the test.

You can't let the traction weights set down on the bed.

Absolutely necessary:

You have to keep your weight off your foot for at least 3 weeks.

You must lie perfectly still for the bone scan.

You mustn't have any metal on your body for the MRI test.

Never remove these screws.

Assume you are giving instructions to a patient with a new leg cast. Use some of the phrases above to give one instruction from each category.

1. Optional:_____

2. Recommended: _____

3. Required: _____

4. Absolutely necessary:_____

Other types of instruction statements:

Expectation or possibility statements:

Should can also mean *expectation* (The discomfort **should** be minimal, meaning that *you expect small discomfort*) or *possibility* (If there **should** be any pain, you can take aspirin, meaning that *if and when pain occurs…*). **Should** is also used to make a request more polite (I **should** think it would be good for you to exercise more often).

Consequence statements:

Consequence statements indicate cause and effect, and have the form of **If you…, then…**

If you get up and move around, **then** you will heal faster.

If you use heat treatments before you exercise, **then** your joint will not be as stiff.

If you get your cast wet, **then** it will have to be replaced.

chapter

The Urinary System

33

Answer Key: Review the related chapter to answer these questions. A complete answer key was provided to your instructor.

REVIEW OF ANATOMY AND PHYSIOLOGY

Labeling

Anatomy of the Kidney

Directions: Label the following structures on the diagram of the kidney.

renal artery
renal vein
fibrous capsule
renal pyramid
calyx
renal pelvis
renal papilla
medulla
cortex
renal column
ureter

SHORT ANSWER

Assessing the Urinary System

Directions: Read the clinical scenario and answer the questions that follow.

Scenario: You are caring for several patients who have actual or are at risk for urinary disorders. In your daily assessment of these patients, you should look for specific kinds of data.

1. List five questions that you might ask a patient who has or suspects a urinary disorder.

   a. _____

   b. _____

   c. _____

   d. _____

   e. _____

2. List five specific physical assessments that should be done on a patient with a urinary disorder.

   a. _____

   b. _____

   c. _____

   d. _____

   e. _____

MATCHING

Diagnostic Testing

Directions: Match the diagnostic test (or test result) on the left with the most appropriate nursing action or assessment finding on the right.

1. _____ RBCs and WBCs in urine
2. _____ Hematuria
3. _____ Urine pH below 4.5
4. _____ Creatinine clearance
5. _____ Ureteral and renal biopsy
6. _____ Urine culture
7. _____ Specific gravity below 1.010 and urine osmolality below 100 mOsm/kg
8. _____ Bladder scan
9. _____ Intravenous pyelogram (IVP)
10. _____ Renal angiography

a. Pink-tinged urine after test; increase fluid intake to minimize discomfort
b. Assess patient for signs of acidosis
c. Dilute urine
d. Instruct patient in steps to follow to collect a clean-catch midstream urine specimen
e. Assess patient for other signs of urinary tract infection
f. Try to determine at what point during urination blood first appears
g. Obtain a 24-hour urine specimen and one blood sample during test
h. Vital signs and popliteal and pedal pulses are checked every 15 minutes for the first hour
i. Verify BUN and creatinine results
j. Palpate for the symphysis pubis and apply gel about 1 inch above

COMPLETION

Urinary Disorders

Directions: Fill in the blanks to complete the statements.

1. An absence of urine is called _____, which rarely occurs, but may be associated with acute renal failure.

2. Urination that occurs during the night is known as _____.

3. _____ is voiding more often than every 2 hours because of inflammation, decreased bladder capacity, psychological disorders, or increased fluid intake.

4. _____ is a delay in starting the stream of urine that may be related to partial obstruction.

5. Emptying the bladder regularly prevents _____ and eliminates toxic substances.

6. Long-term care residents and home care patients are continuously monitored for signs of urinary tract _____.

APPLICATION OF THE NURSING PROCESS

Caring for a Patient with Urinary Incontinence

Directions: Read the scenario and provide the answers to the following questions.

Scenario: Mr. Yakada is an elderly patient who was recently admitted to an extended-care facility. He has chronic urinary incontinence and currently he has an indwelling catheter. The family would like to have the catheter removed as soon as possible.

1. What factors could potentially contribute to Mr. Yakada's incontinence?

   a. Health conditions: _____

   _____

   _____

   b. Medications: _____

   _____

2. List three things to assess when a patient has an indwelling catheter.

   a. _____

   b. _____

   c. _____

3. Write an expected outcome for the nursing diagnosis of Risk for infection related to indwelling catheter.

   _____

   _____

4. List five nursing interventions to prevent infection for a patient with an indwelling catheter.

   a. _____

   b. _____

   c. _____

   d. _____

   e. _____

5. The health care provider writes an order to encourage fluids without restriction. At the end of the shift, the I&O sheet indicates that Mr. Yakada had 8 ounces of water at 8:00 AM, 300 mL of juice for breakfast, 12 ounces of coffee for lunch, 10 ounces of milk for dinner, and 800 mL is gone from his 1000 mL bedside water pitcher. How many mL total do you record for intake for this shift? _____ mL

6. List five nonsurgical alternatives to an indwelling catheter for patients such as Mr. Yakada.

   a. _____

   b. _____

   c. _____

   d. _____

   e. _____

7. Which urinalysis results indicate that the expected outcome (free from infection) is being met?
   a. Color: amber yellow
   b. Odor: aromatic
   c. Specific gravity: 1.030
   d. White blood cells: 0–4 (per low power field)

PRIORITY SETTING

Directions: Read the scenario and prioritize the nursing actions as appropriate.

Scenario A: You are caring for Ms. Popovitch on a rehabilitation unit. She has been doing well and is frequently ambulating off the unit with her family. She tells you that she is having urinary frequency but currently denies any other symptoms.

1. What is your priority action?
   a. Measure and record urinary output every hour.
   b. Check to see if fluid intake is higher than usual.
   c. Obtain an order for a urinalysis.
   d. Notify the health care provider or RN.

Scenario B: You are working with a new nursing assistant who disconnects the catheter from the drainage bag tubing "to collect a fresh urine specimen."

1. What is your priority action?
   a. Report the incident to the nurse manager.
   b. Allow her to continue and later talk to her in private.
   c. Do everything that assists her to maintain asepsis.
   d. Immediately stop her and do the procedure yourself.

Scenario C: The nurse is caring for a patient who is currently en route to have diagnostic testing to include an intravenous pyelogram (IVP) and blood cultures. Which abnormal laboratory result should the nurse deal with first?
   a. Call the primary care provider to report protein in the urine.
   b. Call the nephrologist to report uric acid greater than 750 mg/24 hours.
   c. Call the urologist to report a postvoid residual volume of 250 mL.
   d. Call the radiologist to report a creatinine of 1.6 mg/dL.

TABLE ACTIVITY

Directions: Complete the following table with the action, nursing implications, and patient teaching points for each drug classification.

Classification	Action	Nursing Implications	Patient Teaching
Urinary antispasmodics antimuscarinics oxybutynin (Ditropan) solifenacin (Vesicare) tolterodine (Detrol) trospium (Sanctura) darifenacin (Enablex) fesoterodine (Toviaz)			
Bladder stimulant bethanechol (Urecholine)			
Medication for benign prostatic hypertrophy tamsulosin (Flomax) doxazosin (Cardura) terazosin (Hytrin) alfuzosin (Uroxatral) silodosin (Rapaflo)			
Tricyclic antidepressants imipramine (Tofranil) amitriptyline (Elavil)			

REVIEW QUESTIONS FOR THE NCLEX® EXAMINATION

Directions: Choose the correct answer(s) for the following questions.

1. The patient reports having a color change in the urine. What question should the nurse ask first to collect more information about this symptom?
   1. "Do you have any history of kidney problems?"
   2. "What color is the urine?"
   3. "Are you having any pain with urination?"
   4. "When did you first notice this?"

2. The patient is suffering from glomerulonephritis. Which reaction is most likely to be associated with this disorder?
   1. Dribbling of urine or passing only the overflow
   2. Inability to void after removal of an indwelling catheter
   3. An immune reaction creating antibodies and antigen-antibody complexes.
   4. Passing urine when laughing, sneezing, or coughing

3. A major cause of end-stage kidney disease is:
   1. hypertension.
   2. hyperthyroidism.
   3. prostate enlargement.
   4. kidney stones.

4. The patient is scheduled to have a kidney biopsy. Which laboratory results should be reported to the radiologist before the patient has the procedure?
   1. An elevated INR
   2. An elevated BUN
   3. A decreased RBC
   4. A decreased WBC

5. The nurse is explaining the procedure for a cystoscopy. After the procedure, the patient should expect which set of circumstances?
   1. NPO status for several hours after the procedure
   2. Burning, frequency, and pink-tinged urine
   3. Bedrest with bathroom privileges for 24 hours
   4. Indwelling catheter in place to measure output

6. The patient has returned from renal angiography. What are likely to be the health care provider's orders? *(Select all that apply.)*
   1. Check vital signs q 15 min for the first hour, then q 2 hours x 2.
   2. Check popliteal and pedal pulses q 15 min for the first hour, then q 2 hours x 2.
   3. Perform a neuro check q 15 min for the first hour, then q 2 hours x 2.
   4. Check bowel sounds q 15 min for the first hour, then q 2 hours x 2.

7. The nurse hears in report that the patient is having oliguria, but the etiology is currently unknown. Which intervention is the nurse most likely to incorporate into the plan of care?
   1. Measure and record the output every hour.
   2. Provide extra time and assistance in going to the bathroom.
   3. Obtain an order for urine culture and sensitivity.
   4. Encourage the patient to take extra fluids.

8. The nurse must check the residual urine on a patient who reports urinary frequency. Which instruction should the nurse give to the patient?
   1. Advise the patient to avoid eating or drinking after midnight.
   2. Instruct the patient to void and empty bladder as much as possible prior to the test.
   3. Have the patient drink 2–3 glasses of fluid prior to the test.
   4. Ensure that the patient understands the bowel preparation procedure.

9. The patient had a Foley catheter removed 4 hours ago, but reports inability to void with a subjective sensation of needing to urinate. Which action should the nurse perform *first*?
   1. Notify the RN or the health care provider.
   2. Initiate hourly intake and output.
   3. Use the bladder scanner or palpation to assess fullness.
   4. Put the patient on the toilet and turn on the water.

10. The nurse is looking at the urine results for several patients. Which patient is the nurse most immediately concerned about?
    1. Pregnant woman has bright yellow urine.
    2. A diabetic patient has very pale urine.
    3. A young male athlete has brownish-red urine.
    4. A patient taking amitriptyline (Elavil) has bluish-green urine.

CRITICAL THINKING ACTIVITIES

Scenario: You are caring for Mr. Whipple who is scheduled for a renal biopsy. He is very apprehensive. This is his first biopsy, and he admits that he does not know anything about it; however, he fears the worst about the procedure and the results.

1. List two purposes of a renal biopsy.

   a. _____

   b. _____

2. Write a very brief explanation of how the procedure is done and what Mr. Whipple will experience.

   _____

   _____

   _____

   _____

3. What two interventions could you use to help Mr. Whipple decrease his anxiety?

   a. _____

   b. _____

4. What is the most serious immediate postprocedure complication of a renal biopsy?
   a. Vomiting related to anesthesia
   b. Frank bleeding and hemorrhage
   c. Infection and inflammation
   d. Decreased urinary output

5. Mr. Whipple expresses fear and anxiety while waiting for the results. "I just can't stand this waiting. Call the doctor right now or I am leaving the hospital!" What is the best response?
   a. "It's too dangerous for you to leave. You just had the procedure."
   b. "I'll call the doctor if you agree to calm down and wait."
   c. "You can leave if you want to; it is your right to do as you wish."
   d. "I see that you are anxious. Let me check on the status of the report."

STEPS TOWARD BETTER COMMUNICATION

VOCABULARY BUILDING GLOSSARY

Term	Definition
hy poth' e size	to suggest an answer that explains a group of phenomena
pa' tent	open, unobstructed
pa' ten cy	the condition of being open

PRONUNCIATION SKILLS

Directions: Pronounce the following words.

lithotripsy (lith'o trip' sy)	crushing stones in an organ such as the kidney
plasmapheresis (plas'ma fer ee'sis)	removal of plasma from withdrawn blood and retransfusion in a different form into the donor
oliguria (ol i gu' ree a)	diminished urine secretion in relation to fluid intake
polyuria (pol i u'ree a)	excessive secretion of urine
suprapubic (su' pra pew' bik)	above the pubes
extracorporeal (ex' tra kor po'ree al)	situated or occurring outside the body

COMPLETION

Directions: Fill in the blank with the correct word from the Vocabulary Building Glossary and Pronunciation Skills.

1. Make sure the tube is _____ before you use it.

2. We _____ that the infection is bacterial, but we will need to check it.

3. The physician will perform a(n) _____ on the patient with kidney stones.

WORD ATTACK SKILLS

Directions: Write the meaning of the word element.

1. Olig(o)-: _____
2. Poly-:_____
3. Supra-:_____
4. Extra-: _____
5. Hypo-:_____

COMMUNICATION EXERCISE

1. With a peer, practice performing a urologic assessment and history-taking. Use the Focused Assessment box in the textbook. Each partner should listen for clear pronunciation and may ask for an explanation of a word or procedure.

2. Write a dialogue you could use to ask a patient questions about drug history.

GRAMMAR POINTS

When you are trying to establish a history from a patient, it is very important to use the correct past or present tense. You want to clearly determine what has happened in the past, such as what medications he/she has taken, as opposed to what medications are being used now. Use *tag phrases* or *time words*, to be clear.

Examples:

Have you had frequency of urination *in the past*?

Do you have frequency of urination *now*?

CULTURAL POINTS

There are many commonly used terms for urination, many which are nonmedical and were learned in childhood but are still used by adults. You may need to know these when talking with your patients. For example, I need to *urinate, void, pee, make pee-pee, go pee, make water, take a leak, piss, use the urinal, go to the toilet/ bathroom*, etc. With your classmates, make a list of as many medical and nonmedical terms you can think of.

Care of Patients with Disorders of the Urinary System

Answer Key: Review the related chapter to answer these questions. A complete answer key was provided to your instructor.

COMPLETION

Directions: Fill in the blanks to complete the statements.

1. _____ is the accumulation of nitrogenous products, which is signaled by an increase in BUN and serum creatinine.

2. The patient complaining of burning with urination is experiencing the symptom called _____ _____.

3. You assess an arteriovenous graft by feeling for a(n) _____ over the graft.

4. Having to get up at night more than once to urinate is called _____.

5. _____ commonly occurs about 2–3 weeks after a group A beta-hemolytic streptococcal infection.

6. When the normal flow of urine is obstructed, urine can back up into the urinary tract and fill the kidney pelvis. This is called _____.

SHORT ANSWER

Cancers of the Urinary System

Directions: Provide answers for the following questions.

1. Often, the only sign of cancer of the bladder is _____.

2. What are four risk factors for cancer of the bladder?

   a. _____

   b. _____

   c. _____

   d. _____

3. What are three diagnostic tests used to confirm bladder cancer?

   a. _____

   b. _____

   c. _____

4. How does photodynamic therapy for bladder cancer work? _____

   _____

   _____

5. The primary treatment for cancer of the kidney is _____ before metastasis has occurred.

Urinary Diversion

Directions: Read the scenario and provide the answers to the following questions.

Scenario: You are caring for several patients who have urinary diversions. You recognize that while there are various surgical procedures that the health care provider may perform, there are some commonalities in the nursing care such as I&O and ostomy care.

1. An ileal conduit provides for evacuation of _____.

2. A cutaneous ureterostomy produces _____ urine.

3. The problem with a sigmoid conduit is that _____ frequently occurs.

4. The immediate postoperative nursing care plan for a patient with diversion of urinary flow should include the following nursing actions:

   a. Measurement of: _____

   b. Observation of: _____

5. Write a short-term goal for a patient's disturbance in self-image after urinary diversion.

   _____

   _____

   _____

6. List three common causes of peristomal skin problems *other than* seepage of urinary waste around the stoma.

   a. _____

   b. _____

   c. _____

7. List five nursing interventions that could help a patient prevent or overcome odor from an ureterostomy.

a. _____

b. _____

c. _____

d. _____

e. _____

LABELING

Different Types of Urinary Diversions

Directions: Label the drawings below with the correct name of the procedure depicted using the following list.

ureterosigmoidostomy (sigmoid conduit)

ileal reservoir (Kock pouch)

cutaneous ureterostomy

ileal conduit

APPLICATION OF THE NURSING PROCESS

Caring for a Patient with a Kidney Stone

Directions: Read the scenario and provide the answers to the following questions.

Scenario: You are working in a clinic and Mr. Depp arrives in acute distress and complains of severe left lower back pain. He is restless and pacing and unable to focus on your questions. His wife tells you that he "is peeing small amounts of bloody urine."

1. List at least four risk factors for kidney stones.

    a. _____

    b. _____

    c. _____

    d. _____

2. Which nursing problem is the priority for Mr. Depp?
    a. Possible obstruction of flow due to a blockage created by the kidney stone
    b. Pain from ureteral spasm and probable movement of kidney stone
    c. Risk of urinary tract infection due to urinary stasis
    d. Lack of communication regarding discomfort

3. What are three important nursing actions in the care of a patient who is trying to pass a kidney stone?

    a. _____

    b. _____

    c. _____

4. What are three things you should teach Mr. Depp about the lithotripsy procedure?

    a. _____

    b. _____

    c. _____

5. Which statement by Mr. Depp indicates that he understands the information about lithotripsy?
    a. "The procedure is done on an x-ray table."
    b. "I'll have to remain very still for about 10 minutes."
    c. "I should not feel any pain or discomfort during the procedure."
    d. "I will be given sedation during the procedure."

PRIORITY SETTING

Directions: Read the scenario and prioritize as appropriate.

Scenario: Mr. Wyaksit is postoperative from a kidney transplant and was transferred 5 days ago from the ICU to the general medical-surgical unit. He appeared to be recovering quickly and was independently ambulating. Last night, he tripped and fell to the floor, but appeared uninjured and told the nurse, "No damage done." This morning he is reluctant to get out of bed. Which set of assessment findings is the most critical?

    a. Pulse 110/min, BP 120/60 mm Hg, Hct 30%
    b. Fever 101° F, redness at the incision site
    c. Urinary output of 40 mL/hr, rising BUN
    d. Pain over the iliac fossa transplant area
    e. Bruise and swelling with decreased pulse over right wrist
    f. Decreased appetite with subjective dry mouth

REVIEW QUESTIONS FOR THE NCLEX® EXAMINATION

Directions: Choose the correct answer(s) for the following questions.

1. The nurse is teaching a patient at risk for stone formation how to avoid developing kidney stones. What information should the nurse give the patient?
    1. Drink enough liquids to produce at least 3500 mL of urine every 24 hours.
    2. Fluid intake should approximate urine output every 24 hours.
    3. Eat a well-balanced diet with high-quality protein and fruits and vegetables.
    4. Try to exercise at least four times a week and sleep 8 hours a night.

2. Diagnosing kidney stones sometimes involves several studies to identify and locate stones. These may include: *(Select all that apply.)*
    1. urinalysis.
    2. exploratory surgery.
    3. renal angiogram.
    4. CT of abdomen and pelvis.

3. Hemodialysis is performed for the end-stage kidney disease patient. Data that indicate treatment effectiveness would be:
    1. a rise in hemoglobin and hematocrit.
    2. a fall in glucose and sodium levels.
    3. a fall in potassium, creatinine, and urea levels.
    4. an increased alertness and a sense of well-being.

4. Other than taking baseline vital signs, an important nursing intervention to perform the morning of dialysis is:
    1. keeping the patient NPO until after the dialysis.
    2. administering 1 liter of normal saline to prevent shock.
    3. giving subcutaneous heparin to prevent blood clotting during dialysis.
    4. withholding blood pressure medications until the pressure has stabilized after dialysis.

5. When planning nursing care for the patient who has renal failure, the nurse encourages a diet that is:
    1. high in calories but low in protein and potassium.
    2. high in protein, moderate in calories, and low in sodium.
    3. high in fat and protein but low in potassium and sodium.
    4. high in fiber, with mainly fruits and vegetables and some grains.

6. A nursing intervention for the patient who has just returned from surgery with a new arteriovenous fistula is to:
    1. maintain a heparin drip to prevent clotting in the fistula.
    2. release the elevated extremity and perform range-of-motion exercises every 2 hours.
    3. assess the fistula site for hematoma and check for bruit every 2–4 hours.
    4. assess the fistula for visual signs of clotting every 2–4 hours.

7. The nurse is looking at abnormal results of a urinalysis. Which finding is more specific to chronic glomerulonephritis, and is less likely to be present if the patient has acute cystitis?
    1. Glucose
    2. Red blood cells
    3. Urinary casts
    4. White blood cells

8. Planning nursing care for the patient following surgery for kidney trauma may include: *(Select all that apply.)*
    1. close monitoring for hypovolemic shock.
    2. hourly urine output measurements.
    3. monitoring of the size of the flank hematoma.
    4. neurologic monitoring every shift.

9. Sulfamethoxazole-trimethoprim (Bactrim) is prescribed for the patient's cystitis. When doing discharge teaching, the nurse would be sure to instruct the patient to:
    1. take the medication between meals to enhance absorption.
    2. take 3000–4000 mL of fluid per day to prevent crystallization.
    3. be aware that this medication might turn the urine orange or red.
    4. watch for signs of jaundice associated with liver toxicity.

10. What changes in the urinary system occur with aging that predispose elderly women to urinary frequency and infection?
    1. Decreased fluid intake to prevent incontinence
    2. An increased glomerular filtration rate
    3. Estrogen depletion that results in structural atrophy
    4. An increased bladder capacity due to loss of tone

11. Which signs and symptoms are associated with nephrotic syndrome?
    1. Proteinuria, hyperlipidemia, hypoalbuminemia, and severe edema
    2. Hematuria, frequent and urgent urination, and low back pain
    3. Burning, itching, frequency of voiding, and dysuria
    4. Unilateral flank pain that radiates into the genitalia and inner thigh

12. A patient has acute renal failure and is in the diuretic phase. With an increased output, there is a danger of:
    1. hyponatremia.
    2. hyperkalemia.
    3. fluid overload.
    4. catabolism.

13. A patient with chronic renal failure is receiving epoetin alfa (Epogen). The purpose of this medication is to:
    1. increase urinary output.
    2. bind phosphate; given with meals.
    3. prevent problems of calcium loss.
    4. treat anemia; promotes RBC formation.

14. One of the relevant nursing problems in caring for a patient with renal failure is rapid fatigue upon activity. Which intervention would be appropriate in helping the patient accomplish activities of daily living (ADLs)?
    1. Tell the patient to do as much as he can and then return later to help him finish.
    2. Instruct the nursing assistant to watch him do ADLs and report back on his progress.
    3. Instruct the nursing assistant to do everything for him unless he tells her that he can do it himself.
    4. Assess his energy level in the morning and then direct the nursing assistant to do specific tasks for him.

15. What is characteristic of stage 1 chronic renal failure?
    1. BUN and serum creatinine levels begin to rise.
    2. Glomerular filtration rate falls.
    3. Urine concentration is decreased and polyuria and nocturia occur.
    4. Electrolyte and fluid imbalances are serious; wastes accumulate.

16. Which patient needs counseling about contacting all sexual partners for follow-up care?
    1. Patient diagnosed with chronic glomerulonephritis
    2. Patient diagnosed with hydronephrosis
    3. Patient diagnosed with nephrotic syndrome
    4. Patient diagnosed with urethritis

17. The nurse is caring for a patient with acute glomerulonephritis and observes obvious edema. What is the best rationale for frequent auscultation of the lung fields for this patient?
    1. Assessing the lungs is the standard of care for any acutely ill patient.
    2. The patient is on continuous bedrest and will suffer the effects of immobility.
    3. Observable edema on the body surface suggests congestion in the internal organs.
    4. The patient is likely to have had a preexisting throat infection.

18. The nurse is supervising a nursing student who is preparing to irrigate a nephrostomy tube. Which action would the nurse advise the student to perform *first*?
    1. Talk to the patient and explain the procedure.
    2. Read the health care provider's order to clarify the instructions.
    3. Check the chart and make sure informed consent was signed.
    4. Obtain all the equipment and mentally review the procedure.

19. The health care provider orders a Foley catheter for a patient involved in a serious car accident. The nurse notes that there is bleeding at the urethral meatus. What is the priority action?
    1. Obtain extra supplies to cleanse the meatus.
    2. Get a bedpan and ask the patient to void.
    3. Insert the Foley and closely monitor for hematuria.
    4. Notify the health care provider, because there may be a tear.

20. Which patient has the greatest risk for acute renal failure?
    1. Trauma patient with an episode of prolonged hypovolemia
    2. Patient with chronic renal failure who is noncompliant with dietary restrictions
    3. Patient with frequent kidney stones undergoing nephrolithotomy
    4. Patient with bladder tumor and painless hematuria

CRITICAL THINKING ACTIVITIES

Scenario: Mr. Sounds has chronic renal failure. His health care provider has decided that Mr. Sounds is a good candidate for peritoneal dialysis. This is a new therapy for Mr. Sounds, but he is eager to learn and co-operate.

1. Prepare a brief description of the purpose of peritoneal dialysis and the principle by which it works to help Mr. Sounds understand this new therapy.

    _____

    _____

    _____

2. List five nursing actions specific to the care of Mr. Sounds for his peritoneal dialysis.

    a. _____

    b. _____

    c. _____

    d. _____

    e. _____

3. When administering peritoneal dialysis to Mr. Sounds, you would evaluate him each day. What is the most common complication?
    a. Peritonitis
    b. Clotting of the catheter
    c. Hemorrhage from heparin in the solution
    d. Retention of in-flow solution within the abdomen

STEPS TOWARD BETTER COMMUNICATION

VOCABULARY BUILDING GLOSSARY

Term	Pronunciation	Definition
urgency	er' jen see	a need for immediate action, hurry
linked	link'd	connected, joined
intermittent	in ter mit' ent	happening with stops and starts; periodic
pertinent	per' tin ent	pertaining or related to; important to know in relation to a subject
flank	flaynk	the side of the body between the ribs and ilium
void	voyd	to expel urine from the bladder; to make invalid

COMPLETION

Directions: Fill in the blanks with the correct words from the Vocabulary Building Glossary to complete the statements.

1. A sign of kidney infection is pain in the _____ area.

2. The nurse asks the patient to _____ into a specimen container for a urinalysis.

3. If the patient states that there has been blood in the urine, it is a very _____ piece of information.

4. The patient with cystitis experiences dysuria, but may also have urinary _____.

5. Smoking has been _____ as a risk factor in cancer of the bladder.

6. The male patient with benign prostatic hyperplasia (BPH) may experience a(n) _____ stream when he urinates.

WORD ATTACK SKILLS

Combining Forms

nephr/o-	kidney
glomerul/o-	network of capillaries
ur/o-	urine, urinary tract
ren/o-	kidney
oli/olig/o-	little, few, scanty
poly-	many, much

Directions: Using slash marks, break these words into their word elements or parts. Write the meaning of each word part, then give the meaning of the word.

1. Glomerulonephritis: _____

   _____

   _____

2. Hypoalbuminemia: _____

   _____

   _____

3. Nephrolithotomy: _____

   _____

   _____

4. Pyelonephrolithotomy: _____

   _____

   _____

5. Ureterosigmoidostomy: _____

_____

_____

PRONUNCIATION SKILLS

Directions: Pronounce these abbreviations and write their meanings.

1. ARF: _____

2. CRF: _____

3. GFR: _____

4. ATN: _____

5. UTI: _____

6. NSU: _____

7. ESRD: _____

8. ESWL: _____

9. TURP: _____

10. AV: _____

11. CAPD: _____

Pronunciation Pairs Exercise

Many words are pronounced the same except for the last letter that creates the final sound. It is important that this final sound be pronounced correctly so that the listener will understand the meaning of what is being said. Many of these sounds are difficult for the second language speaker to hear and pronounce.

Directions: With a study partner, take turns pronouncing the word pairs listed below while the other listens without looking at the list. The listener should write down the words heard. Take turns speaking and then listening. Check to see that the words written by the listener are correct. (For extra practice, write the word pairs on small cards and mix up the order. Do the exercise frequently.)

life	live		barf	bark		duct	duck
of	up		ureter	urethra		tape	take
have	had		loop	lose		waste	wake
can	can't		lose	loose		help	health
out	ouch		tube	tooth		holds	holes
track	tract		gland	clamp		stones	stomas
putting	pudding		car	cart		lab	lap

The Endocrine System

chapter

35

Answer Key: Review the related chapter to answer these questions. A complete answer key was provided to your instructor.

COMPLETION

Directions: Fill in the blanks to complete the statements.

1. The _____ is often referred to as the "master gland" of the body.

2. Parathormone acts on the renal tubules to increase the excretion of _____ in the urine and the reabsorption of _____.

3. Parathormone raises the serum calcium level by stimulating _____ and increasing calcium absorption in the _____ tract.

4. A hormone produced by the adrenal cortex that influences sodium and water balance is _____.

5. The adrenal medulla secretes _____ and _____.

6. The adrenal cortex secretes mainly _____ and _____.

7. The mineralocorticoids affect the balance of _____.

8. The glucocorticoids are essential for proper utilization of _____, _____, and _____.

9. The primary glucocorticoid is _____.

10. Primary actions of cortisol are to increase _____ levels and to _____ the inflammatory response.

TABLE ACTIVITY

Hormone Changes that Occur with Aging

Directions: Complete the table below. Add the hormones that increase, decrease, or essentially remain unchanged with aging. The first block is done for you.

Hormones that usually decrease with age	aldosterone, renin, calcitonin, and growth hormone; in the older female, estrogen and prolactin; and in the older male, testosterone
Hormones that may increase with age	
Hormones that remain unchanged or are slightly decreased	

SHORT ANSWER

Hypothyroidism

Directions: Read the clinical scenario and answer the questions that follow.

Scenario: You are working in an endocrinology clinic. Ms. Venucha is an older woman who has been referred by her health care provider for a possible thyroid disorder. Ms. Venucha tells you that she has been slowing down lately and has felt "mildly bloated, sluggish, and constipated." She agreed to have some diagnostic testing done, but she feels she needs some general information about the thyroid and the diagnostic testing.

1. List five effects of thyroid hormones.

    a. _____

    b. _____

    c. _____

    d. _____

    e. _____

2. Name four serum tests that are done to evaluate thyroid function.

    a. _____

    b. _____

    c. _____

    d. _____

3. List four commonly used drugs that can alter the results of thyroid tests.

   a. _____

   b. _____

   c. _____

   d. _____

4. List at least three teaching points to include for a patient who needs a radioactive iodine uptake exam to assess thyroid function.

   a. _____

   b. _____

   c. _____

5. Briefly describe how aging affects the thyroid gland and thyroid hormone levels.

   a. _____

   _____

   b. _____

   _____

   c. _____

   _____

   d. _____

   _____

APPLICATION OF THE NURSING PROCESS

Caring for Patients at Risk for Type 2 Diabetes

Directions: Read the scenario and provide the answers to the following questions.

Scenario: You are working in an ambulatory clinic. Mr. Bob, a middle-aged patient, comes in for a checkup and he reports having mild fatigue and some gradual but progressive weight gain over the past 6 months. He suspects he may have diabetes, "because my father had it."

1. List five or six questions to ask a patient who is suspected of having an endocrine disorder.

   _____

   _____

   _____

   _____

   _____

2. Write an example of an appropriate outcome for the nursing diagnosis Altered nutrition, more than body requirements, related to altered glucose metabolism.

_____

_____

3. List three general nursing interventions that will help a diabetic patient who has Altered nutrition, more than body requirements to maintain a normal body weight.

a. _____

b. _____

c. _____

4. Write an example of evaluation outcome for the following goal: Patient will verbalize beginning understanding of diagnostic testing for diabetes at the end of teaching session.

_____

_____

_____

_____

5. Mr. Bob currently weighs 225 lbs. The health care provider has suggested that he should gradually lose weight to achieve a target goal of 85 kg. Mr. Bob asks you to help him with some calculations.

a. How long will it take him to achieve the target goal if he can lose 2 pounds/month? _____

b. How long will it take him to achieve the target goal if he can lose 5 pounds/month? _____

c. How long will it take him to achieve the target goal if he can lose 8 pounds/month? _____

PRIORITY SETTING

Directions: Read the scenario and prioritize as appropriate.

Scenario: You are the only nurse standing in the nurses' station and the unit secretary hands you computer printouts of several laboratory values.

1. Which patient needs priority attention?
   a. Mr. Jez has positive ketone bodies in the urine.
   b. Ms. Lukic has serum T_4 of 10 mg/dL.
   c. Mr. Doig has a 2-hour postprandial glucose of 150 mg/dL.
   d. Ms. Kost has a fasting blood glucose of 20 mg/dL.

2. You recognize that one of the patients needs immediate attention; however, Mr. Jez, Mr. Doig, and Ms. Kost have been assigned to other nurses. Of the four patients, Ms. Lukic is the only patient that has been assigned to you. What is your priority action?
   a. Check on Ms. Lukic.
   b. Find the nurse assigned to the critical patient.
   c. Inform the charge nurse about the lab values.
   d. Check on the most critical patient.

REVIEW QUESTIONS FOR THE NCLEX® EXAMINATION

Directions: Choose the correct answer(s) for the following questions.

1. The patient is experiencing fatigue with loss of energy and is currently undergoing multiple tests to diagnose a possible endocrine disorder. She states, "I just want to know what is going on. I'm so tired of these tests." What is the most therapeutic response?
   1. "Did you talk to your health care provider about the test results?"
   2. "Let me go look at your chart and find the results."
   3. "You sound really frustrated about the diagnostic testing."
   4. "I'd be tired too, if I had to deal with everything you have."

2. A patient is diagnosed with a thyroid disorder. The nurse anticipates that the patient is mostly likely to have problems with:
   1. metabolic rate.
   2. water reabsorption.
   3. bone fragility.
   4. increased blood glucose.

3. Which patient is most likely to have a nursing diagnosis of Altered nutrition: less than body requirements?
   1. Patient with hyperthyroidism
   2. Patient with decreased estrogen production
   3. Patient who has type 2 diabetes
   4. Patient with hypothyroidism

4. The patient is undergoing a hypertonic saline test to detect diabetes insipidus. One of the nursing responsibilities is to teach the patient to:
   1. produce a urine specimen using a clean-catch technique.
   2. produce a urine specimen in the marked container each hour.
   3. void in the early AM and discard the first urine specimen.
   4. produce a urine specimen at the end of the test period.

5. The health care provider orders a dexamethasone suppression test to assist in the diagnosis of Cushing disease. An appropriate nursing action would be to:
   1. collect a clean-catch urine specimen.
   2. note the start and end time on the laboratory slip.
   3. check orders for drugs to be withheld.
   4. administer vasopressin SC as ordered.

6. A patient is being tested to determine the degree of diabetic control of blood sugar over the preceding 2–3 months. What is the correct test to make this determination?
   1. Fasting blood glucose
   2. 2-hour postprandial blood glucose
   3. Glucose tolerance test
   4. Hemoglobin A_{1C}

7. Which patient has the greatest risk for injury related to bone fracture?
   1. Patient with a thyroid disorder
   2. Patient with a parathyroid disorder
   3. Patient with a pancreatic disorder
   4. Patient with a testicular disorder

8. The health care provider orders laboratory tests for several serum electrolytes. Which set of electrolytes would most likely reflect parathyroid function?
   1. Calcium and phosphorus
   2. Sodium and magnesium
   3. Potassium and chloride
   4. Sodium and potassium

9. The patient needs several diagnostic tests to rule out endocrine disorders. Which task would be appropriate to assign to the nursing assistant?
   1. Note medications that the patient takes on the laboratory order.
   2. Ask the patient if he has any questions or needs anything.
   3. Instruct the patient how to obtain a clean-catch specimen.
   4. Deliver the urine specimen to the laboratory.

10. The health care provider orders an aldosterone urine test for a patient. No one on the unit, including the charge nurse, is familiar with this test. What should the nurse do?
    1. Collect a clean-catch urine specimen and send it to the laboratory.
    2. Call the health care provider and ask for clarification of the order and procedure.
    3. Check the laboratory policy and procedure manual.
    4. Ask the patient not to void until after the procedure is clarified.

CRITICAL THINKING ACTIVITIES

Scenario A: Your neighbor tells you that she is thinking about taking Synthroid to lose weight because a relative has been taking Synthroid that was obtained "through the Internet" and that person lost about 15 pounds very easily.

1. How would you respond to your neighbor? _____

   _____

   _____

   _____

   _____

2. One of the functions of thyroid hormones is to affect tissue response to epinephrine and norepinephrine. Briefly describe to your neighbor the potential effects on blood pressure and heart rate.

   _____

   _____

3. Discuss some of the problems that might occur as people try to save money by using the Internet as a health care resource.

   _____

   _____

   _____

   _____

   _____

Scenario B: Your cousin tells you that she thinks she has hypoglycemia. She wants your opinion about whether she might have diabetes. Her health care provider has reassured her that she does not have diabetes but she doesn't believe him.

1. Write a brief statement that you could use to redirect your cousin back to her provider.

   _____

   _____

   _____

   _____

2. List at least five questions that your cousin could ask her provider.

   a. _____

   b. _____

   c. _____

   d. _____

   e. _____

3. Would you feel comfortable giving her an opinion about the diabetes? Why or why not?

   _____

   _____

   _____

STEPS TOWARD BETTER COMMUNICATION

VOCABULARY BUILDING GLOSSARY

Term	Pronunciation	Definition
alter	al'ter	to change, to make different
aspect	as'pect	area, or part of a surface
assay	ass'ay	a test for purity
elicit	e lis'it	to gather or solicit information from someone
lability	lay bil'ity	instability, likely to change, easily altered
negative feedback	neg' ah tiv feed' bak	a response to a message which is intended to change or stop the message
postprandial	post pran' dee al	after dinner, or after any other meal
render	ren'der	to cause a change
sluggish	slug'gish	slow-moving, inactive
stalk	stawk	1. (noun) a stem or support of a plant or organ. 2. (verb) to follow or pursue secretly
synthesis	sin'the sis	combining of parts to make a whole

COMPLETION

Directions: Fill in the blanks with the correct words from the Vocabulary Building Glossary to complete the statements.

1. The person who has hypothyroidism usually feels _____.

2. A patient should be instructed not to _____ their medication regimen without first consulting a health care provider.

3. When there is too much circulating cortisol in a person's system, he often displays emotional _____.

4. Pituitary problems may _____ a female infertile.

5. When checking for thyroid disease, the examiner pays particular attention to the frontal _____ of the neck.

6. Fructosamine _____ is another test to monitor control of glucose over time.

7. The word *parathormone* is a(n) _____ of the two words *parathyroid* and *hormone*.

8. The patient gave _____ in response to the questionnaire about the new hospital menus.

9. She cut the _____ of the flower so that it would fit the vase.

10. A nap is often the favorite _____ activity of many people.

11. A good history-taking will _____ a lot of information from the patient.

WORD ATTACK SKILLS

hyper-	over, more
hypo-	under, less
endo-	internal
exo-	external
para-	beside, next to; near

PRONUNCIATION SKILLS

Directions: Take turns practicing with a peer the pronunciation of these words to increase your ability to speak English clearly.

adenohypophysis (ad noh hi po' fi sis)	anterior pituitary
adrenocorticotropic (ah dree'no kor'tih ko tro'pik)	a hormone acting on the adrenal cortex
verbalization (ver'bal iz a' shun)	putting into words
antiinflammatory (an' tee in flam'ah tor y)	preventing inflammation
hypopituitary (hi' po pih too' ih tar y)	decreased secretions from the pituitary gland

Care of Patients with Pituitary, Thyroid, Parathyroid, and Adrenal Disorders

chapter

36

Answer Key: Review the related chapter to answer these questions. A complete answer key was provided to your instructor.

COMPLETION

Directions: Fill in the blanks to complete the statements.

1. Simple goiter causes problems when it enlarges to the point of placing _____
   _____.

2. Graves disease is another name given to _____.

3. The danger in an Addisonian crisis is severe _____ and possible shock.

4. Patients with Cushing syndrome may have weakness due to abnormal protein catabolism and have loss
   of _____.

5. Syndrome of inappropriate antidiuretic hormone (SIADH) secretion causes
   _____ of fluid.

6. Pheochromocytoma is a rare tumor of the _____ which secretes catechol-
   amines.

APPLICATION OF THE NURSING PROCESS

Care of Patients with Hyperthyroidism

Directions: Read the clinical scenario and answer the questions that follow.

Scenario: You are caring for a middle-aged woman, Ms. Riata, who has been admitted for treatment of her hyperthyroidism. Ms. Riata has been living with this diagnosis for a period of time; however, she has not had success with conservative therapy, so she is being admitted for a partial thyroidectomy. Although she is knowledgeable about the disease and the impending surgery, she is emotionally labile and appears exhausted.

1. The physical signs and symptoms of hyperthyroidism include:_____

   _____

   _____

2. Psychological or emotional symptoms of hyperthyroidism include episodes of: _____

    _____

    _____

    _____

3. Which diagnosis is likely to be included in the care plan for Ms. Riata?
    a. Unable to perform activities of daily living related to lethargy
    b. Nutrition excess related to decreased metabolic rate
    c. Self-esteem disturbance related to facial puffiness and swelling
    d. Constipation related to decreased gastrointestinal motility
    e. Nervousness related to agitation and difficulty concentrating

4. List three nursing actions that should be included in the postoperative nursing care plan of a patient after partial thyroidectomy.

    a. _____

        _____

    b. _____

        _____

    c. _____

        _____

5. Write an example of an evaluation outcome for the following patient discharge teaching goal. Patient will identify three signs and symptoms to report related to tetany and three for thyroid storm.

    _____

    _____

    _____

    _____

    _____

PRIORITY SETTING

Directions: Read the clinical scenario and prioritize nursing actions as appropriate. Also identify tasks that can be performed by various members of the health care team.

Scenario: You arrive for your shift at the hospital. Before you can even get your coat off, the day shift RN says, "Quick! Come help me! I have a patient who is going down the tubes!" You run to the room and recognize Ms. Dredge who has hypothyroidism. The RN says, "The doctor has just diagnosed her with myxedema coma and wrote these orders. Will you help me and the nursing assistant so that we can take care of this lady quickly?"

1. From the <u>list below</u>, prioritize the **top five** interventions that need to be accomplished first.

    1. _____

    2. _____

    3. _____

    4. _____

    5. _____

2. Identify which tasks (if any) could be assigned to the nursing assistant or the unit secretary and which should be performed by licensed nurses. Identify with the following abbreviations which caregivers should be assigned the different tasks. Place the initials in front of the appropriate task.
   RN—Registered Nurse
   LPN—Licensed Practical/Vocational Nurse
   NA—Nursing Assistant
   UC—Unit clerk or secretary

   _____ a. Assess response to external warming blanket

   _____ b. O_2 at 3 L per N/C

   _____ c. Vital signs q 2 hours and notify health care provider for BP <100/60 or >160/90

   _____ d. Blood glucose STAT

   _____ e. Levothyroxine sodium now 0.5 mg IV push over 5 minutes

   _____ f. IV access × 2 (Saline lock × 1)

   _____ g. IV bolus 250 mL × 1 over 30 minutes STAT

   _____ h. Place on cardiac monitor

   _____ i. Place continuous pulse oximeter

   _____ j. Maintenance IV D_5.45 NS 150 mL/hour

   _____ k. Call for EKG now

   _____ l. Give 1/2 amp D_{10} IV push for BS < 60

REVIEW QUESTIONS FOR THE NCLEX® EXAMINATION

Directions: Choose the correct answer(s) for the following questions.

1. A patient is admitted for a minor elective surgery. He also has a diagnosis of Cushing syndrome. Which physical assessment findings are associated with Cushing syndrome and are likely to be documented in the patient's record?
   1. Dry, scaly skin and brittle nails
   2. Abnormal protrusion of the eyeballs
   3. Enlarged thyroid gland
   4. Buffalo hump and moon face

2. A patient is diagnosed with diabetes insipidus. Which finding is characteristic of this disorder?
   1. Excessive, dilute urine
   2. Increased blood pressure
   3. Tachycardia
   4. Exertional dyspnea

3. The nurse is caring for a patient who has SIADH. Which nursing intervention is appropriate for the care of this patient?
   1. Giving hypotonic fluids as ordered
   2. Restricting fluids to 500–1000 mL/day as ordered
   3. Administering somatropin via subcutaneous injection as ordered
   4. Administering IV calcium gluconate as ordered

4. The nurse is caring for a patient who is receiving large doses of radioactive iodine. The care plan should include which precaution?
   1. No special precautions beyond Standard Precautions
   2. Wearing a lead apron when delivering nursing care
   3. Isolation of the patient for 8 days (half-life of drug)
   4. Having the patient wear a radiation detection badge

5. The patient is diagnosed with a rare tumor of the adrenal gland (pheochromocytoma). The nurse recognizes that the priority vital sign to monitor frequently is:
   1. respiratory rate.
   2. temperature.
   3. blood pressure.
   4. pulse.

6. The nurse is caring for a postoperative patient who has had a hypophysectomy. Which nursing intervention(s) would be appropriate in the care of this patient? *(Select all that apply.)*
   1. Keep the patient flat in bed.
   2. Note and report change in mental status.
   3. Change nasal drip pad as needed.
   4. Instruct patient to cough deeply.
   5. Assist the patient with mouth rinses.

7. The nurse is assessing a patient with simple goiter. What is the first sign usually noticed in this condition?
   1. Difficulty swallowing
   2. Difficulty breathing
   3. Enlargement in the front of the neck
   4. Abnormal protrusion of the eyeballs

8. The nurse is administering an iodine preparation to a patient. What is a nursing implication in administering this drug?
   1. Monitoring the vital signs, especially the blood pressure
   2. Diluting and administering through a straw to prevent staining teeth
   3. Administering the drug SQ in the abdominal area
   4. Monitoring the lab results for hyponatremia or hyperkalemia

9. Which statement by the patient indicates a need for additional teaching about the treatment plan for hyperthyroidism?
   1. "I could be treated with antithyroid drugs and ablation therapy."
   2. "Ablation therapy could possibly cause hypothyroidism."
   3. "I'll have a thyroidectomy first and then get ablation therapy."
   4. "I could get ablation therapy on an outpatient basis."

10. The nurse is administering antithyroid drugs to the patient. Which dangerous adverse effects are a concern with antithyroid drugs?
    1. Agranulocytosis and hepatotoxicity
    2. Hypoglycemia and neurotoxicity
    3. Hyponatremia and renal toxicity
    4. Seizures and ototoxicity

11. The nurse is carefully assessing a postoperative patient who had a thyroidectomy. Which assessment finding is most likely to be associated with one of the potential complications of this surgery?
    1. Blindness
    2. Tetany
    3. Profound diuresis
    4. Hypertensive crisis

12. Thyroid cancer is often not diagnosed in the early stages. The primary reason for this is:
    1. there are no tests available for early thyroid cancer.
    2. diagnosis is delayed to allow for maturing of cells.
    3. the signs and symptoms are common to other disorders.
    4. there are no detectable signs and symptoms until the disease is widespread.

13. Which therapies and medication is the health care provider likely to order for a patient who is experiencing an Addisonian crisis?
    1. Fluid restriction and prazosin (Minipress)
    2. IV glucose and levothyroxine sodium (Synthroid)
    3. Isotonic sodium chloride and calcitonin (Caltine)
    4. Fluid bolus and IV hydrocortisone (Solu-Cortef)

14. When planning care for a patient with hypothyroidism, what would the nurse do?
    1. Provide extra snacks and encourage the patient to eat frequently.
    2. Place the patient in a cool room to avoid overheating.
    3. Provide extra time to avoid rushing the patient.
    4. Provide a calm, quiet atmosphere for episodes of emotional outbursts.

15. Which endocrine disorder is most likely to mimic the symptoms of a cardiac disease?
    1. Hyperthyroidism
    2. Myxedema
    3. Sheehan syndrome
    4. Diabetes insipidus

16. The nurse is caring for a patient with hyperparathyroidism. Which set of laboratory values is the primary concern?
    1. Calcium and phosphorus
    2. Glucose and potassium
    3. White blood cell count
    4. Urinalysis and blood urea nitrogen

17. A patient has recently had a thyroidectomy. The nurse notes that the patient demonstrates sudden onset of muscular twitching and spasms. What is the priority intervention?
    1. Initiate seizure precautions.
    2. Check the patency of the IV site.
    3. Obtain the emergency airway equipment.
    4. Check the patient's temperature.

18. Which patient has the greatest risk for developing Cushing syndrome?
    1. Patient who recently had a subtotal parathyroidectomy
    2. Patient who has diabetes insipidus
    3. Patient on long-term steroid therapy
    4. Patient with low serum calcium

19. The nurse is caring for a patient with diabetes insipidus. Which pattern of urinary output would be the most typical of this disorder?
    1. Usually more than 2.5 L/day
    2. 30 mL/hour
    3. Output will approximate intake
    4. Urine cortisol level will be high

20. The nurse is caring for several patients with endocrine disorders. Which patient is most likely to have desmopressin acetate (DDAVP) ordered as part of the therapy?
    1. Patient with hypoparathyroidism
    2. Patient with Graves disease
    3. Patient with hyperthyroidism
    4. Patient with diabetes insipidus

21. What are signs and symptoms of hypothyroidism? *(Select all that apply.)*
    1. Decreased appetite but increased weight
    2. Bagginess under eyes and swelling of face
    3. Feeling overheated
    4. Pressured speech
    5. Sluggish mental activity, impaired memory, depression
    6. Constipation, abdominal distention, flatulence
    7. Husky voice, thinning eyebrows, hair loss

22. What are signs and symptoms of adrenal cortical insufficiency (Addison disease)? *(Select all that apply.)*
    1. Generalized malaise
    2. Muscle weakness, muscle pain
    3. Orthostatic hypotension and vulnerability to cardiac dysrhythmias
    4. Anorexia, nausea and vomiting, flatulence, and diarrhea
    5. Anxiety, depression, and loss of mental acuity
    6. Hyperglycemia

23. The health care provider orders IV normal saline to infuse 500 mL over 6 hours. What is the pump setting? _____

CRITICAL THINKING ACTIVITIES

Scenario: Your patient is diagnosed with pheochromocytoma. This is a rare condition that can be fatal. The patient was just admitted and the night nurse is not able to give you much information about pheochromocytoma; however, "the patient is stable and did not have any problems for me."

1. What is the most likely complication of this tumor if it is not treated? _____

   _____

2. What are the signs and symptoms that you might see with this condition? _____

   _____

   _____

3. Identify at least three actions (with rationale) that you should immediately take if this patient shows signs of a hypertensive crisis.

   _____

   _____

   _____

4. When you are working on the unit and encounter patient conditions that are unfamiliar to you (and maybe unfamiliar to the rest of the staff), how can you quickly access the necessary information you need to care for the patient?

   _____

   _____

   _____

STEPS TOWARD BETTER COMMUNICATION

VOCABULARY BUILDING GLOSSARY

Term	Pronunciation	Definition
bulge	bulj	to extend outward, stick out, protrude
fidget	fi' djet	to move nervously, especially the hands
hence	hens	for this reason, therefore
husky	hus'ky	low-sounding, rough; sturdy
idiopathic	id' ee o path' ik	the cause is not known
inertia	in er' shah	lack of movement, resisting change
lethargic	lah thar' jik	tired, inactive
moody	moo' dee	changing emotions frequently; often sad
slurred	slur'd	not clear, words run together
taper off	tap'er off	to gradually become smaller or less
tetany	tet' ah nee	muscle cramps or twitching
"think straight"		think clearly and normally
undue	un dew'	excessive, too much
wringing	ring' ing	to twist or squeeze (hands or soft material)

COMPLETION

Directions: Fill in the blanks with the correct words from the Vocabulary Building Glossary to complete the statements.

1. If the parathyroid glands are accidentally removed during a thyroidectomy, the patient may experience

   _____.

2. When cortisone is prescribed to treat a nonhormonal illness, it is important that the patient

   _____ the dosage gradually to prevent a hormone imbalance.

3. The patient with Addison disease becomes very fatigued and may seem to be in a state of

   _____.

4. The patient with the thyroid condition was irritable and _____.

5. Hypoparathyroidism can be caused by a(n) _____ atrophy of the glands.

6. While the patient was still groggy from the anesthetic, her words were _____.

7. Cushing disease is from a(n) _____ amount of cortisol circulating in the blood.

8. The nurse could tell that the patient was nervous because she kept _____ her hands.

9. There was a big _____ in the man's hip pocket where he kept his wallet.

10. Mr. Johnson was confused and kept saying, "I can't _____."

11. The child was restless and she began to _____ in the chair.

12. After I ate that huge meal, I felt sleepy and _____.

WORD ATTACK SKILLS

myx/o-	mucus
-crine, -crin/o	secrete

PRONUNCIATION SKILLS

Directions: Take turns with a peer practicing pronouncing these words to increase your ability to speak English clearly.

ac′romeg′aly (ak′ ro meg′ ah lee)	thickening of lips and nose, enlargement of extremities (hyperpituitarism)
ex′ophthal′mos (ek′ sof thal′ mos)	abnormal protrusion of the eye; eyes bulge or stand out in the face
myx′ede′ma (mik′ sah dee′ mah)	a condition resulting from low thyroid production
phe′ochromocytoma (fe′ o kro′mo si′ to ma)	a small tumor of the adrenal glands

CULTURAL POINT

Some people think that Americans, especially American women, are too concerned about their body images. Do you think this is true? If you are from a different country, is this different in your native country? What is the ideal body image there? Is there a relationship between body image and health?

_____

_____

_____

Care of Patients with Diabetes and Hypoglycemia

Answer Key: Review the related chapter to answer these questions. A complete answer key was provided to your instructor.

COMPLETION

Directions: Fill in the blanks to complete the statements.

1. The long-term consequences of diabetes mellitus are chiefly the result of damage to the large and small _____.

2. It is known that the risk of having some form of diabetes increases in proportion to the _____ of relatives who are affected, the _____ of the relatives, and the severity of their disease.

3. Weight loss in patients with type 1 diabetes occurs partly because of the loss of _____ and partly because in the absence of sufficient _____, the body begins to metabolize its own proteins and stored fat.

4. People with poor control over their diabetes are prone to infection because of decreased function of _____ and abnormal phagocyte function.

5. The older diabetic patient is at risk of developing hypoglycemia even before _____ are obvious.

6. Diabetic _____ occurs directly from changes in the renal blood circulation.

7. When insulin is not present in adequate amounts to meet metabolic needs, the body breaks down _____ and _____ for energy.

8. An abundance of the byproducts of fat metabolism results in potent organic acids called _____.

9. Recommended for all patients with type 1 or type 2 diabetes is _____ _____, a personalized diet plan.

10. Four signs and symptoms of hypoglycemia include _____, _____, _____, and _____.

SHORT ANSWER

Type 2 Diabetes

Directions: Read the clinical scenarios and answer the questions that follow.

Scenario: Mr. Eick is an elderly widower with type 2 diabetes. He has been managing his own diabetic condition for the past 15 years; however, he recently moved in with his eldest daughter because he has been increasingly lonely and forgetful. Mr. Eick's daughter also has diabetes and has a good general knowledge of diabetes, but she asks you for some information specific to diabetes in the elderly.

1. Why is "tight control" not advised for elderly type 2 diabetic patients? _____

    _____

2. Why is weight loss not a priority goal for an elderly diabetic patient? _____

    _____

    _____

    _____

    _____

3. What are two problems concerning exercise for older diabetic patients? _____

    _____

    _____

    _____

    _____

4. Which exercise activities are considered the safest for older diabetic patients? _____

    _____

5. For older patients who are taking oral hypoglycemic agents, list two relevant facts related to aging.

    a. _____

        _____

    b. _____

        _____

SHORT ANSWER

Medications for Diabetes

Directions: Answer the following questions related to insulin injection preparation.

1. When regular insulin and long-acting insulin are to be mixed together for an injection, which insulin is drawn up first? _____

2. How are NPH and Lente insulin "mixed" before being drawn up with the syringe? _____

   _____

3. Why is insulin never given orally? _____

   _____

4. What is the proper way to warm chilled insulin? _____

   _____

5. The patient is to receive 3 units of regular insulin and 11 units of NPH. After both medications are
   drawn up, how many total units will be in the syringe? _____ units

6. Every patient on insulin should be monitored for _____ after insulin injections.

Directions: Answer the following questions related to oral hypoglycemic agents.

7. If a patient is allergic to sulfonamide antibiotics, which group of antihypoglycemic agents could cause a
   similar allergic reaction?

   _____

8. What are the two most common side effects of the second-generation oral hypoglycemic agents?

   _____

   _____

9. How is metformin (Glucophage) thought to work? _____

   _____

10. What disease or condition would be a contraindication for the drug acarbose (Precose)?

    _____

11. Why must you always check for drug interactions when a patient is taking an oral hypoglycemic?

    _____

    _____

    _____

APPLICATION OF THE NURSING PROCESS

Caring for Patients with Diabetic Ketoacidosis (DKA)

Directions: Read the scenario and provide the answers to the following questions.

Scenario: Jason, age 16, is on the school track team and he was able to maintain a B average in his studies. Jason's mother reports that within the past several months, he has lost about 20 lbs, lost interest in his classes at school, and complains of being too tired to study or participate in any sports at school or at home. He began running a fever several days ago with flu-like symptoms and now presents to the emergency department with nausea and vomiting. He is listless, flushed, and dehydrated. The emergency department health care provider makes a medical diagnosis of diabetic ketoacidosis (DKA).

1. Since this is a new diagnosis for Jason and his family, what information will they need in the next few days?

   a. _____

   b. _____

   c. _____

   d. _____

2. List at least six physical assessment findings that are likely to be seen with DKA.

   a. _____

   b. _____

   c. _____

   d. _____

   e. _____

   f. _____

3. List four general treatment goals for patients with DKA.

   a. _____

   b. _____

   c. _____

   d. _____

4. Write an expected outcome for the nursing diagnosis Fluid volume deficit due to hyperosmolar state.

   _____

   _____

5. List three nursing interventions (including assessments) that are appropriate to restore fluid balance.

   a. _____

   b. _____

   c. _____

6. List at least two laboratory tests that would be used to evaluate treatment outcomes for a patient in DKA.

   a. _____

   b. _____

7. Which task would be appropriate to assign to the nursing assistant?
   a. Assist Jason to don a patient gown.
   b. Take the initial set of vital signs.
   c. Gather emergency equipment.
   d. Inform Jason's mother about wait time.

PRIORITY SETTING

Scenario: You are working in an extended-care facility. You walk into Mr. Jipnak's room and the nursing assistant tells you that Mr. Jipnak refused his breakfast this morning and went out for a brisk walk. He appears pale, diaphoretic, and is too lethargic to swallow. His blood sugar is 30 mg/dL. You have standing orders to treat hypoglycemia with 1 mg Glucagon IM if the patient is unable to swallow.

Directions: Prioritize the nursing actions below to assist Mr. Jipnak during this hypoglycemic episode.

_____   a. Turn the patient on his side.

_____   b. Give a fast-acting source of sugar and a longer-acting source, such as crackers and cheese or a meat sandwich if alert enough to swallow.

_____   c. Administer 1 mg of Glucagon by injection after mixing the solution in the bottle until it is clear.

_____   d. If the patient does not awaken within 15 minutes, give another dose of Glucagon and inform a health care provider of the situation immediately.

_____   e. Assess ability to swallow after second dose of Glucagon.

_____   f. Assess level of consciousness and ability to swallow.

REVIEW QUESTIONS FOR THE NCLEX® EXAMINATION

Directions: Choose the correct answer(s) for the following questions.

1. The patient is a type 1 diabetic who has been admitted for ketoacidosis and influenza. Which assessment findings are most likely to be documented in this patient's record?
    1. Headache, thirst, and anorexia
    2. Weight gain, polyuria, and dizziness
    3. Diaphoresis, headache, and nervousness
    4. Weakness, stomach pain, and sweating

2. A patient was recently diagnosed with latent autoimmune diabetes of adults (LADA). According to evidence-based management, which medication is the health care provider mostly likely to prescribe in the early phase?
    1. Metformin (Glucophage)
    2. Glyburide (DiaBeta)
    3. Glipizide (Glucotrol)
    4. NovoLog insulin

3. What is an important safety intervention for type 1 diabetes patients?
    1. Provide an 1800-calorie American Diabetes Association (ADA) diet.
    2. Assess for signs of hypoglycemia after insulin is given.
    3. Monitor intake and output carefully.
    4. Do not allow ambulation without assistance.

4. Evaluation of correct balance of food, exercise, and insulin for a diabetic patient would be to:
    1. assess trends of blood sugar levels.
    2. assess daily weight trends.
    3. determine what the blood pH is now.
    4. determine if electrolytes are in balance.

5. An infection such as influenza can be a cause of DKA because:
    1. patients continue insulin but do not eat properly.
    2. use of over-the-counter decongestants interferes with insulin.
    3. infection causes an increased metabolic rate and release of extra glucose.
    4. the patient does not rest well or sleep because of cough and discomfort.

6. Which diagnostic test would be ordered to evaluate the response to therapy at a 6-month follow-up appointment?
    1. Glucose tolerance test
    2. Fasting blood sugar test
    3. 2-hour postprandial blood sugar test
    4. Hemoglobin A$_{1C}$

7. The reason a patient with uncontrolled type 2 diabetes tends to gain weight is because:
    1. he has a big appetite and experiences polyphagia.
    2. of insulin resistance; the food he eats is not fully metabolized.
    3. the excess glucose in his body makes him retain excess water.
    4. he tends to become very sedentary because of little energy.

8. Whenever a type 1 diabetic patient knows that he is going to exercise heavily, he should:
    1. skip his insulin dose both before and after the exercise.
    2. drink a large quantity of water.
    3. eat an extra high-protein snack to prevent hypoglycemia.
    4. take extra insulin to compensate for that used during the exercise.

9. The diabetic patient undergoing surgery experiences considerable stress, which alters his blood sugar levels. For this reason, he is usually given:
    1. an extra allotment of calories before surgery.
    2. intravenous insulin during surgery.
    3. twice as much IV fluid as the nondiabetic patient receives.
    4. a large dose of long-acting insulin prior to surgery.

10. One problem that occurs fairly often in elderly type 2 diabetic patients is hyperglycemic hyperosmolar syndrome (HHS). It occurs most often after:
    1. abdominal surgery and nasogastric suction.
    2. fractures that cause immobility.
    3. multiple diagnostic tests during which patients have been NPO.
    4. a febrile illness or gastrointestinal flu.

11. For type 1 diabetes, which statement is true?
    1. Usually responds to diet and exercise only
    2. Must receive exogenous insulin
    3. Can be managed with oral hypoglycemics
    4. Islet cell transplantation is a first-line treatment

12. Which factors make diabetic patients prone to infection? *(Select all that apply.)*
    1. Poor control of diabetes
    2. Increased function of leukocytes and phagocyte function
    3. Decreased blood supply to the tissues related to atherosclerosis of blood vessels
    4. Chronic neurologic and vascular changes allow organisms to enter tissues
    5. Diabetic patients are overweight and have poor hygiene

13. The ADA recommends screening all adults, especially if overweight, for type 2 diabetes starting at age:
    1. 21, to be repeated every 5 years.
    2. 45, to be repeated every 3 years.
    3. 50, to be repeated every year.
    4. 60, to be repeated every 2 years.

14. Which statement by a patient most strongly indicates a need for further assessment and possible diagnostic testing to screen for diabetes?
    1. "Typically, I urinate a moderate amount just before I go to bed."
    2. "I seem to be really thirsty, but I guess it could be the heat."
    3. "I like to have a snack after I exercise, but I try to watch my calories."
    4. "I probably have diabetes; most of my friends have it."

15. Which statement by a patient's family member indicates an understanding of the signs and symptoms of hypoglycemia?
    1. "He could refuse to eat because he is angry."
    2. "He could be flushed and look dehydrated."
    3. "He could be irritable because his sugar is low."
    4. "He will urinate a lot and be very thirsty."

16. Which viral agent is thought to attack the beta cells of the pancreas causing an onset of insulin-dependent diabetes mellitus (type 1)?
    1. Herpes simplex
    2. *Staphylococcus aureus*
    3. Cytomegalovirus
    4. Coxsackievirus

17. The patient is receiving rapid-acting insulin before meals. What action by the nurse is correct?
    1. Wait until the food tray is delivered to the patient before giving the insulin dose.
    2. Instruct the patient to report any feelings of nausea.
    3. Perform a fingerstick glucose, administer the insulin dose, and wait 30 minutes before providing the meal.
    4. Assess the patient for increased thirst, hypotension, dry mucous membranes, and deep respirations prior to administering the insulin.

18. Which statement by the patient indicates a need for additional teaching on diabetic foot care?
    1. "I should check both feet daily for cracks, blisters, or abrasions."
    2. "I should cut the nails straight across and smooth with an emery board."
    3. "I should elevate my feet whenever possible to improve circulation."
    4. "I should soak my feet in hot water every day and use mild soap."

19. The nurse is teaching the patient how to manage his diabetes during times of minor illness, such as during mild gastrointestinal upset. What is appropriate information to tell the patient?
    1. Discontinue your insulin if you are vomiting.
    2. Take at least 1 cup of water or calorie-free, caffeine-free liquid each hour.
    3. Test your blood sugar once or twice a day.
    4. If taking an oral hypoglycemic agent, increase the dose for 2–3 days while ill.

20. The nurse is interviewing a patient to establish a database. The patient has reported being excessively thirsty but has never been diagnosed with diabetes. Which questions would be appropriate to ask the patient during this initial interview? *(Select all that apply.)*
    1. Have you had any recent weight loss?
    2. Have you become increasingly hungry over the past few months?
    3. Are you having any trouble sticking to your dietary plan?
    4. Do you have to urinate (go to the toilet) more than you used to?
    5. Have you noticed that you are more tired than you were 6 months ago?
    6. Have you made any plans on how to cope with a chronic illness?
    7. Has anyone in your family ever been told he or she has diabetes?

CRITICAL THINKING ACTIVITIES

Scenario: Ms. Thomas, age 62, has been diagnosed as a type 2 diabetic. She is 50 pounds overweight and leads a very sedentary life. She worked as a secretary until 3 months ago, when she began to feel weak and "tired all the time." Her health care provider has prescribed diet and exercise and Glucophage for the management of her diabetes. Ms. Thomas is reluctant to engage in an exercise program and has many questions about it. How would you answer the following questions?

1. "What does exercise do for a person with diabetes?" _____

_____

_____

2. "What kind of exercise do I have to do?" _____

_____

_____

3. "Do I have to keep a record of exercise, too?" _____

_____

_____

STEPS TOWARD BETTER COMMUNICATION

VOCABULARY BUILDING GLOSSARY

Term	Pronunciation	Definition
sequelae	se kwe′ lay	(plural) consequences
brittle	brit′ el	easily broken; (referring to diabetes: hard to control, with wide daily variations in glucose level)
postprandial	post′ pran′ dee al	after a meal
first generation	first′ jen er ay′ shun	original in a line of creation or descent: families (e.g., *first-generation* American); objects or inventions (e.g., original is *first generation,* further development is *second generation*)
tight control	tyt′ kun trol′	control within a narrow range; carefully regulated control
unmask	un mask′	uncover something hidden
basement membrane	bays′ ment mem′ brayn	a delicate membrane in the secreting glands
susceptible	su sep′ ti bul	likely or liable to develop; to be affected by

COMPLETION

Directions: Fill in the blanks with the correct words from the Vocabulary Building Glossary to complete the statements.

1. The child's glucose level was difficult to keep within normal limits because his diabetes mellitus was very _____.

2. Diabinese is a(n) _____ hypoglycemic agent.

3. The health care provider was trying to _____ what was causing the patient's symptoms of extreme shakiness and headaches that occurred periodically.

4. Blindness and renal failure are _____ of long-term uncontrolled blood glucose levels.

5. Older adults who are obese seem to be more _____ to diabetes mellitus.

6. When screening for diabetes mellitus, the health care provider may order a(n) _____ blood sugar level drawn.

7. The best way to avoid complications of diabetes mellitus is to maintain _____ of blood glucose.

WORD ATTACK SKILLS

Directions: Sometimes words that you find in daily speech are used in a different way in the hospital or medical setting. Can you give the two meanings for each?

1. Brittle
    a. Medical usage: _____
    b. Everyday usage: _____

2. Basement
    a. Medical usage: _____
    b. Everyday usage: _____

PRONUNCIATION SKILLS

melli'tus (mel eye' tus **or** mel ee' tus) (may vary depending on the part of the country where you live)

Somo'gyi (so mo' gee)

Directions: Practice pronouncing the following terms:

HHNK: hyperosmolar hyperglycemic nonketotic

DKA: diabetic ketoacidosis

CULTURAL POINT

Young people in the United States are very sensitive to the opinions of others, especially their peers, about body image, their attractiveness, friends, and capabilities in school and sports. They do not want to appear different. For example, they like to wear the same style of clothing and hair, and eat the same kinds of food. This can make it very difficult for a young person who is diabetic and must eat differently, perform blood sugar checks often, and self-administer insulin.

You must work with the patient and family to help the patient lead as normal a life as possible. Encouraging sports with guidelines for blood sugar checks, extra snacks, and insulin adjustments promotes safe participation. When the patient wishes to sleep over at a friend's house, appropriate snacks can be sent along and the friend's parents can be made aware of the patient's requirements of blood sugar checks, insulin, and meals. You can teach the patient how to make smart food choices when out with friends at restaurants or fast-food places.

COMMUNICATION EXERCISE

When working with diabetic patients, you must assess for problems relating to compliance with prescribed treatment. Trust between you and the patient must be developed before the patient will be open and honest discussing problems related to the diet, exercise program, blood glucose monitoring, and medication schedule. There are certain ways to approach these topics that seem to work better than others.

The following are questions nurses often ask diabetic patients. In italics, there is an example of a better way to obtain the desired explanation in each case.

"Are you sticking to your meal plan?"

"Tell me about any problems you are having with your meals."

"How much are you exercising now?"

"Are you able to exercise as much as you thought you could?"

"Are you checking your blood sugar before meals?"

"Tell me how your blood sugar checks with the glucometer are going."

"Are you taking your insulin at the times it is scheduled?"

"What kind of problems, if any, are you having in giving yourself insulin at the designated times?"

"Are you checking your feet for problems each day?"

"Tell me, when have you have managed to work checking your feet into your daily routine?"

"Are you remembering to take your oral medication each day?"

"How are things going with taking your oral medication?"

This rephrasing allows patients, especially teens, to perceive themselves in charge of the situation and avoid what they see as accusatory questions.

The Reproductive System

Answer Key: Review the related chapter to answer these questions. A complete answer key was provided to your instructor.

REVIEW OF ANATOMY AND PHYSIOLOGY

Terminology

Directions: Match the term on the left with the correct statement, function, or definition on the right.

1. _____ Perineum
2. _____ Fallopian tubes
3. _____ Epididymis
4. _____ Spermatic cord
5. _____ Uterus
6. _____ Menarche
7. _____ Seminal vesicles
8. _____ Prostate gland
9. _____ Lactation
10. _____ Androgens

a. Attaches the testes to the body
b. Hollow pear-shaped organ with a thick muscular wall
c. Milk production
d. Flat muscular surface anterior to the anus
e. Onset of menstruation
f. Tube that conducts sperm from the testes to the vas deferens
g. Form the pathway for the ovum
h. Male sex hormones
i. Produce a fluid that nourishes sperm
j. Located below and to the rear of the bladder

COMPLETION

Directions: Fill in the blanks to complete the statements.

1. The ovarian cycle has two phases: the _____ phase and the _____ phase.

2. The amount of blood loss with normal menstruation is _____ to _____ mL.

3. Signs and symptoms of the climacteric period and menopause include _____, _____, and _____.

4. The length of the menstrual cycle can be influenced by _____, _____, _____, and _____.

5. _____ and _____ are released from the anterior pituitary gland when it is stimulated by gonadotropin-releasing hormone (GnRH).

6. Maturation of the male reproductive organs occurs at _____.

7. The only means to prevent conception 100% is _____.

8. Some medication for emergency contraception can be effective when taken up to _____ days after unprotected sex.

Examination and Diagnostic Testing

Directions: Fill in the blanks to complete the statements.

1. Breast self-examination may be done monthly, about _____ after menstruation begins, or on a specific date each month after menopause.

2. Vulvar self-examination should be performed _____. The woman should report any changes such as _____, _____, or _____ and should be alert to new _____.

3. Testicular self-examination should be done _____.

4. The purpose of testicular self-examination is for early detection of _____.

5. A test that is performed for postmenopausal bleeding is a(n) _____.

6. Regularly scheduled mammograms after age _____ are recommended by the American College of Obstetricians and Gynecologists.

7. A(n) _____ is used to evaluate abnormal cells and lesions, particularly after a positive Pap smear.

8. A vaginal ultrasound may be done to detect the _____ of the uterine lining, _____ of the uterus, the presence of _____, the size of ovaries and the presence of cysts or tumors.

Table Activity

Contraceptive Method	How Method Works	Side Effects/Precautions	Degree of Effectiveness
Abstinence			
Fertility Awareness Methods			
Basal body temperature (BBT)			
Calendar or rhythm method			
Ovulation or Billings method			
Symptothermal method			
Chemical predictor test			
Mechanical or Barrier Contraception			
Intrauterine device (IUD)			

Contraceptive Method	How Method Works	Side Effects/Precautions	Degree of Effectiveness
Male condom			
Cervical cap (FemCap)			
Female (internal) condom			
Diaphragm			
Vaginal sponge			

Contraceptive Method	How Method Works	Side Effects/Precautions	Degree of Effectiveness
Spermicidal Methods			
Gels, foams, creams			
Hormonal Methods			
Oral contraceptives (OCs)			
Injectable contraceptives (Depo-Provera)			
Sustained-release implants (Nexplanon)			
Emergency contraception (EC)			
Vaginal ring			
Skin patch			

Contraceptive Method	How Method Works	Side Effects/Precautions	Degree of Effectiveness
Permanent Contraception			
Tubal ligation (female; surgical)			
Vasectomy (male)			

Menopause

Directions: Read the scenario and answer the questions that follow.

Scenario: Ms. Stahl, age 52, has begun having menstrual irregularity, alternating between a scanty flow and heavy bleeding, and often missing periods. Her gynecologist assures her that she is entering the climacteric and there are no signs of abnormalities of her uterus. Ms. Stahl is an engineer and she works mostly with men at her office. She asks you for more information.

1. Menopause is described as cessation of menses for a(n) _____-month period due to decreased estrogen production.

2. Women may be prescribed vaginal creams containing estrogen to restore

   _____ and _____ to vaginal tissues.

3. In addition to menstrual irregularity, list at least seven other psychological and physiologic symptoms that sometimes accompany menopause.

   a. _____

   b. _____

   c. _____

   d. _____

   e. _____

   f. _____

   g. _____

SHORT ANSWER

Nursing Assessment of the Female Reproductive System

Directions: Read the scenario and answer the following questions about nursing assessment of a patient's gynecologic health status.

Scenario: You are working in a gynecology clinic. Ms. Simmons is a new patient who comes in for a routine pelvic examination and her annual Pap smear. You are collecting information that will contribute to identifying problems and educational needs.

1. Why is the female patient's age relevant to a nursing assessment?

   _____

   _____

   _____

2. Why would you be interested in Ms. Simmons' sexual activities; for example, at what age she became sexually active and how many partners she has had?

   _____

   _____

3. List information that would be included in the patient's menstrual history.

   a. _____

   b. _____

   c. _____

   d. _____

   e. _____

4. List some subjective and objective data that would be useful in assessing a patient with a gynecologic disorder.

   Subjective data:

   a. _____

   b. _____

   c. _____

   d. _____

   e. _____

   Objective data:

   a. _____

   b. _____

   c. _____

   d. _____

PRIORITY SETTING

Directions: Read the scenario and prioritize the steps of assisting with a pelvic exam.

Scenario: Ms. Gian has come in for a pelvic exam and a Pap smear. You are preparing her for examination and will assist the doctor during the procedure.

_____ a. Assemble clean gloves and supplies.

_____ b. Encourage Ms. Gian to void because a full bladder will make the exam more uncomfortable.

_____ c. Stay with Ms. Gian, encourage her, and give information.

_____ d. Orient Ms. Gian to the equipment and the purpose of the exam.

_____ e. Position Ms. Gian appropriately (i.e., lithotomy position).

_____ f. The unit should provide privacy and good lighting.

CRITICAL THINKING ACTIVITIES

Promoting Men's Reproductive and Sexual Health

Directions: Read the clinical scenario and answer the questions that follow.

Scenario: You are participating in a men's health fair. You have been asked to collect information about various topics regarding men's sexual health and disorders of the reproductive system.

1. What are three ways in which disorders of the male reproductive organs might be prevented?

   a. _____

   b. _____

   c. _____

2. Describe when, how, and why a testicular self-examination should be done.

   a. When:_____

   b. How: _____

   c. Why:_____

3. Name four ways that you can be instrumental in the community in promoting male reproductive and sexual health.

   a. _____

   b. _____

   c. _____

   d. _____

REVIEW QUESTIONS FOR THE NCLEX® EXAMINATION

Directions: Choose the best answer(s) for the following questions.

1. Which statement by a patient indicates a need for additional teaching about the "morning-after pill"?
   1. "It has to be taken within 72 hours after unprotected sex."
   2. "It works by preventing ovulation, implantation, or fertilization."
   3. "It may cause nausea and vomiting, so I should take an antiemetic."
   4. "It can be used to terminate a first trimester pregnancy."

2. Male reproductive disorders are commonly treated by a:
   1. specialist.
   2. urologist.
   3. family practice provider.
   4. nurse practitioner.

3. When should a female start having routine pelvic exams and Pap smears?
   1. As soon as she becomes sexually active or at age 20
   2. At age 16, if she has family history of cervical cancer
   3. At age 21
   4. Whenever she starts her menstrual periods

4. A patient is being discharged home after a vasectomy. What teaching should be given? *(Select all that apply.)*
   1. Contraception will still need to be used until two sperm counts are negative.
   2. There may be a decrease in libido or sexual performance postprocedure.
   3. Scrotal pain and swelling can be treated with NSAIDs and ice for the first 12–24 hours postprocedure.
   4. Some form of scrotal support will help with discomfort.
   5. Sexual intercourse may be resumed after 48 hours.

5. Which information should be included when collecting sexual health information? *(Select all that apply.)*
   1. Whether sexually active
   2. Type of contraception used
   3. History of sexually transmitted infections
   4. History of urinary tract infections
   5. Number of sexual partners

6. Pelvic relaxation syndrome may lead to:
   1. abdominal pain.
   2. cervical dysplasia.
   3. metrorrhagia.
   4. a cystocele.

7. The nurse is assessing the sexual health of an elderly woman. Which is the most likely physical symptom that an elderly woman would report?
   1. Does not feel attractive anymore.
   2. Is always too tired for sex.
   3. Has no sexual desire.
   4. Has decreased vaginal lubrication.

8. Older women who are, or have been, on long-term hormone replacement therapy are at increased risk for: *(Select all that apply.)*
   1. metrorrhagia.
   2. breast cancer.
   3. oligomenorrhea.
   4. endometrial cancer.

9. A primary cause of male impotence is related to changes in which body system?
   1. Vascular
   2. Respiratory
   3. Urinary
   4. Neurologic

10. Nurse advocacy for the LGBTQIA+ population includes: *(Select all that apply.)*
    1. assuming the patient is heterosexual until told otherwise.
    2. ensuring a welcoming and safe environment for all patients.
    3. use neutral and inclusive language with all patients.
    4. refer patients to other resources rather than address their needs.
    5. be aware of biases and communication barriers to care.
    6. honor and respect whatever information the patient shares regarding sexual orientation and gender identity.

CRITICAL THINKING ACTIVITIES

Scenario: You are talking to several neighbors about sexual activity and the use of birth control among teenagers and young adults. There are various opinions among the parents and you can tell that it is a very controversial topic. Several of the parents want to know your opinion about the how to deal with their sexually active teens and what they should tell them about birth control.

1. What factors are involved in selecting a method of contraception? _____

   _____

   _____

2. What are the advantages and disadvantages of using a condom? _____

   _____

3. What other types of contraception should be taught? _____

   _____

   _____

4. What is the female condom? Why is it generally not widely used? _____

   _____

   _____

   _____

   _____

STEPS TOWARD BETTER COMMUNICATION

VOCABULARY BUILDING GLOSSARY

Term	Pronunciation	Definition
slough, slough off	sluf	(verb) separating and dropping off of dead tissue; to shed
period	pir' ee ud	a woman's monthly menstrual flow
"the change of life"		psychological response to menopause

COMPLETION

Directions: Fill in the blanks with the correct words from the Vocabulary Building Glossary to complete the statements.

1. During menstruation, the uterine lining will _____.

2. When calculating the estimated date of delivery, the health care provider asks the date of the woman's last _____.

3. With family support and an optimistic outlook for the future, a woman can view _____ as a new transitional period.

WORD ATTACK SKILLS

Directions: Using the word elements listed below, give the meaning of each word.

gyn/o	woman
oo	ovum
orchi/o	testis
andr/o	male
colp/o	vagina
mamm/o	breast

1. Culposcopy: _____

2. Gynecology: _____

3. Mammogram: _____

4. Orchitis: _____

5. Androgen: _____

ABBREVIATIONS

Directions: Write in the meaning for each abbreviation.

1. OC: _____

2. BSE: _____

3. VSE: _____

4. FSH: _____

5. IUD: _____

6. PSA: _____

7. BBT: _____

8. LGBTQIA+: _____

CULTURAL POINTS

Culture and Tradition

Culture and tradition influence attitudes and values toward sex and sexuality. Some cultures are very open about sexual matters, while others are very private and such issues are not discussed with others. Many cultures have attitudes that lie somewhere in between openness and extreme privacy. In any culture, there are acceptable and unacceptable modes of behavior, and there are people who follow the traditions and those who do not.

Think about the traditions you grew up with and what you learned about how to feel toward sexual behavior. How is your attitude toward sexuality different from the traditions you see around you today? How do you feel about these differences? How will such a difference affect your behavior as a nurse? Can you be nonjudgmental about sexuality?

Care of Women with Reproductive Disorders

Answer Key: Review the related chapter to answer these questions. A complete answer key was provided to your instructor.

COMPLETION

Health Promotion

Directions: Fill in the blanks to complete the statements.

1. Lifestyle changes to reduce the incontinence symptoms associated with pelvic relaxation syndrome include increased _____ and a(n) _____ diet to avoid constipation, and maintaining optimum _____.

2. Patients at risk for osteoporosis should be advised to stop smoking and to avoid excessive

   _____, _____, _____, or soft drink intake.

3. _____ measures are designed to decrease the probability of becoming ill. Examples include maintaining a health or nutrition history and providing immunizations.

4. Warning signs of ovarian cancer include _____, _____, or _____ pain; difficulty eating or _____; and urinary _____ or _____.

COMPLETION

Disorders of the Reproductive System

Directions: Fill in the blanks to complete the statements.

1. A diet high in _____ helps decrease the symptoms of _____ _____.

2. Uterine bleeding may be considered abnormal if the interval between menstruation is fewer than _____ days or more than _____ days; the duration of menstrual flow is more than _____ days or the amount of blood loss exceeds _____ mL.

3. A recommendation to decrease the cramping from menstruation is the use of _____.

4. Common symptoms of leiomyoma include backache, a sense of lower _____ pressure, constipation, urinary _____ or _____, and abnormal uterine bleeding.

5. Continuous hormonal contraceptive therapy for endometriosis includes drugs such as _____ or _____, which suppress growth of the endometrial tissue.

6. Toxic shock syndrome (TSS) is a rare, potentially fatal disorder caused by strains of _____ that produce toxins that cause shock, coagulation defects, and tissue damage if they enter the bloodstream.

7. If removal of a tumor from the uterine wall is needed, a(n) _____ is performed.

8. The patient with endometriosis often experiences _____ and excessive _____ with menstruation.

TABLE ACTIVITY

Directions: Complete the boxes in each column.

Comparisons of Two Types of Common Vaginal Infections

	Bacterial Vaginosis	Yeast Infection
Primary causative organism(s)		
Onset		
Odor		
Itching		
Discharge		
Sexually transmitted		
Vulvar signs		
Vaginal signs		
Treatment		

Cancers of the Reproductive System

Directions: Read the scenario and answer the questions that follow.

Scenario: You have been asked to do a community presentation that includes some basic information about gynecologic cancers. You want to share information about the risk factors and signs and symptoms that women should watch for.

1. The most common malignant tumor of the female reproductive tract is _____ cancer.

2. List six risk factors for cervical cancer.

    a. _____

    b. _____

    c. _____

    d. _____

    e. _____

    f. _____

3. List three risk factors for ovarian cancer.

    a. _____

    b. _____

    c. _____

4. What are the signs and symptoms of vulvar intraepithelial neoplasia (VIN)? _____

    _____

5. Explain in your own words why ovarian cancer is known as the "silent cancer." _____

    _____

    _____

    _____

6. Regular pelvic examinations and Pap smears may enable early diagnosis of _____ and provide opportunity for early and more successful intervention.

7. The _____ vaccine given to girls at or before puberty may prevent the type of HPV infection that causes cervical cancer.

APPLICATION OF THE NURSING PROCESS

Care of the Patient with Breast Cancer

Directions: Read the scenario and provide the answers to the following questions.

Scenario: Ms. Donner has been diagnosed with breast cancer and is admitted for a lumpectomy. She has had some preoperative teaching prior to being admitted to the hospital. The RN completed the admission assessment and history.

1. In evaluating preoperative teaching with Ms. Donner, which statement by the patient indicates that she understands what is happening during the lumpectomy procedure?
   a. The surgeon removes only the tumor.
   b. The surgeon removes the entire breast and axillary lymph nodes.
   c. The surgeon removes the tumor and a portion of the surrounding breast tissue and axillary lymph nodes.
   d. The surgeon removes the breast, axillary lymph nodes, and chest wall muscles under the breast.

2. Ms. Donner's maintenance IV is dextrose 5% with normal saline 1000 mL to infuse over 8 hours. What is the pump setting? _____

3. What is your first concern for Ms. Donner when she returns from the operating room?
   a. Risk for depression
   b. Risk for bleeding
   c. Risk for infection
   d. Risk for falls

4. List four specific nursing measures that would be included in the nursing care plan for Ms. Donner immediately after lumpectomy.

   a. _____

   b. _____

   c. _____

   d. _____

5. Which task would be appropriate to assign to the nursing assistant?
   a. Assist Ms. Donner to use the spirometer correctly.
   b. Do bilateral pulse checks on the upper extremities.
   c. Teach Ms. Donner that no blood pressures are taken on affected side.
   d. Assist Ms. Donner to ambulate in the hall.

6. List information that would be helpful to Ms. Donner in planning her discharge after lumpectomy.

   a. _____

   b. _____

   c. _____

   d. _____

REVIEW QUESTIONS FOR THE NCLEX® EXAMINATION

Directions: Choose the best answer(s) for the following questions.

1. A patient presents to the clinic stating that she is having problems with heavy periods with bleeding between periods, painful bowel movements, and painful sexual intercourse. You expect her to be treated for:
    1. an inflammation of the lower genital tract.
    2. leiomyoma.
    3. endometriosis.
    4. menorrhagia.

2. An intrauterine medication to treat dysmenorrhea is:
    1. an intrauterine device.
    2. levonorgestrel-releasing system.
    3. mefenamic acid.
    4. COX-2 inhibitor.

3. Breast cancer that is HER2-positive has shown to be responsive to which adjuvant therapy?
    1. Medroxyprogesterone acetate (Depo-Provera)
    2. Trastuzumab (Herceptin)
    3. Alendronic acid (Fosamax)
    4. Ethinyl estradiol (Lybrel)

4. The nurse is assessing a patient for risk factors for breast cancer. The nurse includes questions about: *(Select all that apply.)*
    1. family history of relatives with breast cancer.
    2. early menarche, late menopause.
    3. late first pregnancy or no children.
    4. abnormal cells in previous breast biopsy.
    5. history of being less than ideal body weight.

5. Osteoporosis (a decrease in bone mass) puts the postmenopausal woman at increased risk for bone fracture. Lifestyle activities that increase this risk include: *(Select all that apply.)*
    1. inadequate lifetime intake of calcium and vitamin D.
    2. taking vitamin C and iron supplements.
    3. smoking.
    4. sleeping 9–10 hours night.
    5. excess alcohol and/or caffeine intake.

6. Pelvic relaxation syndrome may lead to:
    1. abdominal pain.
    2. cervical dysplasia.
    3. metrorrhagia.
    4. a cystocele.

7. A patient is being treated for menorrhagia. In a follow-up appointment, which testing would be appropriate for evaluating the treatment's effectiveness?
    1. Electrolytes
    2. Ultrasound of the ovaries
    3. Hemoglobin and hematocrit
    4. CT scan of the pelvic organs

8. Older women who are, or have been, on long-term hormone replacement therapy are at increased risk for: *(Select all that apply.)*
   1. metrorrhagia.
   2. breast cancer.
   3. oligomenorrhea.
   4. endometrial cancer.

9. In an elderly woman, vaginal bleeding is a possible sign of:
   1. hormone imbalance.
   2. cervical or uterine cancer.
   3. breast cancer.
   4. vaginal-rectal fistula.

10. Measures that may decrease the discomfort of dysmenorrhea include:
    1. doing aerobic exercises when the discomfort first starts.
    2. avoiding foods such as asparagus and watermelon.
    3. using a heating pad and doing pelvic rock exercises.
    4. avoiding use of tampons and douching.

11. Motrin, Anaprox, and Advil are examples of drugs used for dysmenorrhea because they inhibit:
    1. the transmission of pain along nerve pathways.
    2. salt and water retention.
    3. smooth muscle spasm in the uterus.
    4. production of prostaglandins.

12. Two measures that have been found to decrease the discomfort of fibrocystic breast changes are:
    1. taking vitamin C and getting sufficient exercise.
    2. decreasing fat and protein in the diet.
    3. controlled weight loss and wearing a support bra.
    4. taking vitamin E and decreasing caffeine intake.

PRONUNCIATION SKILLS

This exercise gives you practice in speaking and listening for pronunciation of final consonants.

Directions: With a partner, take turns saying the words below. The speaker chooses and pronounces one word in each line, marking the word pronounced. The listener numbers a sheet of paper from 1–11 and writes the words heard (or circles the words in the book). Check for listening accuracy. Switch roles and do the exercise again. Take special care to pronounce the end of each word fully and clearly.

1. birth   burn   bird
2. risk   wrist
3. weight   weighed   wake   wait
4. pain   pale   pay   paid
5. take   tape
6. cost   cot
7. age   aids
8. sigh   sign   sight   side
9. team   teen   teeth   teach
10. you   use   used   youth
11. not   nod

WORD ATTACK SKILLS

Directions: Using the word elements listed below, give the meaning of each word.

a-	lack, none, not, without
dys-	bad, difficult, wrongly
men/o-	month
meta/o-	after, beyond, above
-rrhea	flow, discharge
-rrage	excessive bleeding
-rrhagia	hemorrhage

1. Menorrhea:_____

2. Amenorrhea: _____

3. Dysmenorrhea: _____

4. Metrorrhagia:_____

5. Menorrhagia: _____

ABBREVIATIONS

Directions: Write in the meaning of each abbreviation.

1. ART: _____

2. DUB: _____

3. AUB: _____

4. PCOS: _____

5. TSS: _____

6. D&E: _____

7. PMS: _____

8. HPV: _____

9. PMDD: _____

10. HRT: _____

CULTURAL POINTS

Confidentiality

Confidentiality is a nursing responsibility in all patient situations. When discussing matters of very personal nature such as reproductive problems, it is particularly important to offer the patient reassurance that any information given will remain private. Such information must not be discussed even with other nurses, unless these others are directly involved in the patient's care.

Care of Men with Reproductive Disorders

Answer Key: Review the related chapter to answer these questions. A complete answer key was provided to your instructor.

COMPLETION

Directions: Fill in the blanks to complete the statements.

1. With aging, the decrease in _____ may affect erectile function.

2. Erectile dysfunction has both _____ and organic causes.

3. Whenever examining the genital area, _____ should be provided.

4. Follow-up care for vasectomy includes a second sperm count that should be done _____ later to verify that the vas deferens is not intact.

5. Inflammatory epididymitis is most likely to result after an infection of _____, _____.

6. Hydrocele causes enlargement of the _____ and is usually _____.

7. The patient with epididymitis complains of _____ pain plus _____ and pain in the scrotum.

8. Testicular torsion is commonly caused by _____ levels in young adult males but can also be the result of _____ trauma.

9. _____ is a condition that results in the inability to have a uniform erection of the penis.

10. Men who have had an undescended or partially descended testicle are most at risk for _____ cancer.

11. A man is more likely to experience erectile dysfunction if he has been _____ for some time.

12. _____ is the gold standard of treatment for benign prostatic hyperplasia (BPH) and is performed under spinal anesthesia.

13. An enlarged prostate may eventually cause _____.

14. BPH produces no symptoms until the growth becomes large enough to press against the

    _____.

15. Because hemorrhage always is a danger after prostate surgery, vital signs are taken every _____ hours initially, then every _____ hours.

16. After prostate surgery, a high-fiber diet and stool softeners may be prescribed to prevent straining, which increases _____ pressure and can cause further bleeding.

17. If a postprostatectomy patient reports severe pain in the bladder region, you should check for an obstruction in the _____ or the _____ before administering an analgesic.

18. Bilateral orchitis is serious and very often causes _____.

19. _____ usually is given to lessen the severity of mumps orchitis.

20. Cancer of the penis is rare, occurring mostly in males with _____ infections or males who were not _____.

21. Dilation and clumping of the tributary vessels of the spermatic vein creates a(n)

    _____.

22. All males between the ages of _____ and _____ should practice testicular self-examination regularly on a monthly basis.

23. Men over the age of _____ should have an annual digital rectal exam and prostate-specific antigen (PSA) test to help reduce the death rate from _____.

24. For postoperative self-care, the health care provider instructs the patient to drink 12–14 glasses (8 ounces/glass) of water each day. Convert the range of intake/day into mL. _____ mL

APPLICATION OF THE NURSING PROCESS

Care of the Patient with Epididymitis

Directions: Read the scenario and provide the answers to the following questions.

Scenario: You are working at the university student health center. Mr. Jefferson comes in and tells you he would like to see a health care provider because he thinks he might have an infection. He is reluctant to disclose information to any female nurses or providers and would "rather talk to a guy."

1. Identify four strategies that you can use to help patients of the opposite gender to feel more comfortable in talking about sexual health.

   a. _____

   b. _____

   c. _____

   d. _____

2. List subjective and objective data that should be included in the nursing assessment of a patient with a disorder of the male reproductive system.

   Subjective data:

   a. _____

   b. _____

   c. _____

   Objective data:

   a. _____

   b. _____

   c. _____

   d. _____

3. The health care provider tells Mr. Jefferson that he has epididymitis. What is the treatment for this disorder?

   a. _____

   b. _____

   c. _____

   d. _____

   e. _____

4. Which of the following nursing problems would need to be addressed to help Mr. Jefferson prevent future problems with reproductive organs and maintain good sexual health? *(Select all that apply.)*
   a. Need for education concerning self-care and safe sex practices
   b. Risk for impotence
   c. Nervousness concerning the health care interview
   d. Risk for future infection

5. Which statement by Mr. Jefferson indicates a need for additional teaching about the treatment and prevention of epididymitis?
   a. "My sexual partners should be treated for HPV infection."
   b. "My other testicle could become infected."
   c. "Treatment includes antibiotics and analgesics."
   d. "The scrotum is elevated and I can use an ice pack."

SHORT ANSWER

Care of the Patient with Benign Prostatic Hyperplasia

Directions: Read the clinical scenario and answer the questions that follow.

Scenario: Mr. O'Grady is an older man who has always enjoyed good health. He reports some dribbling after urination and also nocturia that has slowly but progressively become more annoying. The health care provider informs him that he has BPH.

1. Signs and symptoms of BPH include:

   a. _____

   b. _____

   c. _____

   d. _____

   e. _____

2. What drug therapies are used to treat BPH?

   a. _____

   b. _____

3. What are some dietary modifications that you could review with Mr. O'Grady?

   a. _____

   b. _____

PRIORITY SETTING

Directions: Read the scenario and prioritize appropriately.

Scenario: You are working in an emergency department. It is a busy night. Several of the following patients are very uncomfortable and all are anxious to receive care and attention.

1. Which male patient has the condition with the highest priority for attention?
   a. The patient with a testicular torsion
   b. The patient with urinary retention secondary to BPH
   c. The patient with orchitis
   d. The patient with Klinefelter's syndrome

REVIEW QUESTIONS FOR THE NCLEX® EXAMINATION

Directions: Choose the best answer(s) for the following questions.

1. When discussing prostate cancer with a patient who has a strong family history of the disorder and BPH, the nurse tells him that which medication is used to help prevent prostate cancer?
   1. Finasteride
   2. Doxazosin
   3. Terazosin
   4. Tamsulosin

2. When considering complementary and alternative therapy for prostate cancer, which is true?
   1. Plant extracts should not be taken if the patient is receiving hormone therapy.
   2. It is best to train the body to hold urine for an increasingly longer duration.
   3. Research has proven that saw palmetto helps relieve symptoms.
   4. Surgery is the only way to improve symptoms.

3. A patient has been diagnosed with BPH and is asking if surgery is indicated. Identify which are indications for surgical intervention. *(Select all that apply.)*
   1. Hematuria
   2. Incontinence
   3. Elevated PSA
   4. Urinary tract infections
   5. Urinary retention
   6. Pain on urination

4. A patient asks the nurse for information about prostate cancer and how it develops. The nurse answers:
   1. "It is a quick-growing cancer and the nodule is small."
   2. "Prostate cancer is a very slow-growing cancer."
   3. "It is a cancer that is related to sexually transmitted viruses."
   4. "This type of cancer is embryonic and continues to grow slowly after birth."

5. After a transurethral resection of the prostate (TURP), a priority nursing problem in the immediate postoperative period is:
   1. Altered activity tolerance due to required bedrest.
   2. Pain due to bladder spasms.
   3. Potential for bleeding due to surgery.
   4. Anxiety due to sexual function after surgery.

6. Which diagnostic test would most likely be performed on an elderly patient who has a PSA result of 7.2?
   1. Another blood sample for PSA
   2. CT scan of the pelvis
   3. Voiding urethrogram
   4. Prostate needle biopsy

7. Nocturia is a common symptom experienced by males, resulting from:
   1. use of condoms for contraception.
   2. BPH.
   3. a high-fiber diet.
   4. taking an antiestrogen agent.

8. Silodosin (Rapaflo) is prescribed, and the nurse explains to the patient that it:
   1. lowers testosterone levels.
   2. lowers PSA levels.
   3. decreases the prostate size by 50%.
   4. promotes relaxation of smooth muscle.

9. The nurse teaches a patient that a potential side effect of tamsulosin (Flomax) is postural hypotension and that he should:
   1. take his blood pressure each day.
   2. change positions slowly to prevent dizziness.
   3. call the office if he starts having headaches.
   4. rest for half an hour each afternoon.

10. Which instruction(s) would be appropriate to teach a patient regarding self-care following a TURP? *(Select all that apply.)*
    1. Drink 3–4 glasses of water during the day.
    2. Avoid bladder stimulants such as alcohol and spicy foods.
    3. Avoid strenuous exercise for 2–3 weeks after surgery.
    4. Keep follow-up appointments.
    5. Self-catheterize as needed to prevent urinary retention.

11. The elderly patient is unable to pass urine. He is diagnosed with BPH and the health care provider has ordered the insertion of a Foley catheter. Which task would be appropriate to assign to the nursing assistant?
    1. Insert the Foley catheter using sterile technique.
    2. Provide perineal and Foley care after insertion.
    3. Observe the meatus for skin breakdown during hygienic care.
    4. Evaluate the patient's response to the Foley insertion.

CRITICAL THINKING ACTIVITIES

Scenario: Your neighbor confides that she and her husband have been trying to have a baby for several years without success. They suspect that he may have some infertility problems, because she had a successful and uneventful pregnancy when she was a teenager and ultimately the baby was adopted. Your neighbor tells you that they are having trouble talking about it because "Jason doesn't think he is infertile and he is having some trouble with the idea that I was pregnant before. What can I do to convince Jason to get checked out? Is there anything that you know that we should or should not be doing?"

1. Would you feel comfortable giving advice to this neighbor? If so, what would you say? _____

   _____

   _____

   _____

   _____

   _____

2. How is male fertility assessed?

   a. _____

   b. _____

   c. _____

   d. _____

   e. _____

3. What are some of the environmental factors that can affect fertility in males? What are some teaching points that address these factors?

a. _____

_____

b. _____

_____

c. _____

_____

STEPS TOWARD BETTER COMMUNICATION

VOCABULARY BUILDING GLOSSARY

Term	Pronunciation	Definition
cessation	ses sa′ shun	stopping, ceasing
open-ended questions		questions that cannot be answered by "yes," "no," or by a short answer; open-ended questions begin with "Why?" or "How?" or "What can you tell me about…" and open-ended questions do not expect a specific response
gonads	go′ nads	sex glands; the testes and ovaries

COMPLETION

Directions: Fill in the blanks with the correct words from the Vocabulary Building Glossary to complete the statements.

1. Suppressing secretion of testosterone by the _____ is a method of treating prostate cancer.

2. After a TURP, if a clot occludes the urinary catheter, there is a(n) _____ of urine drainage.

3. Using _____ when assessing for sexual dysfunction often elicits the most information.

ABBREVIATIONS

Directions: Write the meaning of each abbreviation. Pronounce each abbreviation.

1. BPH: _____

2. PSA:_____

3. TSE: _____

4. TURP: _____

WORD ATTACK SKILLS

-cele   tumor; hernia

GRAMMAR POINTS

When taking medical histories and performing assessments, use the following phrases to obtain time-specific information from the patient.

Occurring now	Occurred in the past	Continues to occur
Do you feel	Have you felt	Have you been feeling
Do you have	Have you had	Have you been having
Have you noticed	Have you ever had	What have you been noticing
What do you take	What did you take	Have you been taking
Do you use	Did you use	Have you been using
Are you using	Have you used	
Would you describe	Is there a history	
Do you perform	Did you perform	Have you been performing
How much do you drink/eat/sleep		

PRONUNCIATION SKILLS

*Directions: Practice saying these words aloud, giving special attention and emphasis to the syllables with accent marks (') and extra emphasis to the syllables in **boldface**.*

epididymitis (ep' i did' i **my'** tis)

cryptorchidism (krip **tor'** ki dizm)

suprapubic prostatectomy (su' prah **pew'** bic pro' sta **tek'** tow mee)

transure'thral resection of the prostate (trans you **ree'** thral ree sek' shun of the pro stayt') (TURP)

COMMUNICATION EXERCISE

Practice Assessment

With a male partner, practice performing an assessment by asking the questions in the Focused Assessment box in the textbook. The partner should listen for clear pronunciation of the questions and should answer clearly. He may ask for an explanation of a question or procedure.

Popular Slang Terminology

There are other terms your patients may use to name sex organs and functions. Proper medical terms are given below in **boldface**. Nonmedical but polite terms are in parentheses ( ). The others are not medical terms and are not polite, but they are words you should understand when you hear them.

genitals, (private parts), privates, down below

penis, dick, cock, dong, shlong, prick

testes, (testicles), gonads, scrotum, balls, nuts

sexual intercourse, (have sex, make love), do it, fuck, screw, make it, bonk, bang

ejaculate, come, have it off, jack, jack off

Care of Patients with Sexually Transmitted Infections

chapter

41

Answer Key: Review the related chapter to answer these questions. A complete answer key was provided to your instructor.

COMPLETION

Directions: Fill in the blanks to complete the statements.

1. Sexually transmitted infection (STI) can be spread by intimate physical contact, _____ contact, or during the _____ process.

2. The largest population groups affected by STIs are _____ and _____.

3. In men, _____ associated with sexual activity may be the first sign of STI.

4. The Centers for Disease Control (CDC) Advisory Committee on Immunization Practices has recommended routine human papillomavirus (HPV) vaccinations for all _____-year-old males and females.

5. Symptoms of pelvic inflammatory disease (PID) include _____, _____, and _____.

6. Chlamydia is a danger to women because it can cause _____.

7. STIs are primarily passed through intimate contact with _____.

8. The _____ virus can cause _____ in the female.

9. Discharge from the skin lesions of a patient with syphilis is contagious in the primary stage until _____.

10. A mother with hepatitis B virus (HBV) transmits the disease to her fetus via the blood traveling through the _____.

11. STIs are to be reported to the _____.

12. The female patient should be advised not to _____ before a vaginal examination.

SHORT ANSWER

Care of the Patient with Syphilis

Directions: Read the clinical scenario and answer the questions that follow.

Scenario: The incidence of syphilis is increasing. You are working in a downtown STI clinic. Mr. Delmonico, a young man, tells you that he had sexual relations several weeks ago and suspects that he may have contracted an STI. The doctor orders a Venereal Disease Research Laboratory (VDRL) test.

1. List at least four questions that you would ask Mr. Delmonico to collect data regarding his risk for STI.

   a. _____

   _____

   b. _____

   _____

   c. _____

   _____

   d. _____

   _____

2. What are the symptoms of primary syphilis?_____

   _____

   _____

   _____

3. What is the treatment for syphilis? _____

   _____

   _____

4. The doctor orders a STAT dose of benzathine penicillin 1.8 g (2.4 million units) IM. The pharmacy delivers benzathine penicillin 600,000 units/mL. How many mL should you give? _____ mL

5. What follow-up information related specifically to syphilis would be appropriate for Mr. Delmonico?

   a. _____

   b. _____

   c. _____

   d. _____

PRIORITY SETTING

Directions: Read the scenario and prioritize as appropriate.

Scenario: You are caring for several patients with STIs. Prioritize the order in which you will attend to the needs of these patients.

_____ a. Ms. Jones needs a copy of her medical records to take to her primary care provider appointment next week.

_____ b. Ms. Rodriguez needs her first dose of IV antibiotics for acute PID.

_____ c. Mr. Kowolski needs reinforcement of follow-up procedure for syphilis.

_____ d. Mr. Sakai needs an IM dose of ceftriaxone for gonorrhea.

_____ e. Ms. Hantu needs encouragement to identify multiple sexual partners.

APPLICATION OF THE NURSING PROCESS

Care of the Patient with Pelvic Inflammatory Disease

Directions: Read the scenario and provide the answers to the following questions.

Scenario: Ms. Tesoro is admitted for acute PID. She is a young woman and she appears to be very ill and suffering with pain. She tells you that she has been treated for an STI in the recent past.

1. What are two possible causes of PID?

    a. _____

    b. _____

2. Which of the following signs and symptoms would you expect to find in the documentation of a patient with acute PID?
    a. Severe abdominal and pelvic pain and fever
    b. Clear, copious, mucus-like vaginal discharge
    c. Multiple open lesions on the labia and vulva
    d. Back pain and heavy menstrual periods

3. Review the procedure for assessing the abdomen and abdominal pain. _____

    _____

    _____

    _____

    _____

    _____

4. Write a sample outcome for the nursing problem of abdominal pain subsequent to inflammation.

    _____

    _____

Ms. Tesoro feels much better after 2 days of IV antibiotics. She tells you that she has had STIs several times, "but I always bounce back from it after the antibiotics."

5. List four or five education points that you could review with Ms. Tesoro.

    a. _____

    b. _____

    c. _____

    d. _____

    e. _____

6. Write a sample evaluation statement for the following nursing problem and patient goal: Need for education about self-care to prevent recurrence or other STIs; Patient will verbalize three ways to prevent recurrence of STIs after patient teaching sessions.

    _____

    _____

    _____

REVIEW QUESTIONS FOR THE NCLEX® EXAMINATION

Directions: Choose the best answer(s) for the following questions.

1. When teaching a patient who is being treated for *Chlamydia trachomatis,* the nurse should stress that:
    1. medication must be taken every day for a month.
    2. partner(s) must be treated concurrently.
    3. swimming and hot-tubbing are contraindicated while under treatment.
    4. lesions must be kept clean and dry to prevent secondary infections.

2. Doxycycline is prescribed for the patient with a chlamydial infection. The order would most likely say to administer the medication _____ for _____ days.

3. When the nurse teaches about "safer sex" practices, it should be stated that proper use of condoms includes using:
    1. petroleum jelly as a lubricant.
    2. saliva as a lubricant.
    3. a spermicide containing nonoxynol-9.
    4. lambskin condoms.

4. A patient has come to the clinic after having been notified of exposure to gonorrhea. He states that his exposure occurred 11 days ago. If he is infected, signs and symptoms that would be expected are:
    1. headache, rash, stiff neck, irritability, and joint pain and stiffness.
    2. urinary frequency and burning with purulent discharge from the urethra.
    3. nausea, diarrhea, fever, and urinary frequency and urgency.
    4. burning sensation of the penis and swollen lymph nodes in the groin.

5. When teaching about HPV vaccination (Gardasil/Cervarix), which facts should be included? *(Select all that apply.)*
    1. Only one dose is required.
    2. The vaccine should not be given to children under 14 years old.
    3. Two vaccines are effective in preventing genital warts.
    4. The vaccine is effective in preventing STIs.
    5. Three vaccines are available.

6. In females, testing for Chlamydia is done by:
   1. low vaginal swab for culture and identification.
   2. blood test for VDRL.
   3. Pap smear.
   4. vaginal swab for gram stain.

7. Which nursing responsibilities are related to collecting specimens for diagnosis of STIs? *(Select all that apply.)*
   1. If antimicrobials have been started, note this on the lab slip.
   2. Provide appropriate draping and privacy.
   3. Female patients should douche before vaginal cultures or smears.
   4. Document medication history.
   5. Cultures and smears usually are obtained with a clean swab.
   6. Label specimens and deliver to the lab according to facility policy.

8. The patient is reluctant to talk about his sexual history. Which statement by the nurse would be the most appropriate to complete the task of obtaining a sexual history, while considering the psychological comfort of the patient?
   1. "This will only take a few minutes to complete these questions."
   2. "Let's take a short break; then we can continue."
   3. "Don't be embarrassed. I ask everybody these same questions."
   4. "Let's start with your kidneys. Are you having trouble with urination?"

9. A new nursing assistant expresses fear in caring for patients with HIV/AIDS. Later, the nurse observes this assistant helping a menstruating hepatitis B patient with toileting. She is not wearing gloves. Which statement(s) would help the nursing assistant understand infection control precautions in caring for patients with STIs?
   1. "Use Standard Precautions for all patients, especially when body fluids are involved."
   2. "Good hand hygiene is adequate when caring for patients with STIs."
   3. "Hepatitis patients and HIV/AIDS patients deserve equal care and attention."
   4. "Hepatitis virus is actually more virulent than HIV/AIDS, so you should be more afraid of patients with hepatitis."

10. Which statement made by a patient indicates an understanding of the information and teaching about genital herpes?
    1. "It is highly contagious, but it is only transmitted by sexual contact."
    2. "I am cured once vesicles in the genital area crust over and resolve."
    3. "Numbness and tingling may occur 24 hours before lesions appear."
    4. "If lesions are present, it is best to use a condom and spermicide."

11. Which patient statement is true about STIs?
    1. "One nice thing about current medical practice is that there is a cure for every STI."
    2. "Barrier protection should be used during intercourse with new partners, even if pregnancy is not a concern."
    3. "Chlamydia is the most common sexually transmitted viral infection."
    4. "Syphilis has been conquered and it is no longer possible to contract it."

CRITICAL THINKING ACTIVITIES

Scenario: You are talking to a group of young female sex workers at a local community health drop-in center. Most of them report using condoms and they claim awareness of the potential for STIs; however, you decide to take advantage of this teachable moment to reinforce STI information.

1. Explain in your own words why having a treatable STI such as gonorrhea still puts one at higher risk for an untreatable STI such as HIV/AIDS.

   _____

   _____

2. Explain in your own words why young women are at an increased risk for STIs. _____

   _____

   _____

   _____

   _____

3. Explain in your own words the advantage of a single-dose antibiotic treatment for a group such as the sex workers.

   _____

   _____

   _____

STEPS TOWARD BETTER COMMUNICATION

VOCABULARY BUILDING GLOSSARY

Term	Pronunciation	Definition
genital	jen'ah tal	pertaining to the reproductive organs
monogamous	mon og' ah mus	a relationship with only one other person
heterosexual	het' ah ro sek' shoo al	prefers sexual relationships with the opposite sex
homosexual	ho' mo sek' shoo al	prefers sexual relationships with the same sex
draping	dray'ping	covering with a sheet or towel to provide privacy and prevent embarrassment
reluctant	re luk' tant	hesitant; not wanting to do something
assurance	ah shur' ans	self-confidence; certainty
nonjudgmental attitude	non judj men'tal at'ti tood	indicating by words, facial expressions, and body language that you have no opinion, good or bad, about what a person has done or what is happening

COMPLETION

Directions: Fill in the blanks with the correct words from the Vocabulary Building Glossary to complete the statements.

1. One way to practice "safer sex" is to be _____.

2. A person diagnosed with an STI is often _____ to tell his or her partner.

3. A male-female sexual relationship is called a(n) _____ relationship.

4. _____ relationships in our society often meet with community condemnation in this country.

5. It takes practice to perform an assessment for STIs with _____.

6. You should provide appropriate _____ for all examinations and procedures that involve the genital area.

7. You must present a(n) _____ when caring for a patient with an STI.

ABBREVIATIONS

Directions: Write out the meaning of the following abbreviations.

1. OC: _____

2. STI: _____

3. HBIG: _____

4. HPV: _____

5. PID: _____

6. HBV: _____

COMMUNICATION EXERCISE

Obtaining a history of sexual activity requires tact, sensitivity, and an objective attitude to make the history-taking easier for you and the patient. Here are some phrases you could use.

"I know this is a sensitive area, but we need to have this information to help you."

"This information is necessary to protect your baby." *(For a pregnant woman or expectant father)*

"Are you willing to give me the names of your sex partners so they can get the health care they need?"

"I am legally required to ask you about your sex partners, for their protection."

Here is some body language you could use.

Introduce yourself and shake hands when you meet.

Smile, but be businesslike rather than overly friendly.

Sit in an alert but relaxed position. Try to seem at ease yourself. Keep a neutral facial expression.

Do not be apologetic; this is necessary business.

Look the person in the eye when you are talking, but not constantly. You may look at your history form or computer screen some of the time when listening.

Careful, quiet, nonjudgmental listening is helpful.

Maintain an appropriate distance. Getting too close may make the patient uncomfortable; too much distance indicates distaste, formality, or coldness.

A touch on the shoulder or arm at an appropriate time may be reassuring.

Allow sufficient time for the interview so you are not rushed.

Be attentive and quiet; do not fidget.

Make sure to convey acceptance of what is being said even if it conflicts with your personal world view. This is about the patient—not about you.

Offering a tissue to a person who becomes tearful is considerate and shows awareness of the person's feelings.

Use illustrations and models for teaching purposes to help maintain objectivity.

Respect confidentiality and privacy.

Ensure privacy for dressing and undressing; drape the patient for exams.

Knock—and pause—before entering the room.

Interview in a space where others cannot hear.

The Integumentary System

chapter

42

Answer Key: Review the related chapter to answer these questions. A complete answer key was provided to your instructor.

REVIEW OF ANATOMY AND PHYSIOLOGY

Terminology

Directions: Match the term on the left with the correct definition, function, or statement on the right.

1. _____ Dermis
2. _____ Epidermis
3. _____ Subcutaneous tissue
4. _____ Stratum corneum
5. _____ Melanocytes
6. _____ Fibroblasts
7. _____ Glands
8. _____ Nails
9. _____ Skin
10. _____ Ultraviolet light
11. _____ Melanin
12. _____ Nerve receptors
13. _____ Hair follicles
14. _____ Sweat glands
15. _____ Change that occurs with aging

a. Act to excrete water and salt
b. Produce new cells to heal skin
c. Skin becomes thinner and more transparent
d. Corium
e. Contain keratin
f. Provides a barrier to bacteria
g. Consists of squamous epithelium
h. Contribute color to skin
i. Attaches skin to underlying structures
j. Transmit feelings of heat, cold, pain, touch, and pressure
k. Absorbs light and protects tissue from ultraviolet light
l. Cells die and slough off
m. Sebaceous, sweat, or ceruminous
n. Skin molecules convert it to vitamin D
o. Produce hair

COMPLETION

Age-Related Changes in the Skin

Directions: Fill in the blank with the correct word or phrase.

1. Wrinkling and sagging of skin as we age occurs because the _____ decreases and _____ tissue diminishes.

2. The elderly person's skin is more _____ and slower to heal because there is a loss of _____.

3. Skin of the elderly becomes drier and may itch due to reduced _____.

4. Because of changes in the skin with aging, the elderly are more susceptible to _____ and _____.

5. Hair thins as we age because the hair growth rate declines and the number of _____ decreases.

6. Nail characteristics change as we age and this makes the nails more susceptible to _____.

7. Melanocyte production changes make the elderly more susceptible to _____ and causes the appearance of _____.

8. Seborrheic keratoses in the elderly appear as _____ on the trunk, arms, and face.

SHORT ANSWER

Causes and Prevention of Skin Problems

Directions: Write brief statements to answer the questions.

1. List four distinct functions of the skin.

   a. _____

   b. _____

   c. _____

   d. _____

2. What are three ways that a person can help prevent skin problems?

   a. _____

   b. _____

   c. _____

3. What are four ways to protect yourself against damage caused by ultraviolet rays of the sun?

   a. _____

   b. _____

   c. _____

   d. _____

APPLICATION OF THE NURSING PROCESS

Caring for a Patient with Fragile Skin Who Is at Risk for Skin Tears

Scenario: You are making home visits to Ms. Nutrim, an elderly woman who is recovering from surgery. Currently she requires assistance with activities of daily living and moving from bed to chair. She is living with her daughter until she recovers enough to return to her own home. The patient tells you that she takes "quite a few medications for my heart and breathing problems."

1. Skin tears frequently occur in the elderly when they are _____ or

    _____ from bed to chair by nursing personnel.

2. Skin tears are usually the result of the forces of _____ or

    _____.

3. Skin tears are very common among the elderly, cause considerable discomfort, are sometimes difficult to

    heal, and are mostly _____.

4. Describe how you can determine skin turgor for Ms. Nutrim. _____

    _____

    _____

5. List five risk factors for skin tears for Ms. Nutrim.

    a. _____

    b. _____

    c. _____

    d. _____

    e. _____

6. List six measures that could be used to prevent skin tears.

    a. _____

    b. _____

    c. _____

    d. _____

    e. _____

    f. _____

7. While reviewing Ms. Nutrim's discharge summary from the hospital, you see that a category I skin tear was identified using the Payne-Martin classification system. Which intervention is most appropriate for this wound?
    a. Cover with a transparent adhesive dressing.
    b. Remove the moist skin flap with sterile scissors.
    c. Gently cleanse the skin tear with normal saline.
    d. Apply a pressure dressing to areas of bleeding.

8. Despite all precautions and patient teaching, Ms. Nutrim accidentally causes a small skin tear on her right forearm as she is reaching for an item on her food tray. List four things that should be included in the documentation of this new skin tear.

   a. _____

   b. _____

   c. _____

   d. _____

SHORT ANSWER

Directions: Provide a brief answer for each of the following questions.

1. A thorough medication history is important in diagnosing skin disorders because _____
   _____.

2. The two most common complaints of patients with skin disorders are _____
   and _____.

3. Adequate intake of _____ and _____ is essential
   for healthy skin.

4. _____ functions to keep hair and skin soft and pliable, inhibits bacterial growth
   on the surface of the skin, and helps prevent water loss from the skin.

TABLE ACTIVITY

Skin Lesions

Directions: In the table below, write down examples of disorders or conditions where you might see each type of lesion.

Type of Lesion	Description
Macule	Circumscribed, flat area with a change in skin color; <0.5 cm in diameter *Examples:*
Papule	Elevated, solid lesion; <0.5 cm in diameter. If >0.5, it is a nodule. *Examples:*

Type of Lesion	Description
Vesicle	Circumscribed, superficial collection of serous fluid; <0.5 cm in diameter *Examples:*
Plaque	Circumscribed, elevated, superficial, solid lesion; >0.5 cm in diameter *Examples:*
Wheal	Firm, edematous, irregularly shaped area; diameter variable *Examples:*
Pustule	Elevated, superficial lesion filled with purulent fluid *Examples:*

REVIEW QUESTIONS FOR THE NCLEX® EXAMINATION

Directions: Choose the best answer(s) for the following questions.

1. The nurse is reviewing the documentation of a patient's skin assessment. Which piece of data causes the most immediate concern?
   1. Presence of patches of senile purpura
   2. Skin stays tented after several seconds
   3. Some seborrheic keratoses on the face
   4. Formation of a keloid over a surgical site

2. The health care provider is preparing to examine the patient for a probable fungal infection using a Wood's lamp and a culture may be obtained. What nursing care may be required? *(Select all that apply.)*
   1. Make sure the patient's questions have been answered.
   2. Check to see if an informed consent has been signed.
   3. Label any specimens properly and send to the lab.
   4. Use a bright examination lamp.

3. Environmental factors that could be responsible for a skin disorder include: *(Select all that apply.)*
   1. cold weather.
   2. tropical climates.
   3. exposure to chemicals and other irritants.
   4. exposure to dust and mold.
   5. ultraviolet light exposure.

4. Significant objective data in the assessment of a patient with a skin disorder include:
   1. appearance of skin adjacent to the lesions.
   2. having difficulty eating meals, especially breakfast.
   3. localized or generalized edema of the skin.
   4. complaints of itching sensation in the affected area.

5. Self-assessment of the skin should take place every few months. The patient should be: *(Select all that apply.)*
   1. examining the entire body, including the back.
   2. looking for warts or moles that have decreased in diameter.
   3. assessing warts and moles that have become more uneven in color.
   4. making note of any lesions that have become flat.

6. When itching is a problem, the patient may be instructed to take which type of bath?
   1. Oatmeal
   2. Oil
   3. Tar
   4. Calamine

7. The health care provider tells the nurse that the patient had a positive reaction to a skin patch test. Which manifestation would the nurse expect to observe?
   1. Patient has mild shortness of breath.
   2. Patient has a generalized rash.
   3. Patient has a wheal at the test site.
   4. Patient has localized exudate.

8. Which diagnostic test would be used to differentiate benign versus malignant skin lesions?
   1. Culture and sensitivity test
   2. Cold light examination
   3. Diascopy
   4. Skin biopsy

9. The nurse advises the patient that tanning salons are not recommended. The patient states, "I have talked to a bunch of people who have been using a tanning salon for years without any problems." What is the best response?
   1. "They may not be having problems now, but there will be consequences in the future."
   2. "Professional dermatologists are convinced that tanning has adverse long-term effects."
   3. "It seems like you are interested in doing your own research. Let me get you some additional resources."
   4. "I can tell that you don't believe me, but I would like you to talk to some patients with skin cancer."

10. Your patient is suffering from poison ivy and the health care provider has prescribed a steroid injection. The order reads: methylprednisolone (Solu-Medrol) 35 mg with dexamethasone (Decadron) 2 mg IM. On hand are Solu-Medrol 25 mg/mL and Decadron 4 mg/mL. You will give one combined injection of _____ mL.

CRITICAL THINKING ACTIVITIES

Scenario: Ms. Weiskoff, age 86, is visiting the clinic for a blood pressure check. She has areas of excoriation on her arm and when you ask her about them, she says that her skin itches and the excoriation is from scratching.

1. What would you teach this patient about skin care?

2. What would you recommend she do to prevent excoriating the skin?

3. Should you advise this patient to see a health care provider for this problem? Discuss your rationale for the advice that you decide to give.

STEPS TOWARD BETTER COMMUNICATION

VOCABULARY BUILDING GLOSSARY

Term	Pronunciation	Definition
exasperating	eg zas' pah ray ting	frustrating, psychologically irritating, making one lose patience
trauma	traw' mah	a physical wound or emotional shock

COMPLETION

Directions: Fill in the blanks with the correct words from the Vocabulary Building Glossary to complete the statements.

1. A bad burn causes emotional as well as physical _____.

2. A skin problem that does not clear up easily can be very _____ for a patient.

WORD ATTACK SKILLS

Word Roots

Root words in English can have several meanings and can be used in many forms. You may need to think about which meaning is being used. It may be a new meaning for you, or it may be a new way to use a word you know. One example from this chapter is the word *compromise* (kom' pro miz). *Compromise* is a verb with two meanings:

1. Take an action that endangers health: *Inadequate fluid replacement may compromise the patient's recovery.*

2. Make a decision by mutual consent where both sides get something they want but neither side gets everything: *The family compromised on the hours they would assist with their father's care.*

Compromise is also a noun, meaning "the decision that is made by this method": *The compromise called for fewer hours but less pay for the nurses.*

Compromised is an adjective from the first verb meaning and means "endangered" (it is also the past tense form of the verb): *The patient's health was compromised by the nurse's action.*

PRONUNCIATION SKILLS

wheal (hweel)   itchy, raised, skin area

psori'asis (so ri' ah sis)   skin disorder with patchy areas of silvery scales

es'char (es' kar)   leathery layer of dead tissue resulting from a full-thickness burn or within a pressure ulcer

CULTURAL POINT

In some time periods and cultures, fair, pale, untanned skin implied wealth and leisure, with no need to be out in the sun working. Today in the United States, it is the opposite. Pale skin to some people indicates the pallor of ill health, or the necessity of working inside. Tanned skin means the person has leisure time and money to be outside at the beach, tennis court, or golf course. A tan is looked upon as more "healthy." Therefore, many people want to look tanned. How can you teach people that tanning can be dangerous to their health?

_____

_____

_____

_____

_____

_____

_____

_____

_____

Care of Patients with Integumentary Disorders and Burns

Answer Key: Review the related chapter to answer these questions. A complete answer key was provided to your instructor.

SHORT ANSWER

Integumentary Disorders

Directions: Supply a brief answer or fill in the blank(s).

1. An infection with _____ appears as lesions on the lips and nares that are commonly called *cold sores* or *fever blisters*.

2. Herpes virus infection can be spread from one area of the body to another by _____
_____.

3. Herpes zoster is caused by _____ and is transmissible from one person to another.

4. Fungal infections of the skin can be prevented by _____
_____.

5. Scabies mites burrow under the top layers of the skin and cause _____.

6. Lice are acquired by contact with infested people or their _____,
_____, and _____ have also been known to carry lice and the scabies mite.

7. The treatments most often used for persistent psoriasis are:_____
_____
_____

8. The best preventive measure for skin cancer is _____
_____.

9. A common skin change in the elderly that can precede cancerous skin lesions is _____
_____.

SHORT ANSWER

Caring for a Patient with Nail Fungus

1. Fungal infections flourish in _____, _____, _____ environments.

2. Older adults are prone to develop fungal infections of the _____ or _____. This is called _____.

3. Discuss ways to prevent nail fungal infections. _____

_____

_____

_____

_____

_____

MATCHING

Skin Cancers

Directions: Match the type of skin cancer on the left with the characteristics on the right that best describe it. (More than one answer may apply.)

1. _____   Basal cell epithelioma

2. _____   Squamous cell epithelioma

3. _____   Malignant melanoma: superficial, spreading

4. _____   Malignant melanoma: nodular

5. _____   Malignant melanoma

a. Arises from a lesion that resembles a large, flat freckle
b. Larger lesions are treated with radiation
c. Occurs mainly on head, neck, and hands
d. Horizontal growth can continue for years, vertical growth worsens prognosis
e. Rarely spreads; easily treated
f. Small tumor nodules may ulcerate and bleed
g. Crusted or ulcerated center has a pearly border
h. Itching, oozing, and bleeding may be present
i. Can appear in a variety of colors
j. Has an irregular surface and notched border
k. Is uniformly blackish-grayish color; resembles a blackberry
l. Is somewhat rare
m. Spreads rapidly

COMPLETION

Directions: Fill in the blanks to complete the statements.

1. Is there an age group in which skin cancer is more common? _____

2. What is the method of diagnosis for a suspected skin cancer? _____

_____

3. What is included in the treatment for melanoma?_____

_____

_____

_____

TABLE ACTIVITY

Burn Care

Directions: Complete the following table correlating the pathophysiology and clinical management of a major burn.

Pathophysiology	Medical Management	Nursing Interventions
Dilatation of capillaries and small vessels in area; increase in capillary permeability; plasma seeps out; edema		
Fluid loss; hemoconcentration; reduced efficiency of circulation		
Fall in blood pressure; hypovolemic shock; cellular dehydration		
Sloughing of dead tissue; large open wounds; infection		
Pulmonary and respiratory changes due to inhalation injury, pulmonary edema, obstructed airway		
Pain in response to injury		
Emotional shock due to pain, long-term therapy, changed body image; depression, boredom		

APPLICATION OF THE NURSING PROCESS

Caring for a Patient with Poison Ivy

Directions: Answer the following questions in the spaces provided.

1. An appropriate nursing problem for the patient who has contracted poison ivy on his arms would be:

    _____

    _____

2. An expected outcome for the above nursing problem for this patient might be: _____

    _____

    _____

3. Appropriate nursing measures for the patient who is experiencing exposure to poison ivy and considerable itching are:

    a. _____

    b. _____

    c. _____

    d. _____

    e. _____

TABLE ACTIVITY

Caring for Patients with Pressure Injury

Directions: Complete the following table and describe the characteristics of pressure injury stages.

Stage	Characteristics
Suspected deep tissue injury	
Stage I	
Stage II	
Stage III	
Stage IV	
Unstageable	

SHORT ANSWER

1. The use of a lifting device, a lift sheet, or a trapeze bar to reposition is beneficial to prevent skin damage from _____.

2. Patients with limited mobility need to utilize a(n) _____ device on the bed or in the wheelchair.

3. Whenever a patient is turned, the _____ that were against the bed should be assessed.

4. The way to tell if a reddened area on the skin is a beginning pressure injury is _____ _____.

5. List at least five measures to use that would help in the prevention of pressure injuries.

    a. _____

    b. _____

    c. _____

    d. _____

    e. _____

6. An expected outcome for the nursing diagnosis of Impaired skin integrity related to presence of a pressure injury would be:

    _____

    _____

7. What data would you use to evaluate whether the above expected outcome is being met?

    _____

    _____

REVIEW QUESTIONS FOR THE NCLEX® EXAMINATION

Directions: Choose the best answer(s) for the following questions.

1. Contact dermatitis can be caused by any number of substances. When considering whether a skin problem is contact dermatitis, you would look for which sign(s) and/or symptom(s) indicating that disorder? *(Select all that apply.)*
    1. Erythema and swelling
    2. Ulcerated lesions
    3. Scaling
    4. Pruritus
    5. Vesicular lesions

2. Stevens-Johnson syndrome (SJS) may occur around 14 days after beginning drug therapy. Some of the differences between SJS and contact dermatitis are: *(Select all that apply.)*
   1. SJS is painful, where contact dermatitis itches.
   2. SJS lesions are larger and not localized.
   3. contact dermatitis lesions have necrotic centers.
   4. SJS can be lethal.

3. The main difference between a furuncle and a carbuncle is the:
   1. furuncle is infectious, the carbuncle isn't.
   2. furuncle involves a single hair follicle and the carbuncle involves a group of hair follicles.
   3. carbuncle is an allergic reaction, the furuncle isn't.
   4. carbuncle is caused by ineffective thermoregulation.

4. What is an important teaching point for a patient about self-care for a carbuncle?
   1. A clean washcloth and towel should be used for bathing each day.
   2. Use a cold compress for comfort and to promote drainage.
   3. Take sedatives as prescribed for relief of discomfort.
   4. Avoid injury of any kind to surrounding skin.

5. The nurse is caring for several patients on a surgical floor. Which patient needs to be placed in contact isolation?
   1. Patient has psoriasis with adherent silvery-white scales.
   2. Patient has stasis dermatitis with petechiae and hyperpigmentation.
   3. Patient has herpes zoster with small groups of vesicles along nerve pathways.
   4. Patient has actinic keratoses with small, scaly, grayish papules.

6. Select statements that are true about tinea pedis. It: *(Select all that apply.)*
   1. is a fungal disease.
   2. displays with cracks between the toes with peeling and itching.
   3. is often contracted in public showers and spas.
   4. is treated by keeping the foot moisturized and covered.
   5. is treated with antibiotic ointments and systemic drugs.
   6. is a bacterial infection.

7. A high-priority intervention for the patient with serious burns is:
   1. cooling the burn areas every 2 hours with running water.
   2. beginning intravenous fluid administration as soon as possible.
   3. cleansing the burn areas thoroughly as quickly as possible.
   4. administering a tetanus immunization within the first hour of treatment.

8. What is the highest priority when caring for the burn patient?
   1. Preventing contractures from forming
   2. Grafting to cover open burn areas
   3. Preventing infection or controlling it
   4. Providing psychosocial support to the patient

9. The patient arrives by EMS after being rescued from a house fire. The patient sustained minor burns on the hands and forearms and demonstrates a dry hacking cough. She is upset and weeping, but vital signs are currently stable. The health care provider orders admission for 23-hour observation. What is the priority nursing diagnosis?
   1. Anxiety related to traumatic life-threatening event
   2. Impaired skin integrity related to burns of hands and forearms
   3. Risk for ineffective breathing pattern related to smoke inhalation
   4. Risk for fluid imbalance related to fluid shifting and edema formation

10. Fluid resuscitation is a high priority during the emergent stage of a serious burn. Your patient weighs 182 lbs. His burn percentage is calculated to be 40% of body surface. You are to infuse Ringer's lactate. Using the formula provided in the chapter, within the first 8 hours after the burn, he should receive _____ mL of Ringer's lactate.

CRITICAL THINKING ACTIVITIES

Scenario A: Mr. Marshall is a 27-year-old truck driver who was burned in a vehicular accident. He has been brought to the emergency department of the community hospital. He has burns over the anterior and posterior surface of both arms, chest, and back.

1. According to the rule of nines, what is his total burn percentage?

2. One of the burns on his chest is a full-thickness burn. What are the characteristics of a full-thickness burn?

3. What are the two major concerns during the first hour after a burn injury?

4. How would you assess whether Mr. Marshall has a respiratory injury?

5. What measures would you expect to be carried out to reduce the risk of infection for Mr. Marshall?

Scenario B: Mr. Marshall has progressed and débridement and grafting on his chest and arms has been carried out. He is undergoing physical therapy; however, he has become progressively withdrawn and less willing to have visitors.

1. When he expresses concern about the scars that are beginning to form, what would you tell him about scar maturation?

2. When he resists performing his physical therapy exercises, how would you encourage him to continue them?

3. What can you do to help him cope with the psychosocial effects of his injuries?

Scenario C: Ms. Ruiz, age 78, is being discharged from the long-term care facility following convalescent care and rehabilitation for a fractured hip. She has a healing stage 2 pressure injury on her left buttock.

1. What equipment would you make certain that the patient has at home to help prevent further injury from pressure ?

2. What teaching would you provide as to the care of the skin and of the healing pressure injury?

Scenario D: Mr. Torres is admitted to your unit from the long-term care facility. He is being treated for pneumonia. You discover an area on the right hip that is raw-looking with serous drainage.

1. How would you correctly document this skin problem?

2. How would you "stage" this ulcer? What stage is it (considering the information above)?

3. What skin care measures should be instituted?

STEPS TOWARD BETTER COMMUNICATION

VOCABULARY BUILDING GLOSSARY

Term	Pronunciation	Definition
proliferation	pro lif' ah ray' shun	rapid increase or multiplication; the reproduction of similar forms, usually meaning cells in medicine
traumatic	traw mat' ik	very emotionally unpleasant

COMPLETION

Directions: Fill in the blanks with the correct words from the Vocabulary Building Glossary to complete the statements.

1. Receiving a diagnosis of melanoma would be a _____ experience.

2. A squamous cell skin carcinoma is composed of a _____ of abnormal cells.

WORD ATTACK SKILLS

Word Elements

auto-	self
allo-	other (same species)
homo-	same, similar
hetero-	different (individual, tissue)
xeno-	foreign, unlike (different species)
epi-	above, on, upon
derm/a-, dermat/o-	skin
-logy	study or science of
-ist	a person who
-graft	to implant or transplant tissue

Using Word Elements

Directions: Fill in the word described by the following phrases.

1. Study of the skin: _____

2. On the skin: _____

3. A person who studies the skin: _____

4. Transplant tissue from another person: _____

5. Transplant tissue from oneself: _____

PRONUNCIATION SKILLS

débride'ment (da breed' maw)	removal of dead tissues and foreign material from a wound
xen'ograft (zen'o graft)	graft of tissue between animals of different species

COMMUNICATION EXERCISES

A.   If you noticed a skin lesion that looked as if it might be a skin cancer on someone you didn't know well, how would you bring it to the person's attention without offending him or her? Americans normally do not like to have attention called to personal matters, especially any deformities that might be considered negative or personal. However, this is such an important matter that you might want to find a way to approach the person. It would be best to catch the person's attention and speak to him or her in a manner that cannot be overheard by others. Write out what you would say to the person.

B. Describe:

1. The attitude you should take with a patient who has a long-term recovery ahead. _____

_____

2. The diversional and occupational activities you could suggest. _____

_____

C. Write a short dialogue explaining to an elderly patient why it is important for him to turn or shift his position in bed and in his chair so that he doesn't develop skin injury from pressure. Make some suggestions to help him remember. (Turn when the TV commercial comes on, when he turns the page in his magazine, when he hears people in the hall, when he returns from a trip to the bathroom.)

_____

_____

_____

_____

_____

Care of Patients in Disasters or Bioterrorism Attack

Answer Key: Review the related chapter to answer these questions. A complete answer key was provided to your instructor.

COMPLETION

Directions: Fill in the blanks to complete the statements.

1. A disaster exists when the number of _____ exceeds the resource capabilities of the area.

2. _____ or _____ are terms used to describe the maximum services a facility can offer when every resource is used.

3. Triage for a disaster is based on first saving those with life-threatening conditions and a likelihood of _____.

4. _____ is a top priority when large groups of people are together in a shelter because the incidence of communicable disease is much greater.

5. In a disaster situation, it may take several days for rescuers to arrive so it is recommended that a(n) _____ supply of food and water is available.

SHORT ANSWER

Disaster Management Planning

Directions: Read the clinical scenario and answer the questions that follow.

Scenario: You have been asked to sit on a hospital committee to review and update the hospital's disaster management plan. You have been assigned to investigate the roles and responsibilities of the nursing staff and to develop a list of topics that are relevant to disaster nursing.

1. Under disaster conditions, what may nurses be asked to do?

   a. _____

   b. _____

   c. _____

2. Give four examples of procedures or tasks that you might be expected to perform in the emergency department for patients who may have sustained injury or illness during a disaster.

   a. _____

   b. _____

   c. _____

   d. _____

3. Identify at least five nursing responsibilities in case of a disaster.

   a. _____

   b. _____

   c. _____

   d. _____

   e. _____

4. What are five categories of chemical agents that might be used in a terrorist attack?

   a. _____

   b. _____

   c. _____

   d. _____

   e. _____

5. What are the six pathogens that are most likely to be used as bioterrorism agents?

   a. _____

   b. _____

   c. _____

   d. _____

   e. _____

   f. _____

6. List four general guidelines for your role in bioterrorism preparedness and response.

   a. _____

   b. _____

   c. _____

   d. _____

APPLICATION OF THE NURSING PROCESS

Caring for a Patient with Botulism

Directions: Read the scenario and provide the answers to the following questions.

Scenario: Ms. Kelso is admitted for botulism. She became sick after eating some home-preserved vegetables. Fortunately, she was the only one to eat the vegetables and her family quickly helped her to seek medical attention.

1. What are the early symptoms of botulism?

    a. _____

    b. _____

    c. _____

2. What is the classic triad of symptoms for this disorder?

    a. _____

    b. _____

    c. _____

3. What is the priority diagnosis for Ms. Kelso?
    a. Potential for altered breathing pattern related to flaccid paralysis
    b. Confusion related to botulism toxin
    c. Diarrhea related to food poisoning
    d. Altered physical activity related to decreased strength

4. List at least four interventions (including assessments) to ensure safety for a patient who is having difficulty swallowing.

    a. _____

    b. _____

    c. _____

    d. _____

5. Which statement by the family indicates an understanding of the treatment plan for Ms. Kelso?
    a. "The antitoxin will reverse the muscular paralysis."
    b. "She can be treated with gentamicin (Garamycin)."
    c. "Supportive therapy may be needed for several weeks."
    d. "The drug of choice is ciprofloxacin (Cipro)."

PRIORITY SETTING

Disaster Triage

Directions: Read the scenario and correctly tag the disaster victims.

Scenario: You are participating in a disaster drill and have been assigned to assist in the triage area. The drill instructor gives you the following instructions: "An LPN/LVN would not ordinarily be responsible for making initial triage decisions; however, in this scenario, 250 victims have just converged on the hospital and you must do your best to correctly tag patients. You should ask for help in decision-making if you feel that you are unable to accurately assess and appropriately tag the patient. You will have to use your critical thinking skills in each situation." *Correctly tag each patient (RED, YELLOW, GREEN, WHITE, or BLACK) or refer to RN/MD.*

_____   a. Middle-aged man who is having symptoms of myocardial infarction

_____   b. Child with swollen ankle, decreased range of motion, good peripheral pulses

_____   c. Young woman with vomiting, low-grade fever, and mild abdominal pain

_____   d. Young man with dislocated shoulder and decreased peripheral pulses

_____   e. Child with 90% total body burns

_____   f. Teenager with blunt force abdominal trauma, denies distress, but is diaphoretic

_____   g. Elderly man with insect bite, reports tightness in throat, has angioedema

REVIEW QUESTIONS FOR THE NCLEX® EXAMINATION

Directions: Choose the best answer(s) for the following questions.

1. The nurse is assigned to assist in triage. The purpose and goal of triage is to:
    1. sort patients by priority of need for treatment.
    2. ensure that all patients receive treatment.
    3. ensure that medical equipment is available.
    4. identify the need for supplies and support.

2. The nurse is advising a community group about what to do in the event of a natural disaster such as an earthquake, tornado, or flood. What is appropriate information and advice?
    1. Evacuate the area and leave immediately.
    2. Take refuge in the basement during a tornado warning.
    3. During an earthquake, drop to the floor and crawl to an exit.
    4. For flood warnings, push towels into the cracks under the doors.

3. There are multiple victims during a disaster. The majority of these victims will be triaged and identified with which color of tag?
    1. Red tag
    2. Black tag
    3. Yellow tag
    4. Green tag

4. A patient is being treated for radiation exposure. A chelating agent functions to reduce radiation damage by:
    1. binding the radioactive material.
    2. blocking specific isotopes.
    3. mobilizing radioactive material.
    4. reducing concentration of radioactive material.

5. What is a simple way to purify water when the supply has been disrupted?
    1. Rolling boil for 3–5 minutes
    2. Adding 16 teaspoons of household liquid bleach
    3. Water that drips from a source into a clean cup
    4. Low-boil the water for 20 minutes

6. Victims who may have residual particulate after radiation or chemical exposure should be decontaminated. Victims should be instructed to:
    1. remove and burn clothing.
    2. wear protective gear and double gloves.
    3. scrub skin with water and soap and rinse well.
    4. brush off and vacuum residual particulates.

7. A patient is admitted with radiation sickness. What would the nurse expect to find documented in the patient's chart?
    1. Cardiac arrhythmias and low blood pressure
    2. Nausea, vomiting, diarrhea, and hair loss
    3. Lethargy, constipation, and blurred vision
    4. Renal failure and electrolyte imbalances

8. The patient is admitted for a diagnosis of anthrax. What is the health care provider most likely to order to treat this patient?
    1. IV fluids and oxygen therapy
    2. Ciprofloxacin (Cipro)
    3. Gentamicin (Garamycin)
    4. Antitoxin type A or B

9. Which task related to disaster management would be appropriate to assign to a nursing assistant?
    1. Assisting victims to shower after exposure to toxin
    2. Debriefing others during a critical incident
    3. Triaging incoming green-tag victims
    4. Moving black-tagged victims to designated areas

10. The nurse is assisting in a temporary housing shelter that has been created for displaced victims of a hurricane. What is the priority diagnosis for this group?
    1. Potential for grief related to loss of property, friends, family, etc.
    2. Limited coping ability related to sudden catastrophic event
    3. High potential for infection related to crowding, poor hygienic conditions
    4. Fatigue related to unfamiliar surroundings and stress

11. The nurse is caring for multiple victims who are rapidly arriving from a nearby disaster site. Which communication strategy is the nurse most likely to use?
    1. Active listening
    2. Short directive statements
    3. Therapeutic touch
    4. Silence and reflection

12. The nursing staff is participating in a discussion about practical measures to prepare for a possible pandemic flu event. Which comment by a staff member indicates an understanding of what should be done?
    1. "The hospital needs to get more ventilators for the intensive care unit."
    2. "None of the nurses with children should have to come under those conditions."
    3. "We need to review respiratory isolation precautions and reinforce handwashing."
    4. "This is not a third-world country; we will be okay if we just use common sense."

13. Based on a patient's answers to interview questions, the nurse suspects that the patient may have been exposed to a possible Category A infectious agent. What should the nurse do *first*?
    1. Notify the supervisor about the possibility of contagion.
    2. Don an N-95 or P-100 respirator mask.
    3. Have the patient and family perform hand hygiene.
    4. Isolate the patient in a negative-pressure room.

14. The nurse is assigned to assist the health care provider with "reverse" triage during a disaster event. What information is most relevant to this process?
    1. Identifying the patient's blood type and history of transfusions
    2. Knowing the pattern of pain and vital signs over the past few days
    3. Reviewing the past and present medication history
    4. Evaluating the patient's emotional response to the disaster event

15. Which statement by the nurse indicates that the goals of critical incident stress debriefing are being met?
    1. "I still have nightmares about the disaster, but I don't think about it during the day."
    2. "I am surviving, although I guess I am still drinking more than I should."
    3. "I went out with friends the other night and we talked about how we were all doing."
    4. "I am super-prepared now. I check the disaster equipment every day."

CRITICAL THINKING ACTIVITIES

Scenario A: Your supervisor asks you to work some extra shifts. There has been an unexpected influx of patients with flu-like symptoms. These patients are rapidly progressing into severe respiratory distress. She tells you that your help is really needed; however, you should be aware that relatively healthy young people with no previous health problems are getting sick and the health care providers are not exactly sure what is going on with these patients.

1. Discuss how you might feel about being asked to help under these circumstances and/or expose yourself (and your family) to potentially serious communicable disease.

    _____

    _____

    _____

    _____

    _____

2. When you are comfortable in your first nursing job, what are some things that you could do (or ask) that would prepare you to face a similar scenario?

    _____

    _____

    _____

    _____

    _____

Scenario B: You are working in a downtown walk-in clinic. Typically, the clinic serves low-income families and the homeless population and provides routine health services such as immunizations for children, treatment for minor illness or accidents, or prescription service for blood pressure medications, etc.

1. Explain in your own words why you would need to have a working knowledge of bioterrorism for this work setting.

   _____

   _____

   _____

   _____

   _____

   _____

2. List seven signs or events that suggest a bioterrorism incident has occurred.

   a. _____

   b. _____

   c. _____

   d. _____

   e. _____

   f. _____

   g. _____

Scenario C: You are working in small emergency department in a rural town. There is an explosion in a nearby factory and multiple victims (adult workers) begin to arrive. The health care provider instructs you to start peripheral IVs (with at least an 18-gauge catheter) on all the patients as they arrive and hang normal saline unless ordered otherwise at 125 mL/hour. The hospital runs out of IV pumps, so you must calculate the flow rate using ordinary IV tubing. Calculate the gtts/min using various tubings.

1. Drop factor 20 gtts/mL _____ gtts/min.

2. Drop factor 15 gtts/mL _____ gtts/min.

3. Drop factor 10 gtts/mL _____ gtts/min.

4. Drop factor 60 gtts/mL _____ gtts/min.

5. The charge nurse tells you not to use mini-drip (60 gtts/mL) tubing unless there is nothing else available. Why would they say this?

   _____

   _____

   _____

   _____

   _____

STEPS TOWARD BETTER COMMUNICATION

VOCABULARY BUILDING GLOSSARY

Term	Pronunciation	Definition
catastrophe	ka tas' tro fee	a terrible event, a disaster
disparity	dis par'itee	difference, inequality
duress	du ress'	forced hardship or difficulty
improvise	im'pro viz	to use whatever is available
triage	tree ahzh'	a system for determining priority of need and order or location of treatment

COMPLETION

Directions: Fill in the blanks with the correct words from the Vocabulary Building Glossary to complete the statements.

1. The people who had their homes destroyed in the tornado were experiencing considerable

   _____.

2. The man's leg was badly fractured, so the nurse had to _____ a splint at the scene of the accident.

3. When Ms. Lyons was admitted, there was evident _____ between the appearance of one leg and the other.

4. Hurricane Katrina was a major _____.

5. The nurse was assigned to _____ for the victims of the tornado.

WORD ATTACK SKILLS

Word Meanings

Directions: For each word on the left, circle the word or phrase with the same meaning on the right.

1. mitigate: reduce   add water   delay

2. acuity: distance   perception   lack of water

3. lethargy: fatal   lack of energy   skin condition

4. aerosolize: spray with a liquid   suspend solid particles in a gas   blow dry

ABBREVIATIONS

Directions: Pronounce and give the meaning of each abbreviation.

1. OES:_____

2. FEMA:_____

3. DMAT: _____

4. CSC:_____

5. NOAA: _____

6. CDC: _____

7. CISD (team):_____

8. PTSD: _____

9. EPA:_____

10. EMS: _____

11. HEPA (filter mask): _____

COMMUNICATION EXERCISE

Idioms

Directions: Recall that idioms are usages of language that cannot be translated literally. Idioms are specific to a culture and are often imaginative uses of language. Explain to a partner what the following idioms mean:

1. Telephone tree: _____

   _____

   _____

2. Ground rules:_____

   _____

   _____

Care of Patients with Emergent Conditions, Trauma, and Shock

chapter
45

Answer Key: Review the related chapter to answer these questions. A complete answer key was provided to your instructor.

TERMINOLOGY

Emergent Conditions

Directions: Match the condition or term on the left with the description on the right that is most likely to be associated with it.

1. _____ Choking emergency
2. _____ Carbon monoxide poisoning
3. _____ Heatstroke
4. _____ Index of suspicion
5. _____ Hypothermia
6. _____ Mechanism of injury
7. _____ Pneumothorax
8. _____ Triage
9. _____ Penetrating trauma
10. _____ Shock

a. Labored respirations and decreased breath sounds on one side of the chest
b. Hot, dry skin; victim working outside in summer
c. Vigilance to detect problems that are not obvious
d. Unable to cough or speak, gasping respirations; victim was eating in a restaurant
e. Patient jumped from third-story window
f. Cherry-red skin; victim found unconscious in garage
g. Cool, dry skin; impaired mental ability; elderly victim found at home in winter
h. Presence of knife wound in the abdominal area
i. Decreased perfusion related to depleted blood volume or decreased cardiac output
j. Assessing and sorting to determine order of priority for care

COMPLETION

Directions: Fill in the blanks to complete the statements.

1. _____' laws protect medical personnel from liability when rendering emergency medical care for victims of accidental injury.

2. The purpose of immobilizing the neck of a trauma patient is to keep it as straight as possible, preventing it from _____ or _____.

3. _____ produces paradoxical chest movement.

4. The amount of _____ and current involved, the length of _____ _____, and the condition of the skin determine how much damage may have occurred as a result of an electric shock.

5. The person who sustains a tick bite in a mountainous area may contract

_____ or _____.

6. The heart is extremely sensitive when cold and the patient must be handled carefully to prevent

_____.

CARING FOR A TRAUMA VICTIM IN THE EMERGENCY DEPARTMENT

Directions: Read the clinical scenario and answer the questions that follow.

Scenario: The nurse is working in the emergency department (ED) and several patients have just arrived from the scene of the same accident. All of the victims have been transported by EMS and arrive on stretchers and backboards with C-spine precautions in place. You are asked to help with one of the patients who appears to be less critical than the others at first glance.

1. What are the ABCDEs of assessment?

   A: _____

   B: _____

   C: _____

   D: _____

   E: _____

2. Describe the head-to-toe assessment (secondary survey). _____

   _____

   _____

   _____

   _____

   _____

   _____

   _____

   _____

3. What kinds of information would you try to get from EMS before they leave the ED?

   _____

   _____

   _____

   _____

4. The patient tells you she has to urinate and asks you to remove the C-collar so that she can get up and go to the bathroom. What should you do?
   a. Tell her that you can't remove the C-collar and obtain an order for an indwelling Foley.
   b. Remove the C-collar and help her to maintain the neck in a straight position.
   c. Ask the health care provider if spinal injury has been cleared and if it is okay to remove the C-collar.
   d. Instruct the nursing assistant to help the patient use the bedpan.

5. The ED health care provider tells you that the patient appears to be stable with just a bruise on the lower abdomen, but asks you to check vital signs on the patient every 15 minutes for 1 hour and to repeat the abdominal assessment and to obtain a repeat hemoglobin and hematocrit q hour x 3. Why has the provider asked you to do these assessments and what should you be watching for?

   _____

   _____

   _____

   _____

   _____

SHORT ANSWER

Domestic and Intimate Partner Violence

Directions: Read the clinical scenario and answer the questions that follow.

Scenario: You are working in an outpatient clinic and Ms. Luten comes in for treatment of a broken wrist. She tells you that she slipped and fell. While you are taking her blood pressure you notice bruises on her upper arms and around her neck. Her medical records show that she has been treated for injuries twice within the past year.

1. You suspect that Ms. Luten may be a victim of domestic/intimate partner abuse. What are five questions that you could ask to assess for abuse?

   a. _____

   b. _____

   c. _____

   d. _____

   e. _____

2. List eight physical signs of battering.

   a. _____

   b. _____

   c. _____

   d. _____

   e. _____

f. _____

g. _____

h. _____

3. A clue to the need for an assessment for abuse is _____ in various stages of healing.

4. What are four potential psychological signs of abuse?

a. _____

b. _____

c. _____

d. _____

5. Which task would be appropriate to assign to the nursing assistant?
   a. Take photos of Ms. Luten's bruises.
   b. Sit with Ms. Luten to provide support.
   c. Collect evidence such as torn clothes.
   d. Obtain an ice pack for her wrist.

APPLICATION OF THE NURSING PROCESS

Allergic Reaction

Directions: Read the scenario and provide answers to the following questions.

Scenario: You are outside with your children and you hear your neighbor, Ms. Andrews, calling for help. She tells you that she was just stung by a bee and "last time I had a really bad reaction to it." Currently, she is anxious, and you can see the sting mark with some redness on her forearm around the immediate area.

1. What is the *first* action you should take?
   a. Call 911 and encourage her to stay calm.
   b. Remove the stinger by gently scraping the skin with a credit card.
   c. Elevate the arm and apply an ice pack.
   d. Assess for hives and general weakness.

2. What are eight signs and symptoms of a systemic reaction to a bee sting?

a. _____

b. _____

c. _____

d. _____

e. _____

f. _____

g. _____

h. _____

You have assessed Ms. Andrews and she does not appear to be having the signs or symptoms of a systemic reaction to the sting; however, she tells her daughter to run into the house and get the anaphylaxis kit so that you can see it "because you are a nurse and I don't really remember anything about what's in the kit, or how to use it."

3. What are the name, the strength, and the dosage of the emergency drug in the anaphylaxis kit?

   _____

4. What is the name and dose of a typical over-the-counter medication that could be used after the emergency drug is given? _____

5. Identify four additional self-care measures for bee stings that Ms. Andrews could do at home.

   a. _____

   b. _____

   c. _____

   d. _____

6. Ms. Andrews comes over to your house in the evening to thank you for your help. "I really feel silly about making such a fuss and not knowing anything about that kit." You recognize that while she is not really your patient, she does have some health issues that you can assist her with. What is the priority nursing diagnosis at this point?
   a. Altered skin integrity related to scratching
   b. Insufficient knowledge related to bee sting kit
   c. Potential for altered breathing related to throat constriction
   d. Anxiety related to future allergic exposures

PRIORITY SETTING

Directions: Read the scenario and prioritize as appropriate.

Scenario: You are at a community swimming pool and there is no lifeguard on duty. Suddenly, one of the women says, "My son is in the water! Please help him! I can't swim!" Prioritize the actions for assisting a drowning victim.

_____   a. Transport to a medical facility promptly for evaluation and treatment.

_____   b. The rescuer (you) should direct a bystander to call 911.

_____   c. If the child is breathing, place him on his side.

_____   d. Assess for breathing and pulse.

_____   e. Try to reach the victim without going in deep water.

_____   f. Instruct a bystander to assist you in bringing the child out of water.

REVIEW QUESTIONS FOR THE NCLEX® EXAMINATION

Directions: Choose the best answer(s) for the following questions.

1. Implementation of nursing care for the emergency patient who is admitted with frostbite of the foot includes:
    1. applying a heating pad to the frostbitten area.
    2. giving the patient hot fluids to drink.
    3. wrapping the foot in warmed blankets.
    4. immersing the foot in warm water.

2. A toddler is brought to the ED alert and crying; however, EMS reports that the child was pulled from a neighbor's swimming pool and resuscitated at the scene. The toddler is admitted for 23-hour observation. What is most important observation that the nurse makes during the assessment of this child?
    1. Observing for signs of previous injury that suggest potential child neglect
    2. Monitoring the pulse oximetry readings and auscultating the breath sounds
    3. Assessing the quality of the pulse and rhythm of the heartbeat
    4. Assessing the need for education related to child's developmental needs

3. To evaluate the effectiveness of Lasix and morphine for the treatment of pulmonary edema in an emergency patient, the nurse would:
    1. monitor intake and output.
    2. assess respiratory status.
    3. assess for decreased pain.
    4. check the strength of peripheral pulses.

4. The priority goal when planning the care of the emergency patient admitted in shock would be to:
    1. maintain the patient's body warmth to prevent vasodilation.
    2. decrease the patient's pain to lessen vasoconstriction.
    3. restore the patient's circulating blood volume to promote perfusion.
    4. restore the patient's acid-base balance to aid respiration.

5. A high priority in the immediate treatment of burns of the hands is:
    1. cool burned areas quickly with cool water.
    2. assess ROM of joints and circumferential burns.
    3. cover with blankets or sheets to prevent chilling.
    4. determine the area and degree of the burns.

6. The nurse is at a restaurant and observes a person who appears to be choking. He is conscious and partially able to speak. What is the priority action?
    1. Have a bystander call 911 and stay with patient.
    2. Encourage him to cough and breathe as deeply as he can.
    3. Get behind him and perform abdominal thrusts.
    4. Strike him sharply between the shoulder blades.

7. There is a multi-car accident and several people stop to assist. Under Good Samaritan laws, what applies to voluntary rescuers who assist at the scene?
    1. All rescuers are equally protected against liability.
    2. Rescuers are only protected if they can prove they acted in good faith.
    3. Physicians who stop are held to a higher standard of care than others.
    4. Bad outcomes usually result in liability suits.

8. The patient sustains a venomous snakebite. What is included in the current emergency first-aid treatment?
   1. Wash the wound and lower the extremity.
   2. Apply suction to the area immediately after the bite.
   3. Make an incision over the wound with a sterile tool.
   4. Place a tourniquet above the wound and check the pulses.

9. A group of excited teenagers come to the walk-in clinic; they drag in an adolescent who is unresponsive. There are no obvious signs of injury or bleeding, but his skin is pale and clammy. What questions should the nurse initially ask? *(Select all that apply.)*
   1. "Where are his parents?"
   2. "What school does he attend?"
   3. "What is his name?"
   4. "What happened to him?"
   5. "How long has he been like this?"
   6. "Why didn't you call 911?"
   7. "What was the group doing before he passed out?"

10. The nurse is at a community event and a child accidentally sustains a laceration with apparent arterial bleeding. The nurse's immediate action to control the bleeding is to:
    1. apply pressure directly over the wound with the covered palm of the hand.
    2. tape a sterile or clean dressing over the open wound.
    3. elevate the injured part and immobilize the child and the wound.
    4. periodically remove the original dressing to assess for active bleeding.

11. The nurse is making a home health visit to an elderly patient. The temperature in the house is very hot. The elderly patient is responsive but confused. His skin is hot and dry and he says he feels weak and nauseous. What is the priority action?
    1. Take the patient's temperature and administer an antipyretic.
    2. Notify the health care provider and update the home health agency.
    3. Remove extra clothing and wipe the skin with cool water.
    4. Start an IV infusion of cool fluids and a cool saline lavage.

12. The patient is in cardiogenic shock secondary to a myocardial infarction. Which emergency treatment will the health care provider most likely order for this patient?
    1. Fluid bolus and volume expanders
    2. Epinephrine and bronchodilators
    3. Norepinephrine, dopamine, or dobutamine
    4. Fluid bolus and corticosteroids

13. An elderly patient is at high risk for septic shock. Which symptom is more frequently associated with septic shock in elderly patients compared to younger patients?
    1. Decreased urinary output
    2. Tachycardia
    3. Hypothermia
    4. Slightly elevated temperature

14. The staff is attempting to deescalate the behavior of a patient who is becoming increasingly upset and frustrated. What is the best approach?
    1. Several staff members should surround the patient.
    2. Allow a family member to privately speak to the patient.
    3. Restrain the patient to give a tranquilizing drug.
    4. Explain the purpose of any planned procedures.

15. The nurse has just completed a community presentation about ways to prevent hypothermia during cold-weather outings. Which statement from an audience member demonstrates a need for additional teaching?
    1. "Wearing a hat prevents heat loss through the head."
    2. "I should carry high-energy snacks in case I get lost."
    3. "I should wear or take layers of warm clothing."
    4. "If I get lost I should sit quietly to conserve energy."

CRITICAL THINKING ACTIVITIES

Scenario: You are working in the ED. The health care provider orders IV fluids for several patients. The RN instructs you to hang the fluids and calculate the pump settings.

1. Ms. Sharon needs a maintenance IV of $D_5$0.45 NS 1000 mL to infuse over 8 hours. What is the pump setting? _____

2. Mr. Swan needs a fluid bolus 300 mL of normal saline over 30 minutes. What is the pump setting?
   _____

3. Ms. Phillo needs a fluid bolus 100 mL of 5% dextrose to infuse over 20 minutes. What is the pump setting? _____

4. Mr. Damon needs to receive 500 mL before he goes home to infuse at 125 mL/hour. What is the pump setting? _____
   How many hours will it take to complete the infusion? _____

5. When you are using an IV pump, how can you maximize the "volume to be infused" (VTBI) feature to increase the safe delivery of fluids?

   _____

   _____

   _____

   _____

STEPS TOWARD BETTER COMMUNICATION

VOCABULARY BUILDING GLOSSARY

Term	Pronunciation	Definition
aspirate	as pi rayt′	foreign material becomes lodged in the airway of the respiratory system
battering	bat′ter ing	hitting often and repeatedly
combative	com bat′iv	wanting to fight or argue
corrosive	cor ro′siv	wearing away by chemical action
extremities	eks trem′ ah teez	arms and hands, legs and feet
perfusion	per few′shun	passage of fluid through the organs or tissues
triage	tree ahzh′	a system for determining priority of need and order or location of treatment

COMPLETION

Directions: Fill in the blanks with the correct words from the Vocabulary Building Glossary to complete the statements.

1. The nurse must _____ patients carefully to determine priority and the correct area of treatment.

2. Children frequently _____ hot dogs or hard candy.

3. The patient who had sustained a head injury in the accident became _____ and started to fight with the nurse.

4. The nurse carefully checked all four _____ to see if there were any fractures.

5. There were bruises in various stages and cuts on the woman's body indicating that she was a victim of _____.

6. The child was brought in by the emergency medical team because he had taken a drink of drain cleaner, which is _____.

7. A warm feeling to the foot, pinkish color, and the presence of a pedal pulse indicated that _____ was occurring in the leg and foot.

WORD ATTACK SKILLS

Word Meanings

Directions: For each word on the left, circle the word or phrase with the same meaning on the right.

1. cessa'tion: a period of time   stopping   hard and fast

2. deter'iorate: increase rapidly   change into bad condition   become smaller

Word Elements

circum-   around

oral   mouth

Directions: Write the meaning of the word.

1. circumoral: _____

PRONUNCIATION SKILLS

Directions: Practice pronouncing the words with a partner.

a'queous epineph'rine (ay' kwee us e pin eh' freen)

ven'omous (ven' oh muss)

COMMUNICATION EXERCISE

Directions: Use the information from Box 45-1 and talk to a friend or a family member about how to improve safety in the home. First try using the exact wording in Box 45-1, then try paraphrasing the same information. (Use your own words and style to give the same information.)

Care of Patients with Cognitive Function Disorders

Answer Key: Review the related chapter to answer these questions. A complete answer key was provided to your instructor.

TERMINOLOGY

Directions: Match the term on the right with the meaning on the left.

1. _____ Delirium
2. _____ Cognition
3. _____ Dementia
4. _____ Confabulation
5. _____ Global amnesia
6. _____ Delusion
7. _____ Wandering
8. _____ Sundowning

a. New or increased confusion and disorientation at night
b. Making up conversation to fill gaps in memory
c. Acute confusion
d. Deficit in memory and other cognitive areas
e. Leaving a place or moving with no plan
f. Unable to recall events or remember friends and family
g. Belief in a false idea
h. Mental processes of perception, memory, judgment, and reasoning

COMPLETION

Delirium and Dementia

Directions: Fill in the blanks to complete the statements.

1. The patient experiencing delirium may demonstrate disorganized and distorted thinking and incoherent

   _____.

2. One of the first things you should assess in a patient who is exhibiting signs of delirium is what

   _____ the patient is receiving.

3. A difference between delirium and dementia is that dementia occurs over a(n)

   _____.

4. The most common degenerative disease of the brain is _____.

5. For elders, medications should be given in the _____ amounts possible and increased when the symptoms indicate.

SHORT ANSWER

Caring for a Patient with Acute Confusion

Directions: Read the clinical scenario and answer the questions that follow.

Scenario: Mr. Freed is an elderly man who resides at an assisted-living facility. Although he is occasionally forgetful, he is usually alert and cheerful and enjoys telling stories about his family and his career in the military. He is able to function with minimal assistance. The nursing assistant tells you that today Mr. Freed seems drowsy, disoriented, and extremely irritable.

1. Name four types of medications that could be causing Mr. Freed's change in behavior.

    a. _____

    b. _____

    c. _____

    d. _____

2. What five areas are involved in a quick assessment for delirium and dementia?

    a. _____

    b. _____

    c. _____

    d. _____

    e. _____

3. What are five possible causes of acute confusion?

    a. _____

    b. _____

    c. _____

    d. _____

    e. _____

4. List five things you can do to help decrease Mr. Freed's confusion using reality orientation.

    a. _____

    b. _____

    c. _____

    d. _____

    e. _____

APPLICATION OF THE NURSING PROCESS

Caring for a Patient with Alzheimer Disease

Directions: Provide the answers to the following questions.

Scenario: Mr. Vollander, age 83, lives with his daughter Sylvia. He was diagnosed with Alzheimer disease several years ago. Sylvia is concerned because her father left the house last week and he was missing for several hours before the neighbor helped him back to the house. Sylvia also reports that her father has not recognized her on several occasions.

1. The doctor has told Sylvia that her father may be progressing into moderate Alzheimer stage. List four of the behaviors associated with moderate Alzheimer.

    a. _____

    b. _____

    c. _____

    d. _____

2. Sylvia reports that her father has been losing weight and that she has to remind him to eat and sometimes she even has to feed him. She tells you that, "When Dad was younger, he used to weigh over 250 lbs, and now he is down to about 145 lbs." Convert Mr. Vollander's current weight to kg. _____

3. Which patient problem statement would be a priority for Mr. Vollander?
    a. Confusion due to slow progressive memory loss
    b. Confusion due to biochemical changes in the brain
    c. Altered social interaction due to inability to recognize friends and family
    d. Potential for injury due to faulty judgment
    e. Wandering due to restlessness
    f. Potential for caregiver strain due to prolonged 24-hour responsibility for care

4. List three ways in which you can help Sylvia reduce her own stress.

    a. _____

    b. _____

    c. _____

5. For a patient who is confused or tends to wander, list five teaching points to share with the caregiver to ensure the patient's safety.

    a. _____

    b. _____

    c. _____

    d. _____

    e. _____

6. Which statement indicates that Sylvia understands how to manage her father's confusion?
    a. "If I repeat time, date, and year every morning, he will become oriented to time."
    b. "I'll use several different caregivers; he will be stimulated by other faces."
    c. "I'll provide general orientation to the year by using holiday decorations."
    d. "We'll have big family parties every weekend, just like we used to."

PRIORITY SETTING

Directions: Read the scenario and prioritize as appropriate.

Scenario: You are working in an extended-care facility. You have just received shift report on your six patients. Indicate the order in which you would attend to the needs of these patients.

_____   a. It is the scheduled time for Mr. Russell's AM insulin.

_____   b. Ms. Eoyang is more confused today than she usually is.

_____   c. Mr. Murray has a complaint about the night-shift nurse.

_____   d. Mr. Tosh has a low-grade fever.

_____   e. Ms. Peters has fallen in the bathroom.

_____   f. Mr. Husein is asking for his scheduled pain medication.

REVIEW QUESTIONS FOR THE NCLEX® EXAMINATION

Directions: Choose the best answer(s) for the following questions.

1. The nurse is caring for a patient with who is having difficulty with short-term memory. Which are other signs and symptoms of beginning Alzheimer disease?
    1. Increased forgetfulness, difficulty learning new things, inability to concentrate
    2. Unable to speak or ambulate and profound memory loss
    3. Social withdrawal and decreased ability to perform usual activities of daily living
    4. Outbursts of anger, hostility, paranoia, and wandering

2. What factors cause elderly patients to be at risk for substance-induced delirium?
    1. Increased metabolism and reduction in cardiac and liver function
    2. Decreased metabolism and reduction in cardiac and respiratory function
    3. Decreased metabolism and reduction in kidney and liver function
    4. Increased metabolism and reduction in neurologic and immune function

3. During data collection, the patient's son tells the nurse, "Mom can remember her name, but she doesn't seem to know where she is." Based on this information, which question should the nurse ask *first*?
    1. "How does she like to be addressed?"
    2. "When did you first notice this?"
    3. "What kind of medications does she take?"
    4. "When did she last see the health care provider?"

4. The patient is suffering acute delirium related to a systemic infection. During the evening, the patient appears to be very frightened by the IV tubing. The nurse recognizes that the patient might be experiencing which disturbance?
    1. Hallucination
    2. Illusion
    3. Delusion
    4. Confabulation

5. A 25-year-old patient is brought to the emergency department by the police. He is a poor historian but the police tell the nurse that they were called because he was wandering down the middle of the freeway. He appears confused, disheveled, and malnourished. Which problem statement on the care plan would be of highest priority for this patient?
   1. Altered self-care ability
   2. Wandering due to disorientation to time and place
   3. Potential for injury due to impaired decision-making
   4. Altered nutrition

6. The nurse is caring for a patient in the moderate Alzheimer stage. In planning care, the nurse should anticipate the need for which intervention?
   1. Repeat the date and time frequently.
   2. Restrain the patient to protect from falls and wandering.
   3. Vary routine and provide unstructured environment.
   4. Allot extra time for grooming and toileting.

7. The nurse is working on a busy medical-surgical unit. An elderly patient has fallen out of bed twice, despite repeated verbal instructions to call for assistance. What are appropriate interventions to ensure safety? *(Select all that apply.)*
   1. Encourage family members and friends to stay with the patient.
   2. Obtain an order for an anxiolytic medication.
   3. Keep the patient close to the nurses' station.
   4. Check on the patient frequently to offer nutrition, fluids, pain relief, and toileting.
   5. Place the bed in the lowest position with three side rails up.
   6. Temporarily place restraints and secure knots to the bedrails.
   7. Advise the patient that the hospital is not liable if he refuses to cooperate.

8. The health care provider has ordered that the patient be restrained for 24 hours because he is a danger to himself or others. Which task is appropriate to assign to the nursing assistant?
   1. Selecting the type of restraint.
   2. Checking the circulation in the area distal to the restraint.
   3. Performing 1:1 observation.
   4. Obtaining consent from the patient's family to use restraints.

9. The nursing student is assisting the nurse to apply restraints to a patient. Which action by the student indicates that she understands the procedure?
   1. She checks the circulation and then applies the restraints.
   2. She ties the knot so that it is not readily visible to the patient, family, or staff.
   3. She states that she will check on the patient every 2–4 hours.
   4. She documents the care that was given while the patient was in restraints.

10. The patient is prescribed memantine (Namenda). Common side effects to instruct the patient about are:
    1. insomnia, nervousness, and anxiety.
    2. weight gain, increased thirst, and gastrointestinal upset.
    3. blurred vision, dizziness, and hypotension.
    4. gastrointestinal bleeding, anorexia, and nausea.

11. The nurse is planning care for patients with cognitive disorders. Which task can be assigned to the nursing assistant?
    1. Determine which patients need assistance with hygienic care.
    2. Evaluate the patients' responses to reality-orientation therapy.
    3. Assist patients to ambulate in the hall or enclosed courtyard.
    4. Observe patients for changes in mental status during the shift.

12. A patient is experiencing acute delirium with confusion related to medication side effects. What is the best environmental intervention to use with this patient?
    1. Turn on a favorite television program to provide a familiar distraction.
    2. Ask several family members to come and talk about everyday topics.
    3. Put the patient close to the nurses' station with the door open.
    4. Assign a nursing assistant to observe 1-to-1 in a quiet room.

13. The nurse is making a home visit to an elderly patient with Alzheimer disease. The patient's wife says, "Jim is more confused compared to usual." What is the best response?
    1. "It's hard to see someone that you love deteriorate."
    2. "What kind of changes are you seeing?"
    3. "When was the last time your husband saw a health care provider?"
    4. "With Alzheimer disease, the symptoms do worsen."

14. The nurse hears in report that a patient has global amnesia. The nurse will allot extra time for which intervention?
    1. Talking about family members and their recent visits
    2. Reminiscing about family holidays and past events
    3. Reorienting to person, place, and time
    4. Placing signs and arrows to the bathroom and dining room

15. An elderly patient with mild dementia has demonstrated ability to feed himself, perform toileting independently, and dress himself; however, he frequently says, "You do it for me." What should the nurse do to encourage independence?
    1. Instruct him to try first, and then come back later to see what he has accomplished.
    2. Verbally coach him through the task and observe his performance.
    3. Point out to him that he needs to be independent for as long as possible.
    4. Ask him why he frequently does not want to do things for himself.

CRITICAL THINKING ACTIVITIES

Scenario A: You are working at an extended-care facility. In report, you hear that Mr. Kolanski was restrained during the night for "inappropriate behavior." When you check the chart, you cannot find any order for restraints and the documentation does not include any details about the behavior, the type of restraints, or the care given while the patient was in the restraints.

1. What is your first action?
   a. Call the health care provider and obtain an order for restraints.
   b. Call the nurse at home and ask for details.
   c. Report the incident to the nursing supervisor.
   d. Assess the patient and remove the restraints.

2. During the report, what information should be clarified with the nurse before he or she leaves?

_____

_____

_____

_____

_____

3.   What are your ethical obligations in this situation? What are the ramifications of following through?

_____

_____

_____

_____

_____

Scenario B: Ms. Stoltz is exhibiting behaviors of moderate cognitive decline.

1.   Her daughter, with whom Ms. Stoltz lives, asks what she might do at home to make life easier for her mother. What could the nurse suggest?

_____

_____

2.   What safety interventions would be appropriate to initiate for Ms. Stolz? _____

_____

_____

STEPS TOWARD BETTER COMMUNICATION

VOCABULARY BUILDING GLOSSARY

Term	Pronunciation	Definition
cognition	kog ni′ shun	the mental process of thinking, perceiving, and remembering
confabulation	kon fab u la′ shun	inventing or making up untrue or exaggerated stories and answers to questions
abstract	ab strakt′	not concrete, not material, or not physical; (noun) ideas or theories with no specific application
respite care	res′pit care	short-term care to give relief to the family caregiver for an afternoon or weekend
insight	in′ site	ability to see and understand the truth about something
blunted	blun′ted	not sharp; not perceptive; plain and flat
remote memory	ree mot′ memory	distant in time, long ago
advance directives	ad vans′ di rek′ tivz	instructions about what to do in case of medical emergencies, incapacity, and death; may include power of attorney
confront	kon front	to talk face to face about difficult problems, sometimes argumentatively

COMPLETION

Directions: Fill in the blanks with the correct words from the Vocabulary Building Glossary to complete the statements.

1. A patient suffering from advanced Alzheimer disease generally has a(n)
    _____ affect.

2. When dementia is present, the patient has difficulty comprehending _____ ideas.

3. When patients begin to have great difficulty with memory, they tend to make things up to fill gaps; this
    is called _____.

4. As dementia worsens, _____ decreases, although long-term memory may
    remain intact.

5. The family caregiver of an Alzheimer disease patient badly needs occasional
    _____ for the patient.

6. A patient who frequently loses his way does not usually have any _____ as
    to why this is happening to him and is frightened.

7. The dementia patient often has difficulty with recent memory but can remember things from childhood
    that reside in _____.

8. All adults should have _____ in place, in case an accident or ill-
    ness incapacitates them.

SHORT ANSWER

Memory Examples

Directions: Give two examples each of immediate memory, recent memory, and remote memory.

1. Immediate memory:

    Example: I just drank a cup of coffee.

    a. _____

    b. _____

2. Recent memory:

    a. _____

    b. _____

3. Remote memory:

    a. _____

    b. _____

WORD ATTACK SKILLS

Word Meanings

Directions: Match the adjectives on the left with their correct meanings on the right.

1. _____ Impaired
2. _____ Fragmented
3. _____ Incoherent
4. _____ Disturbed
5. _____ Disoriented
6. _____ Distorted
7. _____ Disorganized
8. _____ Diminished

a. Changed from its true nature or shape
b. Damaged
c. Divided in pieces
d. Less, smaller
e. Not certain of time, place, or identity
f. Not making sense
g. Upset, worried; not normal
h. Without an order or system

PRONUNCIATION SKILLS

Directions: Put the following words in the correct column depending on whether the pronunciation of "-ed" in the word is -id, -d, or -t.

blunted, diminished, disorganized, disoriented, distorted, disturbed, fragmented, impaired

-id	-d	-t

COMMUNICATION EXERCISE

Scenario: Mr. Jones is trying to leave the unit. He repeatedly walks toward the door, saying that he has to go to work. The nursing assistant has called you to intervene because Mr. Jones is becoming increasingly agitated and will not move away from the door.

Distraction is the first method to be used, then negotiation.

Nurse:	"Mr. Jones, I'm Sandra, the charge nurse on this unit. Did you enjoy your breakfast this morning?"
Mr. Jones:	"Well, I guess it was OK."
Nurse:	"Let's talk a walk together down to the common room. There is a group activity going on."
Mr. Jones:	"That would be nice, but I have to go to work now."
Nurse:	"Well, there are some people here who really need your help and advice. They would like to see you now."
Mr. Jones:	"Okay, I guess I could see them now."
Nurse:	"I know they will appreciate seeing you."

CULTURAL POINT

The elderly often have difficulty with recent memory but like to talk about pleasant memories from the past. Conversation with them might be directed at childhood memories of holidays and special vacations or events. Various foods, smells, and pieces of music may remind them of such times. The nurse's own life can be enriched by sharing memories.

Care of Patients with Anxiety, Mood, and Eating Disorders

chapter

47

Answer Key: Review the related chapter to answer these questions. A complete answer key was provided to your instructor.

COMPLETION

Directions: Fill in the blanks to complete the statements.

1. A nursing action that is helpful when a patient is experiencing anxiety is to be _____ and _____.

2. Persons diagnosed with posttraumatic stress disorder (PTSD) have experienced _____ _____ that produce intense horror and recurrent symptoms of anxiety.

3. Dysthymic individuals feel a sense of _____ and _____ that cannot be alleviated by usual means.

4. The individual who switches from being extremely depressed to becoming manic has a(n) _____ disorder.

5. Two hallmarks of mood disorders are the _____ and _____ _____.

6. The depressed patient may have _____ retardation.

7. A diagnosis of generalized anxiety disorder can only be made when the anxiety is present for at least _____ months.

8. Benzodiazepines are used cautiously for anxiety disorders because they are highly _____.

9. _____ often mimics depressive symptoms.

10. _____ is a speech pattern where the speaker quickly switches from topic to topic and there is little or no connection or linkage of ideas.

11. The person with an obsessive-compulsive disorder experiences a(n) _____, which causes _____.

12. The rituals of obsessive-compulsive disorder often take _____ and can interfere with _____.

APPLICATION OF THE NURSING PROCESS

Anxiety

Directions: Read the clinical scenario and answer the questions that follow.

Scenario: A bus full of senior citizens is involved in a minor traffic accident in front of the clinic where you work. The emergency medical personnel have asked to use the clinic as a triage area and have also asked the clinic staff to assist by providing emotional support to the passengers until more help can arrive. One passenger appears to have a broken arm. The others have no obvious physical injuries; however, many of the passengers are very upset.

1. What are six physical signs of severe anxiety that you might expect to find?

    a. _____

    b. _____

    c. _____

    d. _____

    e. _____

    f. _____

2. List five feelings associated with severe anxiety that these passengers could be experiencing.

    a. _____

    b. _____

    c. _____

    d. _____

    e. _____

3. In the elderly, signs of severe anxiety are often somatic. What three signs might indicate severe anxiety in an elderly person?

    a. _____

    b. _____

    c. _____

4. What are three medical conditions that should be considered because they can mimic the signs of severe anxiety?

    a. _____

    b. _____

    c. _____

5. Write a patient goal with outcome criterion for the following problem statement: Severe anxiety due to real or perceived threat.

    _____

    _____

6. List three interventions that could be used to assist a passenger who is experiencing severe anxiety.

   a. _____

   b. _____

   c. _____

7. Which behavior indicates that a passenger is responding to interventions for anxiety?
   a. Passenger cries, but is able to answer questions appropriately.
   b. Passenger cries and repeatedly asks, "What happened to me?"
   c. Passenger is quiet and calm, but will not respond to any questions.
   d. Passenger is wandering around looking for his car keys.

8. Factors that can contribute considerably to positive mental health are:

   a. _____

   b. _____

   c. _____

9. One alternative therapy that may have a calming effect for the anxious person is _____ _____ such as _____ _____.

SHORT ANSWER

Depression

Fill in the blanks with the correct information.

1. Candidates for electroconvulsive therapy (ECT) are those who:

   a. _____

   b. _____

   c. _____

2. ECT works by causing _____ .

3. Side effects of ECT may include _____ .

4. Planning for the patient with depression involves:

   a. _____

   b. _____

   c. _____

5. The priority nursing action for the depressed patient is to _____ _____ .

6. The risk for self-harm for the depressed patient increases when _____ _____ .

7. Risk factors for suicide include: _____

_____

_____

_____

8. When assessing for suicide risk, ask questions concerning:

    a. _____

    b. _____

    c. _____

COMPLETION

Posttraumatic Stress Disorder

Fill in the blanks with the correct information to complete the statements.

1. PTSD may occur after an event that _____

_____.

2. Hallmark signs that indicate a person is experiencing PTSD are _____

_____

_____.

3. Four examples of experiences that might result in PTSD are _____,

_____, _____, and

_____.

4. Flashbacks are _____

_____.

5. Therapies that are helpful for PTSD are _____

_____.

PRIORITY SETTING

Directions: Read the scenario and prioritize as appropriate.

Scenario: You are caring for several patients in an acute psychiatric admission ward. Mr. Canale was admitted for major depression and demonstrates marked psychomotor retardation. Ms. Phillips has bipolar disorder, and this morning she is very intrusive and loud. Mr. Souza was admitted for a severe episode of generalized anxiety disorder and suicidal ideations. Ms. Tobin has a long history of anorexia nervosa; she denies suicidal thoughts but she has attempted suicide in the past. Mr. Buchanan was admitted for major depression. Prioritize the order in which the nurse should address the needs of these patients.

_____ a. Mr. Canale had a bowel movement while sitting in the dayroom, but he will not get up and go to the shower.

_____ b. Ms. Phillips is standing at the nurses' station yelling at the unit secretary.

_____ c. Mr. Souza appears secretive as he walks down the hall; he is carrying something large under his shirt.

_____ d. Ms. Tobin is doing jumping jacks and jogging around the unit.

_____ e. Mr. Buchanan is quiet and appears to be on the verge of crying.

REVIEW QUESTIONS FOR THE NCLEX® EXAMINATION

Directions: Choose the best answer(s) for the following questions.

1. When a patient is showing signs of severe anxiety and it is time for him to bathe and dress, it is best if the nurse:
   1. leaves the patient alone.
   2. asks the patient why he is feeling so anxious.
   3. explain the rationale for practicing good hygiene.
   4. gives simple directions.

2. Which symptoms are most characteristic of depression?
   1. Lack of interest, loss of libido, and flight of ideas
   2. Insomnia, poor hygiene, and grandiose ideas
   3. Overeating, hyperactivity, and rapid speech
   4. Insomnia, anorexia, and lack of energy

3. When communicating with a severely depressed patient, what is the most therapeutic approach?
   1. Be quiet while assisting with activities of daily living.
   2. Interact and talk with the patient and engage him in activities.
   3. Make an extra effort to be cheerful and positive.
   4. Speak in simple, direct sentences when necessary.

4. When planning care for a patient with a mood disorder, what is the highest priority?
   1. Encourage the expression of feelings.
   2. Engage in therapeutic interaction.
   3. Provide a safe environment.
   4. Orient the patient to time and place.

5. The nurse is doing discharge teaching for a manic patient. The patient asks, "Will I have to take lithium forever?" The best answer would be:
   1. "No, only until your symptoms are under control."
   2. "Yes, you will most likely need to take it for your lifetime."
   3. "Possibly your health care provider will let you discontinue after 4–6 months."
   4. "No, most patients can usually do without it after about a year."

6. Which medication is mainly used to treat anxiety?
   1. Paroxetine (Paxil)
   2. Alprazolam (Xanax)
   3. Phenelzine (Nardil)
   4. Amitriptyline (Elavil)

7. In planning care for the depressed patient, the nurse is aware that the risk for self-harm actually increases when the:
   1. patient is discharged and has to care for himself.
   2. antidepressant medications begin to take effect.
   3. family promises, but fails, to visit him in the hospital.
   4. patient is first admitted and does not trust the staff.

8. An MAO inhibitor such as phenelzine (Nardil) may cause life-threatening:
   1. respiratory distress.
   2. gastrointestinal bleeding.
   3. cardiac arrhythmias.
   4. hypertensive crisis.

9. The patient is admitted for anorexia nervosa. Which behaviors are most associated with this disorder? *(Select all that apply.)*
   1. Shifts food around the plate.
   2. Collects recipes.
   3. Makes elaborate meals for others.
   4. Has superstitions about food.
   5. Uses laxatives and vomits in secret.
   6. Practices excessive exercise.

10. Which statement by the patient's family indicates the need for more teaching about the treatment of anorexia nervosa?
    1. "If she'll just eat more, we can take her home and she'll be okay."
    2. "She will have to be hospitalized if she has dehydration or electrolyte imbalance."
    3. "Therapy could take between 1–6 years for this disorder."
    4. "Support groups and family therapy are important aspects of treatment."

11. The patient has bulimia nervosa. Which task would be appropriate to assign to the nursing assistant?
    1. Observe for marks on the knuckles during AM hygiene.
    2. Listen outside the bathroom door for sounds of induced vomiting.
    3. Check the patient's belongings for secret caches of snacks and food.
    4. Escort the patient to group therapy or to occupational therapy.

12. A nurse is assessing a patient who has just returned to the unit after receiving ECT. Which assessment finding is of greatest concern?
    1. Patient complains of a headache.
    2. Patient does not remember having ECT.
    3. Patient displays a cardiac dysrhythmia.
    4. Patient is disoriented to time.

13. The nurse is talking to an elderly patient who states, "Sometimes I wish that I just would fall asleep and never wake up again." What is the most therapeutic response?
    1. "Oh, don't say things like that, everyone would really miss you."
    2. "Are you thinking about committing suicide?"
    3. "Many people would agree that dying during sleep is the best way to go."
    4. "You seem a little sad today, is there anything I can do to help?"

14. The patient was given an SSRI about 60 minutes ago and is now having change of mental status, a rapid pulse, loss of muscular coordination, and hyperthermia. Which action should the nurse take *first* to address this life-threatening condition?
    1. Ensure that there is a patent IV access.
    2. Initiate seizure precautions.
    3. Obtain an order for anxiolytic medication.
    4. Prepare the emergency respiratory equipment.

15. A patient is in the manic phase of bipolar disorder. He is talking very loudly and starting to argue with other patients. Which intervention is the most appropriate to try *first*?
    1. Instruct him to go sit down and watch television.
    2. Take him for a walk down a quiet corridor.
    3. Invite him to play cards or board games.
    4. Advise him to lower his voice or lose privileges.

16. The nurse is teaching the patient about lithium carbonate. What information is appropriate to include in the teaching? *(Select all that apply.)*
    1. It takes 3–4 days to reach therapeutic levels.
    2. It helps decrease the manic behavior.
    3. There is a small margin of safety between a therapeutic level and a toxic level.
    4. Maintain salt intake and drink adequate fluids; salt depletion may cause toxicity.
    5. Take the medication on an empty stomach.
    6. Do not become dehydrated.

17. The patient who is taking an SSRI medication must be monitored for:
    1. weight loss.
    2. hypernatremia.
    3. kidney dysfunction.
    4. gastrointestinal bleeding.

CRITICAL THINKING ACTIVITIES

Scenario A: Mr. Dell is brought to the clinic by a friend. He has been awake for 2 days and has ridden over 200 miles on a bicycle. Although he appears exhausted, he continues to pace around the waiting room, talking loudly, with rapid pressured speech and wild gestures.

1. Which problem is a priority for Mr. Dell?
    a. Altered nutrition due to shortened attention span while trying to eat
    b. Altered sleep pattern due to hyperactivity
    c. Altered communication ability due to flight of ideas and pressured speech
    d. Potential for injury to self or others due to impulsivity and hyperactivity

2. What are three therapeutic communication interventions that can be used in dealing with a patient in the manic phase?

    a. _____

    b. _____

    c. _____

3. What are two ways you may be able to prevent further escalation of manic behavior in a patient?

    a. _____

    b. _____

4. What strategies can you use to maintain your own patience, understanding, and therapeutic efficacy with patients such as Mr. Dell?

_____

_____

_____

_____

_____

Scenario B: Your coworker, Ms. Jones, is 33 years old. She appears to be slightly overweight and suffers from low self-esteem. After lunch, you and other coworkers can frequently hear her vomiting in the bathroom; however, she says she is okay and becomes embarrassed if anybody shows concern. You suspect that she might be bulimic.

1. Write a brief script that could be used to approach Ms. Jones about your concerns. _____

_____

_____

_____

_____

_____

2. What ethical obligations do you have toward a coworker with health problems? _____

_____

_____

_____

_____

_____

STEPS TOWARD BETTER COMMUNICATION

VOCABULARY BUILDING GLOSSARY

Term	Pronunciation	Definition
differentiate	dif er en' shee ate	to see differences
overwhelming	o ver whelm'ing	more than a person can cope with
lethargy	leth'ar jee	extreme tiredness, lack of energy or interest
debilitating	de bil'i tay ting	weakening
elation	ee lay' shun	extreme happiness
recur	re kur'	happen again
somatic	so ma'tik	physical, referring to the body
mimic	mim'ik	act like, imitate
hypervigilant	hy per vij' ah lant	always watchful
escalate	es'ca layt	increase, go to higher levels
frivolity	frih vol' ah tee	light-hearted fun, silliness, gaiety
precipitate	pree sip' ah tayt	to cause to begin
deprivation	dep rah vay' shun	a condition of want and need
conducive	kon doo' siv	helping to cause or produce
lethality	lee thal' ah tee	degree of ability to cause death

COMPLETION

Directions: Fill in the blanks with the correct words from the Vocabulary Building Glossary to complete the statements.

1. Martha was experiencing _____ anxiety after her son was seriously injured and went to surgery.
2. People who are highly anxious may express more _____ complaints than others.
3. Psychotherapy is _____ to resolving moderate depression.
4. During the manic phase, the patient experiences _____.
5. The death of her husband seemed to _____ a period of depression.
6. The depressed patient usually shows signs of _____ and is not interested in exercising.
7. Sometimes it is difficult to _____ between moderate and severe anxiety.
8. Side effects of some of the antidepressant drugs can _____ signs of a neurologic disorder such as Parkinson's disease.
9. When interacting with a patient who has expressed a plan for suicide, you must determine the _____ level.
10. Severe anxiety or severe depression can be _____ to a person's life.
11. Episodes of depression may _____.
12. The very anxious person often becomes _____, studying everyone in the immediate environment.
13. In a person with bipolar disorder, the manic phase can _____ quickly.
14. Patients with anxiety disorders may have experienced periods of _____ as children.

15. The patient who can once again engage in _____ is on the way to being well again.

WORD ATTACK SKILLS

Word Elements

The following word elements appear frequently in this chapter:

-thymia	condition of mind, mood
som/a-, somat/o-	body (physical versus mental)

CULTURAL POINT

Attitudes toward suicide vary. Some religions prohibit suicide, while others do not approve of suicide but feel it is an individual's choice, particularly if one is terminally ill and suffering. There is even an organization called the Hemlock Society that provides information and support for those considering suicide. The Hemlock Society's position is that a person has a right to control his or her own life and death. Their concern is "death with dignity." Some states allow physician-assisted suicide. The nurse needs to explore his or her own feelings about suicide. When a patient's views differ from the nurse's views, the nurse must try to be nonjudgmental. It is important to recognize the differences in attitudes and beliefs that are found among various people.

COMMUNICATION EXERCISE

The following dialogue is an example of one way to interact with a person who is expressing suicidal thoughts.

Patient: "I just can't live like this anymore. I'm going to escape this world and get out of this pain."

Nurse: "It sounds as if you might be planning to take your life. Is that what I am hearing you say?"

Patient: "Yes, I am thinking about it. I'm just not sure yet."

Nurse: "Do you have a plan in mind?"

Patient: "Pills would probably be the easiest way."

Nurse: "Do you have sufficient pills on hand to accomplish your plan? What do you have?"

Patient: "At the moment, I only have a couple of pain pills I and ran out of my antidepressants. I'll have to get some more."

The nurse determines that lethality is not high at the moment.

Nurse: "Have the antidepressants helped you at all?"

Patient: "Not much, and I have been taking them for about 3 weeks."

Nurse: "Antidepressants can take several weeks to work and depression may not resolve for several months. How about talking to your health care provider about your medications?"

Patient: "Okay, I'll talk to him today. If I can get even a little pain relief, I'll be okay."

Nurse: "Let's talk tomorrow and you can tell me what the provider says."

Care of Patients with Substance-Related and Addictive Disorders

Answer Key: Review the related chapter to answer these questions. A complete answer key was provided to your instructor.

COMPLETION

Directions: Fill in the blanks to complete the statements.

1. It takes the body about _____ hour(s) to metabolize one standard drink.

2. In addition to alcohol, other central nervous system depressants include _____ and _____.

3. The greatest danger related to an opioid overdose is _____.

4. For successful rehabilitation of a heroin addict, in addition to long-term treatment, a change in _____ and _____ is essential.

5. Examples of commonly abused inhalants include glue, _____, _____, _____, and other types of solvents.

6. _____ are most frequently abused by teens and children because they are inexpensive and easily accessible.

SHORT ANSWER

Caring for a Patient with Cocaine Use

Directions: Read the clinical scenario and answer the questions that follow.

Scenario: Ms. Jackson, a 25-year-old secretary, started using cocaine as a recreational drug on weekends "just for fun." Within a very short time, she started using cocaine after work and spending more time with friends who were also using increasingly larger amounts. On several occasions, her mother has called in sick for her. Ms. Jackson's mother brings her to the clinic for vitamins and information about cocaine abuse "for a friend." You should collect data to determine Ms. Jackson's baseline knowledge about cocaine and to assess for signs and effects of substance abuse.

1. What are three effects of cocaine that Ms. Jackson could be experiencing?

    a. _____

    b. _____

    c. _____

2. You are aware that different methods of using cocaine create different health issues. In what four ways is cocaine used?

   a. _____

   b. _____

   c. _____

   d. _____

3. What are two teaching points to share with Ms. Jackson about the risks of using cocaine?

   a. _____

   b. _____

4. What are four common feelings of family members who live with a substance-dependent person?

   a. _____

   b. _____

   c. _____

   d. _____

5. What two enabling behaviors has Ms. Jackson's mother demonstrated?

   a. _____

   b. _____

APPLICATION OF THE NURSING PROCESS

Caring for a Patient with Chronic Alcohol Use

Directions: Read the clinical scenario and answer the questions that follow.

Scenario: Mr. Borgatti is a 54-year-old homeless man who frequently comes to the walk-in clinic and shelter for health care, and sometimes for food or a place to rest. He admits to chronic alcohol use and has expressed some thoughts of quitting, but has never followed up on referrals. Today, he is admitted to the hospital for severe malnutrition and electrolyte imbalances. He admits to drinking heavily just before going to the clinic.

1. The diagnosis of alcohol use disorder is based on what criteria?

   a. _____

   b. _____

   c. _____

   d. _____

   e. _____

2. When assessing Mr. Borgatti for a substance use problem, what are three things you should ask about substance usage during history-taking?

   a. _____

   b. _____

   c. _____

3. Name three goals of care for a patient with a substance use disorder.

   a. _____

   b. _____

   c. _____

4. What is the priority problem for Mr. Borgatti?
   a. Absence of compliance due to abstinence from substance
   b. Potential for injury due to alcohol consumption/withdrawal
   c. Lack of home management due to homelessness
   d. Altered nutrition due to excessive alcohol consumption and self-neglect

5. Early symptoms of alcohol withdrawal (anxiety, irritability, and agitation) may manifest as early as:
   a. 1–2 hours after the last drink.
   b. 6–12 hours after the last drink.
   c. 24–48 hours after the last drink.
   d. 2–3 days after the last drink.

6. Write a sample outcome statement for Potential for injury due to complications of withdrawal from alcohol.

   _____

   _____

7. Give three nursing interventions to prevent injuries related to complications of withdrawal from alcohol.

   a. _____

   b. _____

   c. _____

8. The health care provider orders a 500-mL fluid bolus of dextrose 5% with normal saline to infuse over 90 minutes for Mr. Borgatti. What is the pump setting? _____ mL

9. Which task would be appropriate to assign to the nursing student in providing care for Mr. Borgatti?
   a. IV insertion with your supervision
   b. Telephoning the health care provider to give lab results
   c. Assessing Mr. Borgatti for risk for injury
   d. Talking to Mr. Borgatti about the alcohol use

PRIORITY SETTING

Prioritizing for a Patient with Alcohol Withdrawal

Directions: Read the clinical scenario and prioritize as appropriate.

Scenario: You are caring for a patient who has a history of chronic alcohol use. It has been approximately 8 hours since the patient last had a drink. You are vigilant for the signs of withdrawal. The patient currently has a blood pressure of 160/85 mm Hg, pulse 110. Place the interventions in the order of priority.

_____   a.   Orient the patient to person, place, and time.

_____   b.   IV fluids are administered to correct dehydration as ordered.

_____   c.   Encourage a balanced diet high in proteins and multivitamins.

_____   d.   Give chlordiazepoxide HCl (Librium) as ordered.

_____   e.   Establish IV access.

REVIEW QUESTIONS FOR THE NCLEX® EXAMINATION

Directions: Choose the best answer(s) for the following questions.

1. What are the two main defense mechanisms used by substance users?
    1. Repression and regression
    2. Sublimation and splitting
    3. Denial and rationalization
    4. Displacement and identification

2. The patient is taking lorazepam (Ativan) for anxiety. The nurse advises him not to drink alcohol while taking this drug for which reason?
    1. There is an increase in blood pressure caused by frequent use.
    2. There is an additive effect on the nervous system.
    3. There is a decrease in therapeutic response caused by frequent use.
    4. There is increased risk for insomnia and gastrointestinal distress.

3. The nurse is caring for an elderly patient who is prescribed triazolam (Halcion) for insomnia. Benzodiazepines must be used cautiously in the elderly because:
    1. they have a long half-life and are not excreted readily.
    2. they are toxic to the aging endocrine system.
    3. tolerance causes use of increasing doses.
    4. they may be used along with alcohol.

4. The nurse is caring for a patient with a history of substance use. What is the most important intervention in the initial treatment of the substance-dependent patient?
    1. Careful detoxification procedures
    2. Sympathetic care by all health professionals
    3. Medical diagnosis of dependence on the substance
    4. Regular participation in a 12-step program

5. Which assessment should the nurse perform to prevent a life-threatening complication of CNS stimulant withdrawal?
    1. Observe frequently for respiratory depression.
    2. Monitor for cardiac dysrhythmias.
    3. Monitor urinary output.
    4. Watch for bleeding signs.

6. During the physical assessment, the nurse notices bruises and needle marks on the patient's antecubital space. What is the best therapeutic response?
   1. "What are these marks? Are you injecting IV drugs?"
   2. "I am going to ask the health care provider to look at your arms."
   3. "I see you have some bruises. Can you tell me what happened?"
   4. "Let me clean and bandage your arm to prevent infection."

7. The nurse is talking to the patient's mother about enabling. Which statement by the mother indicates that additional intervention is needed for the enabling behavior?
   1. "I am going to let her take responsibility for her decisions."
   2. "I'm her mother. I'll always be there for her no matter what."
   3. "We have all been denying the problem for a long time."
   4. "I will support her recovery by attending Al-Anon."

8. A patient with CNS stimulant use displays agitation and aggression. Which medication is the health care provider most likely to prescribe to address these symptoms?
   1. Methylphenidate (Ritalin)
   2. Lorazepam (Ativan)
   3. Ondansetron (Zofran)
   4. Naloxone (Narcan)

9. A father states to the nurse that he knows his son is using some marijuana. Which would be a therapeutic response by the nurse?
   1. "Tell me about your concerns regarding this issue."
   2. "Marijuana is considered a gateway drug to other recreational drugs."
   3. "How much marijuana is he using?"
   4. "Do you know if he has tried other recreational drugs?"

10. The nurse is assisting the patient with alcohol use to plan activities that will help him to maintain a healthy lifestyle after he is discharged from the hospital. Which are appropriate actions by the nurse? (*Select all that apply.*)
    1. Remind the patient that the physical symptoms of withdrawal will not last forever.
    2. Help him to make a list of activities that would distract him from the cravings.
    3. Ask him to contact old drinking buddies to tell them that he has stopped using alcohol.
    4. Encourage him to socialize with an old drinking buddy and talk about happier times.
    5. Encourage him to participate actively and frequently in a 12-step program.

11. The nurse believes that another nurse is "stealing" narcotic doses from patients and self-injecting the medication. What should the nurse do *first*?
    1. Follow the nurse around to verify suspicions.
    2. Confront the nurse and ask for an explanation.
    3. Ask the patients if they are getting pain relief.
    4. Ask a supervisor to give advice about the situation.

12. A patient with a chronic substance use has a problem of denial of psychological dependence. Which outcome statement is most appropriate?
    1. Patient will stop denying dependence on substances.
    2. Patient will list three negative effects that substances have on his life.
    3. Patient will decrease substance use in 2 weeks.
    4. Patient will talk to his wife about reasons for substance use.

13. Which social situation most strongly indicates that a recovering alcoholic needs to be advised to call his Alcoholics Anonymous sponsor?
    1. There is an after-work get-together where alcohol will be served.
    2. A friend is getting married and the toasting will be done with champagne.
    3. A weekend hunting trip with friends will include beer and other liquors.
    4. A niece is having a birthday party and her father always drinks.

14. A husband indicates to his wife's nurse in the hospital that he is worried she has been drinking too much lately. What is the best response?
    1. "Oh my, I'm really sorry to hear that."
    2. "How is the drinking affecting her?"
    3. "You seem upset by this; tell me about your concerns."
    4. "How long do you think this has been happening?"

15. The nurse is talking to a teenager who says, "Marijuana is not a big deal. It should be legalized." What is the best response?
    1. "Actually marijuana is a gateway substance that can lead to more serious drug use."
    2. "Well, marijuana does help control nausea for chemotherapy patients."
    3. "You should really talk to your parents about this and get their opinions."
    4. "So it sounds like you have some firsthand experience with marijuana."

CRITICAL THINKING ACTIVITIES

Scenario A: You are asked to help develop a community presentation about smoking cessation. One of your tasks is to collect some accurate information that can be used in the presentation.

1. Two serious long-term results of smoking nicotine that may occur are:
   a. addiction to nicotine and impaired coordination.
   b. low blood pressure and cardiac arrhythmias.
   c. stained teeth and bad breath.
   d. lung cancer and emphysema.

2. What are three physical changes that nicotine causes? _____
   _____

3. What are the withdrawal symptoms? _____
   _____
   _____

4. What treatments are available for nicotine addiction? _____
   _____
   _____

Scenario B: Mr. Williams has been admitted with a diagnosis of heroin addiction and detoxification.

1. Recovery from heroin addiction is difficult unless the person: _____
   _____

2. Essential to success for Mr. Williams' recovery are: _____
   _____
   _____

3. Two drugs that may be used during treatment for heroin addiction are _____
   and _____.

STEPS TOWARD BETTER COMMUNICATION

VOCABULARY BUILDING GLOSSARY

Term	Pronunciation	Definition
alleviate	ah lee' vee ayt	make easier or less severe
arousal level	ah row' zel lev' el	ease with which a person can be awakened
denial	dee ny' al	a defense mechanism in which a person will not admit unpleasant or painful realities
diminish	di min' ish	become less, get smaller
eradicate	eh rad'i cayt	get rid of; remove
foster	fos'ter	encourage and help
withdrawal	with drawl'	a group of symptoms that are present when a person stops using a drug
enabling	en ayb'ling	making something easier; doing something for someone that he could do for himself; acting so that one person supports another person's behavior
self-righteous	self ry' chus	very sure that oneself is right and has the correct answers
stigma	stig'ma	a mark of shame

WORD ATTACK SKILLS

Word Meanings

Directions: Underline the correct word in each pair to complete the sentence with the correct meaning.

1. Buying alcohol for an alcoholic spouse who has drunk too much is an example of (self-righteous / enabling) behavior.

2. Extreme jumpiness and nervousness can be a symptom of (denial / withdrawal) from alcohol in the hospitalized patient.

3. Joining a 12-step group such as Alcoholics Anonymous will help (foster / eradicate) a person's decision to stop drinking.

Number Words in Order

Directions: Number these words in order, with the strongest word first.

_____   a.   alleviate

_____   b.   diminish

_____   c.   eradicate

Word Elements

Directions: The following words from Chapter 48 end in the word element -tion. This ending usually indicates the result of an action. In each word defined below, identify the base word, define the base word, and give the whole word's part of speech.

1. Predisposi'tion—being more vulnerable or likely to attain something:

   _____

   _____

2. Rationaliza'tion—an unconscious defense mechanism in which a person finds logical reasons for his actions while ignoring the reality:

   _____

   _____

3. Valida'tion—showing approval, agreeing to the correctness or appropriateness of an action:

   _____

   _____

PRONUNCIATION SKILLS

Directions: Beneath each "s" in the following words write "s" or "z" to show how the letter "s" should be pronounced.

1. predisposition

2. arousal

COMMUNICATION EXERCISE

With a partner, practice asking and answering the questions in the Focused Assessment box in the textbook. Ask for clarification if you do not understand the pronunciation or meaning of what your partner is saying.

Care of Patients with Thought and Personality Disorders

Answer Key: Review the related chapter to answer these questions. A complete answer key was provided to your instructor.

TERMINOLOGY

Thought Disorders

Directions: Match the term on the left with the correct definition or statement on the right.

1. _____ Psychotic features
2. _____ Delusions of grandeur
3. _____ Hallucination
4. _____ Word salad
5. _____ Ideas of reference
6. _____ Neologisms
7. _____ Illusion
8. _____ Flat affect
9. _____ Delusion
10. _____ Alogia

a. Person has an inflated notion of self-importance despite logical reasoning
b. Absence or near-absence of emotional expression
c. Misinterpretation of reality
d. Sensory perception without a corresponding stimulus
e. The person feels that objects, events, or people in his environment have an unusual significance only for him
f. Disorganized mix of words, phrases, and fragments that do not make sense
g. Hallucinations, delusions, and disorganized speech or behavior
h. Made-up new words for expressing confused thoughts
i. False fixed belief
j. Poverty of thoughts

COMPLETION

Schizophrenia

Directions: Fill in the blanks to complete the sentences.

1. When assessing thought disorders, the interview must be _____ because it is difficult for the individual to _____ for very long.

2. Schizophrenia usually develops between the ages of _____.

3. Examples of atypical antipsychotic medications which are used to treat schizophrenia include

   _____, _____, _____,

   and _____.

4. Because of the negative symptoms of _____ and

   _____, elderly schizophrenics are not as likely to seek help.

SHORT ANSWERS

Thought Disorders

Directions: Read the clinical scenario and answer the questions that follow.

Scenario: Ms. Stoddard, age 38, was diagnosed with schizophrenia at age 21. She is frequently admitted to the psychiatric unit for relapse. Currently, she is delusional and verbally hostile. Her appearance is disheveled and she wears layers of clothes inside out and backward. She has a flat affect and sits by herself, talking and gesturing to the air. In the past, she has been prescribed the conventional antipsychotic medication thioridazine (Mellaril). The doctor is trying to give her ziprasidone (Geodon) to see if her symptoms can be controlled by one of the newer medications.

1. List six desirable outcomes for the negative symptoms of schizophrenia.

   a. _____

   b. _____

   c. _____

   d. _____

   e. _____

   f. _____

2. What are four assessment findings for Ms. Stoddard that suggest that she has a thought disorder?

   a. _____

   b. _____

   c. _____

   d. _____

3. Which problem statements would be appropriate for Ms. Stoddard and are likely to be included in her plan of care? *(Select all that apply.)*
   a. Altered communication ability
   b. Altered sensory perception
   c. Altered activity tolerance
   d. Altered socialization
   e. Altered self-care ability
   f. Potential for violence toward self or others
   g. Potential for grief

4. What are three nursing interventions for patients displaying evidence of paranoia?

   a. _____

   b. _____

   c. _____

5. What signs and symptoms should you look for when assessing for extrapyramidal or neuromuscular side effects that are associated with antipsychotic medications?

    a. Pseudoparkinsonism: _____

    _____

    b. Dystonic reaction: _____

    _____

    c. Akathisia: _____

    _____

    d. Tardive dyskinesia: _____

    _____

    _____

    _____

    _____

6. List six common anticholinergic side effects that are seen with the use of antipsychotic medications.

    a. _____

    b. _____

    c. _____

    d. _____

    e. _____

    f. _____

7. The health care provider orders a maximum fluid intake of 2500 mL of water/24 hours, because Ms. Stoddard is known to drink excessive water and this puts her at risk for hyponatremia. Convert 2500 mL into the total number of 8-ounce glasses of water that Ms. Stoddard is allowed to drink. _____ glasses

APPLICATION OF THE NURSING PROCESS

Caring for a Patient with Schizophrenia

Directions: Read the scenario and choose the best answer(s) for the following questions.

Scenario: Mr. Horton is a 23-year-old patient who was recently admitted with the diagnosis of schizophrenia. The police were called to a local restaurant because Mr. Horton had barricaded himself in the men's room and was yelling about terrorists. He is disheveled and appears suspicious and distrustful.

1. In report, the nurse states that Mr. Horton displays positive symptoms of schizophrenia. Which symptoms are considered positive symptoms?
    a. Delusions and hallucinations
    b. Self-care deficits and lack of motivation
    c. Blunted affect and poverty of speech
    d. Social withdrawal and manipulative behavior

2. You observe Mr. Horton. He is standing in a corner by himself and suddenly he puts his hands over his ears and begins to sway back and forth. You hear him say "Shut up, just stop it, shut up!" What does this behavior suggest? Mr. Horton is:
   a. seeking attention.
   b. displaying echolalia.
   c. experiencing a drug side effect.
   d. having an auditory hallucination.

3. Mr. Horton insists that terrorists once kidnapped him. He is afraid that they will return to "finish the job." What is the best response?
   a. "Tell me more about why you think terrorists are after you."
   b. "I can see that you are afraid, but I believe that we are safe here."
   c. "You seem very afraid, but we will protect you from those people."
   d. "Your story about this kidnapping is frightening, but it's illogical."

4. In the acute phase, which is the priority problem for Mr. Horton?
   a. Acute confusion due to a chemical imbalance
   b. Altered socialization due to fear and feelings of persecution
   c. Potential for violence toward self or others due to delusional thinking
   d. Altered self-care ability due to cognitive impairment

5. Mr. Horton loudly argues with the medication nurse and refuses to take his morning medications. "She is a terrorist and is trying to poison all the patients!" What is your first action?
   a. Point out to Mr. Horton that other patients are taking the medicines without ill effects.
   b. Call the health care provider and ask for a temporary emergency order to administer medications.
   c. Support the authority of the medication nurse by gathering four or five other staff members.
   d. Distract Mr. Horton and then later see if he will accept the medication from another nurse.

6. Which activity would be most appropriate for Mr. Horton in the early acute phase of hospitalization?
   a. Attending a music therapy class
   b. Walking in an enclosed patio garden
   c. Playing cards or checkers in the dayroom
   d. Sleeping in his room undisturbed

SHORT ANSWER

Borderline Personality Disorder

Directions: Read the clinical scenario and answer the questions that follow.

Scenario: You are working on a medical-surgical unit. You hear in report that all of the nurses are having trouble dealing with Ms. Arsburg, who was admitted several days ago. One of the RNs suggests a psychiatric consult be obtained because the patient is extremely manipulative, demanding, and "unlikely to follow the treatment plan." Old medical records show that Ms. Arsburg has been previously diagnosed with borderline personality disorder.

1. What are the four main characteristics of borderline personality disorder?

   a. _____

   b. _____

   c. _____

   d. _____

2. What are four things to assess in a patient whom you think might have a personality disorder?

   a. _____

   b. _____

   c. _____

   d. _____

3. Write an outcome for the problem statement: Decreased self-esteem due to past failures and negative responses from significant others.

   _____

   _____

   _____

4. What are two nursing interventions used to deal with manipulative behavior of patients who have personality disorders?

   a. _____

   b. _____

PRIORITY SETTING AND ASSIGNMENT

Directions: Read the scenario and prioritize as appropriate.

Scenario: You are caring for Mr. Richman. He has been rocking and fidgeting and refuses to interact with the staff or other patients. You have observed him talking to himself and you suspect that he may be having command hallucinations.

1. What is the priority patient problem?
   a. Acute confusion with delusions
   b. Altered sensory perception with hallucinations
   c. Potential social isolation
   d. Potential for violence toward self or others

Mr. Richman is now pacing. He yells at one of the other patients and then comes to you and says, "That blearsoning boop is rounding, rounding! Get her down! Stick her with a knife and glass and dead her head!"

2. What is the priority intervention?
   a. Try to figure out what he is saying and empathize.
   b. Firmly instruct him to calm down and go sit down.
   c. Gently tell him his behavior is inappropriate.
   d. Redirect him to a quiet and isolated area.

3. Mr. Richman is unable to follow your verbal instructions. His pacing increases and he begins to wildly gesture. What is the priority action?
   a. Remove the other patients and allow him to pace.
   b. Gather several staff members to stand behind you.
   c. Call the health care provider for an order for chemical restraints.
   d. Repeat your verbal instructions and state the consequences.

4. The nursing assistant is available to help you with Mr. Richman. What task would be appropriate to assign to the assistant?
    a.   Ask the assistant to try to calm him down.
    b.   Ask the assistant to go call the health care provider.
    c.   Have the assistant do one-on-one observation as ordered by the health care provider.
    d.   Assign the assistant to put the patient in four-point restraint.

5. The next day, Mr. Richman is calm and quiet. Which task would be appropriate to assign to the nursing assistant?
    a.   Sit with Mr. Richman and ask him how he is feeling.
    b.   Encourage Mr. Richman to take a shower.
    c.   Talk with Mr. Richman about his future plans.
    d.   Observe Mr. Richman for any agitated behavior.

REVIEW QUESTIONS FOR THE NCLEX® EXAMINATION

Directions: Choose the best answer(s) for the following questions.

1. A patient is experiencing anticholinergic side effects from the drug to counter side effects of his antipsychotic medication. The nurse should suggest which interventions to relieve dry mouth?
    1.   Chew gum, perform mouth hygiene, and increase fluids.
    2.   Encourage fluids, increase fiber in diet, and suck on hard candy.
    3.   Decrease the medication dosage and perform mouth hygiene every 2 hours.
    4.   Track fluid intake, drink milkshakes, and chew gum.

2. The patient is taking an antipsychotic medication, fluphenazine (Prolixin). Which side effect, if noted, should the nurse identify as most significant, requiring immediate intervention?
    1.   A fixed upward gaze
    2.   A shuffling gait
    3.   Tapping of the foot
    4.   Irritability

3. The patient whose family says he is very picky about things in the house such as constantly straightening the fringe on the throw rugs, picking up everyone's dirty dishes right away, and dictating what everyone should do is considered:
    1.   paranoid.
    2.   schizophrenic.
    3.   manipulative.
    4.   obsessive-compulsive.

4. The patient tells the nurse that there are a several men in dark coats who are watching her and planning to steal her belongings. The best response from the nurse is:
    1.   "There are no men watching you."
    2.   "Tell me more about these men."
    3.   "I do not see any men."
    4.   "They won't hurt you."

5. The nurse is working in an acute admission ward in a psychiatric facility. Which safety precautions should the nurse take when caring for these acutely ill patients? *(Select all that apply.)*
    1.   Avoid wearing flashing or dangling jewelry.
    2.   Do not wear a white coat or white uniform.
    3.   Avoid wearing a stethoscope, scarf, or tie around the neck.
    4.   Avoid casual touching without asking permission.
    5.   Stay away from doorways and exits.
    6.   Do not interact with any patients who appear sullen or depressed.

6. The patient is taking olanzapine (Zyprexa) as prescribed. Which patient comment suggests that the medication is successfully treating the patient's positive symptoms of schizophrenia?
   1. "I can leave the hospital whenever I want to."
   2. "Nurse, I am ready to go home. Would you call my mother?"
   3. "I can still hear the voices, but they are very distant."
   4. "The angel stopped talking; now she just sits and waves."

7. The patient is ready to be discharged. The nurse teaches him about his antipsychotic medication and he asks, "What will happen if I stop taking my medication when I go home?" Which is the best reply?
   1. "You should never stop taking your medication."
   2. "Someday you may be able to do without the medication."
   3. "If you can get organized and reduce stress, perhaps you can get along without it."
   4. "If you stop taking your medication, the symptoms will probably return."

8. The patient will be discharged within a day or two. Which statement by the patient's family indicates a need for further discussion about the diagnosis of schizophrenia?
   1. "A stable home environment will help to prevent relapse."
   2. "He might always hear voices, but the medications will help."
   3. "Medication will eliminate his blunted affect and social isolation."
   4. "If he fails to take his medication, it will probably lead to readmission."

9. A patient with schizophrenia comes to the nurse and says, "Here we go, got flacks and sacks and jib-bogny tomorrow. Would you like some?" What is the best response?
   1. "Say that again. I couldn't understand what you are saying."
   2. "Sure thing, flacks and sacks and jibbogny sound great to me."
   3. "I don't quite understand, but I do appreciate you including me."
   4. "You are not making any sense. Try to speak clearly."

10. The nurse is assessing a new patient who was just admitted for schizophrenia. The patient is easily distracted and is rocking back and forth. What strategy should the nurse try *first*?
    1. Get as much information from the chart as possible.
    2. Attempt to get a phone number for a family member.
    3. Use short sentences that can be answered with a yes or no.
    4. Delay the assessment until the patient is more coherent.

11. What is a potential complication of residual negative symptoms that do not respond to medication?
    1. Apathy results in failure to adhere to medication regimen.
    2. Bizarre behavior such as public nudity results in social stigma.
    3. Tardive dyskinesia is permanent and debilitating.
    4. Auditory hallucinations continue, but are less problematic.

12. A patient is admitted to the unit with a diagnosis of borderline personality disorder. Which behavior most typifies this disorder?
    1. Cannot decide what to eat for breakfast without help
    2. Eyes are cast downwards when speaking to others
    3. Suddenly gives her favorite blouse to another patient
    4. Glares at strangers when they enter the room

13. The nurse is talking with a patient who has a borderline personality disorder. The patient says, "I'll tell you a secret because you are the best nurse here." Which comment should the nurse identify as most significant, requiring immediate notification of the supervisor?
    1. "I lied to get in here because I was sick of living with my mother."
    2. "The charge nurse is a lesbian. I've seen her in the lesbo clubs."
    3. "I am going to give myself a little superficial cut so that the doctor will see me."
    4. "I stole some money from my father and he might hurt me when I get out."

14. The problem statement for a patient is altered self-esteem. The nurse instructs the patient to do which activity to promote self-esteem? *(Select all that apply.)*
    1. Make a list of things that she is good at.
    2. Give and receive positive feedback.
    3. Set small, realistic goals.
    4. Describe personal failures in detail to a friend.
    5. Critique personal performance for errors.
    6. Keep a journal of success stories.

CRITICAL THINKING ACTIVITIES

Scenario: You have talked to Ms. Sutton and feel that rapport has been established. She has shared personal information with you, and she states, "I really like talking to you." You leave Ms. Sutton to admit a new patient. Later, when you return, Ms. Sutton hits you and tries to run out the door.

1. What are your initial thoughts about this scenario? _____

   _____

   _____

   _____

   _____

2. What factors may have triggered Ms. Sutton's aggressive behavior? _____

   _____

   _____

   _____

   _____

3. What types of things should you do to protect yourself, patients, and others? _____

   _____

   _____

   _____

STEP TOWARD BETTER COMMUNICATION

VOCABULARY BUILDING GLOSSARY

Term	Pronunciation	Definition
trigger	trig'ger	start a reaction, cause to begin
de-escalation	dee esk ah lay' shun	process of coming back down, as in the calming of a nervous, hyperactive patient
extrapyramidal	eks' trah pir ram' i dal	symptoms outside the pyramidal tracts of the nervous system
erratic	eh rat'ik	inconsistent, not performing normally; irregular

Term	Pronunciation	Definition
odd	awd	something or someone different, strange, unusual, or surprising
eccentric	ek sen' trik	showing unusual behavior; unconventional, peculiar
impulsive	im puhl' siv	acting on sudden urges or desires without thinking of the consequences
boundaries	bown'dreez	limits to behavior or movement
recur	ree ker'	happen again
rationale	rah shun al'	the reason for doing something; the thoughts about why to do something
acting out	ak' ting owt	expressing feelings through nonverbal behavior
borderline	bor' der lyn	on the edge or boundary; precarious
"get under the skin"		causing a reaction, such as irritation or attraction
traits	trayts	characteristic actions or behaviors
subsequent	sub' see kwent	later, following, after a previous event

CHOOSING THE CORRECT WORD

Directions: Underline the word in parentheses that correctly completes the thought.

1. The patient would often take things from stores; this is an example of (eccentric/impulsive) behavior.

2. The patient was removing her clothes in the dayroom after her husband came to visit; this is an example of (subsequent/acting out) behavior.

3. The patient demonstrated (impulsive/odd) behavior by weaving pieces of Styrofoam and old milk cartons into her hair.

4. The nurse was firm with the patient with borderline personality disorder, setting (boundaries/rationale) for acceptable behavior.

5. The family did not know what would (trigger/recur) manic behavior in the patient.

6. Lying and manipulative behaviors are characteristic (traits/de-escalation) of people with borderline personality disorders.

COMMUNICATION

The following is a sample dialogue showing how a nurse can intervene when a patient is becoming agitated. The patient, Anna, is speaking in a loud voice and waving her hands in her daughter's face.

Anna: "You must accept Jesus as your savior or you won't go to heaven. Why haven't you been going to church? You'll be damned forever. I'm saved. Why can't you save yourself?"

Nurse (to patient): "Anna, I see your daughter is here to visit. I like the dress you have on, Anna. You have on your new shoes too!"

Nurse (to daughter): "Anna chose this outfit because she knew you were coming today."

Daughter:	"You look really nice, Mom."
Nurse:	"Yes, she is all ready to have lunch with you in the garden room. Anna, are you hungry? Let's go down to lunch."

The nurse has used distraction to de-escalate Anna's behavior. At the same time, the attention to Anna and the sincere compliments help increase Anna's self-esteem and establish that the nurse is caring and empathetic.

DESCRIPTIVE TERMS

Directions: Place the characteristic behaviors listed below with the correct type of disorder in Cluster A, B, or C as listed in Box 48-3 in the textbook.

clinging	impulsive	perfectionist	socially inhibited
attention-seeking	submissiveness	suspicious	eccentric
distrustful	need for admiration	fears rejection	feels inadequate
lacks empathy	odd	need for control	needy
grandiosity	disregards rights of others	extremely emotional	distorted feelings
lability of emotions	distorted thinking		

Cluster A (Odd/Eccentric)	Cluster B (Dramatic/Erratic)	Cluster C (Anxious/Fearful)
1.	1.	1.
2.	2.	2.
3.	3.	3.
4.	4.	4.
5.	5.	5.
6.	6.	6.
	7.	7.
	8.	8.